Textbook of
Head and
Neck Anatomy

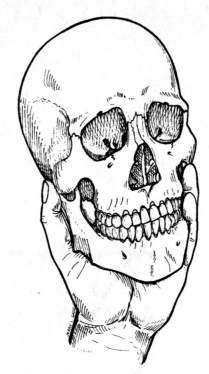

Alas, poor Yorick! I knew him well Horatio, a fellow of infinite jest, of most excellent fancy. He hath borne me on his back a thousand times.
■ **Shakespeare, Hamlet**

Textbook of
Head and
Neck Anatomy

Fourth Edition

James L. Hiatt, Ph.D.

Professor Emeritus
Department of Biomedical Sciences
Baltimore College of Dental Surgery
Dental School, University of Maryland
Baltimore, Maryland

Leslie P. Gartner, Ph.D.

Professor of Anatomy (Ret.)
Department of Biomedical Sciences
Baltimore College of Dental Surgery
Dental School, University of Maryland
Baltimore, Maryland

Original Illustrations by Jerry L. Gadd

 Wolters Kluwer | Lippincott Williams & Wilkins
Health

Philadelphia • Baltimore • New York • London
Buenos Aires • Hong Kong • Sydney • Tokyo

Acquisitions Editor: John Goucher
Managing Editor: Andrea M. Klingler
Marketing Manager: Allison Noplock
Senior Production Editor: Sandra Cherrey Scheinin
Designer: Karen Quigley
Compositor: Maryland Composition/Absolute Service, Inc.

Fourth Edition

351 West Camden Street   530 Walnut Street
Baltimore, MD 21201   Philadelphia, PA 19106

Printed in China

9 8 7 6 5 4 3 2 1

Library of Congress Cataloging-in-Publication Data

Hiatt, James L., 1934–
    Textbook of head and neck anatomy / James L. Hiatt, Leslie P. Gartner.—4th ed.
      p. ; cm.
    Includes bibliographical references and index.
    ISBN 978-0-7817-8932-5
    1. Head—Anatomy. 2. Neck—Anatomy. I. Gartner, Leslie P., 1943– II. Title.
    [DNLM: 1. Head—anatomy & histology. 2. Neck—anatomy & histology. WE 705 H623t 2009]
    QM535.H48 2009
    611'.91—dc22

                                                            2008041276

Care has been taken to confirm the accuracy of the information present and to describe generally accepted practices. However, the authors, editors, and publisher are not responsible for errors or omissions or for any consequences from application of the information in this book and make no warranty, expressed or implied, with respect to the currency, completeness, or accuracy of the contents of the publication. Application of this information in a particular situation remains the professional responsibility of the practitioner; the clinical treatments described and recommended may not be considered absolute and universal recommendations.

The authors, editors, and publisher have exerted every effort to ensure that drug selection and dosage set forth in this text are in accordance with the current recommendations and practice at the time of publication. However, in view of ongoing research, changes in government regulations, and the constant flow of information relating to drug therapy and drug reactions, the reader is urged to check the package insert for each drug for any change in indications and dosage and for added warnings and precautions. This is particularly important when the recommended agent is a new or infrequently employed drug.

Some drugs and medical devices presented in this publication have Food and Drug Administration (FDA) clearance for limited use in restricted research settings. It is the responsibility of the health care provider to ascertain the FDA status of each drug or device planned for use in their clinical practice.

To purchase additional copies of this book, call our customer service department at **(800) 638-3030** or fax orders to **(301) 223-2320**. International customers should call **(301) 223-2300**.

Visit Lippincott Williams & Wilkins on the Internet: http://www.lww.com. Lippincott Williams & Wilkins customer service representatives are available from 8:30 am to 6:00 pm, EST.

Dedicated to

my wife Nancy
and my children, Drew, Beth, and Kurt.
JLH

Dedicated to

my wife Roseann,
my daughter Jen,
and my mother Mary.
LPG

Preface

The *Textbook of Head and Neck Anatomy* was first published in 1982. This textbook was written with the thought in mind that students come to this subject with varying backgrounds; therefore, the regional approach to the study of anatomy was selected over the tedious systems approach. Since that first edition, the textbook has been through two subsequent editions. During these two latter editions we received suggestions from faculty and students that served to improve the quality of the text and its illustrations, tables, and Clinical Considerations. In preparing each new edition, our primary goal remained to present a text designed and written for the student, incorporating all of the requisites of optimal learning. These included succinct, concise writing; well-developed tables that digested information for student understanding; profuse, well-designed illustrations that accommodated learning; identification of new terms; a Glossary and Suggested Readings; and a cross-referenced Index.

We were gratified to learn that the editorial group responsible for the development of the 4th edition of our *Textbook of Head and Neck Anatomy* at Lippincott Williams & Wilkins agreed to the major change to using full color and enlarging the format. Now the tables are larger and more accessible to the reader. Perhaps more important, the illustrations also are larger and in full color, which greatly facilitates anatomical appreciation, understanding, and learning. We have incorporated a number of figures from other Lippincott Williams & Wilkins publications, and we've colorized most of the original art created for the text over the years by our original illustrator, Jerry Gadd. We have also added many new tools for the student to facilitate learning and to broaden one's understanding of the clinical importance of learning anatomy.

Organization

After careful consideration, we adopted an organization of the text that accommodated our teaching styles and the student's learning methods. Thus we have maintained the organization of the previous version for this edition. The first three chapters introduce the basics of anatomy to the student, namely its long history and the specialized terminology that the student must master. Over the years we have found that many students come to anatomy with varied backgrounds, therefore we present a chapter on the body systems, specifically as they apply to head and neck anatomy. This is followed by a chapter designed to introduce the student to anatomical concepts in the oral cavity, palate, and pharynx presented from the standpoint of an oral examination. The next chapter, describing the Embryology of the Head and Neck, is followed by a chapter detailing the osteology of the skull. The succeeding ten chapters are devoted to regional anatomy, ending with the discussion of the Brain and Spinal Cord. Although all of the cranial nerves were presented in the respective chapters, a particular chapter is devoted to the cranial nerves, their associations with the autonomic nervous system, and with their distributions in the head and neck. This is followed with a chapter on the anatomical basis for local anesthesia. There are summarizing chapters on lymphatics, the vascular supply of the head and neck, and the fascia of the head and neck.

Many of our former students have suggested that the posterior neck is not of much value to those preparing for a career in the dental profession. We, therefore, reduced much of the written material in this segment but, for those interested, we have retained the tables and some of the illustrations.

Key Features

Many important relevant *Clinical Considerations* are incorporated within each chapter. These were placed at the end of each chapter in previous editions, whereas in this edition we have placed them at the appropriate position within the text where the subject is discussed. A list of all 139 Clinical Considerations by chapter, title, and page number is presented in the front of the text in order to provide the reader easy access to them for reference and study.

In an effort to assist the student to identify the material contained in major headings, we have incorporated the *Summary Bite.* The Summary Bite is a synopsis of the main points in the text under the heading. Students may find these summary bites useful in preparing for exams.

Tables have been added to each new edition of the text, including the present edition, because they organize and summarize large amounts of information that assist students in mastering information in a minimum amount of time. A list of all 29 of the tables by chapter, table number, and page number is presented in the front of the text to assist the student in finding the table of interest.

Chapter Outlines on the opening page of each chapter highlight the major subjects discussed. This is followed by a section of *Key Terms* that provides brief definitions and/or short descriptions that the student is expected to master.

We use a specific color scheme to indicate the three, and occasionally four, levels of headings within the text, though frequently the fourth level was replaced by bullets. The student should remember that bullets are not above or below the paragraph order, but are merely used to indicate some importance to that particular entry or paragraph.

We have retained the Glossary in this edition to aid the student in grasping the language of anatomy as it relates to the head and neck, as well as an extensive cross-referenced Index. Students seeking additional information concerning the subjects covered in this text will find a current Suggested Readings section in the back of the book helpful. Included are references to textbooks and atlases of Gross Anatomy, Developmental Anatomy, and Neuroanatomy.

Ancillaries

Two new educational tools are being introduced in this 4th edition. We have developed a bank of approximately 200 USMLE Type I examination questions with answers (approximately 10 per chapter) that tests comprehension of the material presented in each chapter.

Available to instructors with this new edition are PowerPoint presentations that provide an overview of each chapter and offers the faculty teaching and/or review resources for use with the textbook. Also available is an image bank of all figures and tables within the text.

A complete, searchable version of the full text is available on thePoint as well at http://thePoint.lww.com/Hiatt4e. thePoint provides dedicated flexible learning solutions and resources for students and faculty using our *Textbook of Head and Neck Anatomy.*

Reviewers

Pamela L. Alberto, DMD
Director of Predoctoral Surgery
Clinical Associate Professor
Department of Oral & Maxillofacial Surgery
New Jersey Dental School—U.M.D.N.J.
Newark, New Jersey

William Bird, RDH, MA
Director
Allied Dental Education Department
Santa Rosa Jr. College
Santa Rosa, California

Alan W. Budenz, MS, DDS, MBA
Professor, Director of Oral Diagnosis and
    Patient Intake
Department of Anatomical Sciences
Department. of Dental Practice
University of the Pacific
San Francisco, California

Susan J. Crim, PhD, MSEd, RDH
Associate Professor and Department Chair
Dental Hygiene
University of Tennessee
Memphis, Tennessee

Karen Kulikowski, DMD
Professor
Department of Allied Dental Education
The University of Medicine and Dentistry of
    New Jersey
Scotch Plains, New Jersey

Acknowledgments

We wish to express our sincere thanks to our colleagues and students for their constructive criticisms as well as their suggestions aimed at improving our *Textbook of Head and Neck Anatomy*. Their comments have been valuable to us and we incorporated many of them into this fourth edition.

We wish to thank Lippincott Williams & Wilkins for affording us the opportunity of borrowing many of the excellent anatomical images from their publications to illustrate the didactic material of our text.

We would especially like to thank Dr. Robert Jaynes, Department of Radiology at Ohio State University College of Dentistry, for his exquisite panographic radiograph; Dr. Stuart Josell, Chairman of Orthodontics, University of Maryland Dental School, for the clinical photographs of a cleft lip and cleft palate; and Dr. Christine Ferrell, Department of Orthodontics, University of Maryland Dental School, for lending us the cephalometric radiograph. We would like to thank one of our students, Kari Moss for permitting us to photograph her eyes. We would especially like to thank Dr. Radi Masri, Research Assistant Professor in the Deparment of Endodontics, Prosthodontics, and Operative Dentistry for Photographing the clinical subjects of the oral cavity in Chapter 4.

Finally we would like to thank our friends at Lippincott Williams & Wilkins for assisting us through every step of the way in the production of the current edition of this book. We extend our gratitude to Jessica Schulteis, temporary Managing Editor; Terry Mallon, Design Coordinator; and Rachelle Detweiler, Ancillary Editor. Special thanks go to Andrea Klingler, our Managing Editor, and Jen Clements, Art Director. These two individuals were always there when we needed them.

Although we have made every effort to ensure care and accuracy, we realize that some errors and omissions may have escaped our attention. Therefore, criticisms, suggestions, and comments that would help to improve this textbook will be appreciated. Comments may be addressed to *jhi34@yahoo.com* and *lpg21136@yahoo.com*.

James L. Hiatt, PhD
Leslie P. Gartner, PhD

List of Tables

List of Clinical Considerations

Contents

Introduction

A natomy has always fascinated humans, not only because of our interest in the delivery of children but also because of the importance of understanding anatomy in healing wounds and caring for the sick. Mankind's interest in anatomy is ancient because it has been learned from archeological evidence that even brain surgery was performed with considerable success as early as 7000 BC in Europe, 3000 BC in Africa, and 2000 BC in the pre-Incan civilizations.

Although anatomic representations and the study of anatomy have been noted in almost every culture, occidental medicine traces its origin to philosophers in the golden age of Greece and the Arabic physicians, who studied, instructed, and wrote about anatomy and attempted to relate it to function and disease. They also named observed structures, and their students expanded this knowledge by discovering and naming yet other structures. Students of anatomy during the Middle Ages—even as late as the 18th century—used Greek and Latin, the *lingua franca* of learned men. Hence, most of the structures named during those centuries of discoveries were named in those languages, a practice continued into modern times.

The earliest written treatise on anatomic studies was set down by the Greek physician Alcmaeon approximately 2500 years ago. He discovered and dissected the optic nerves, tracing them back to the optic chiasma, and deduced their role in binocular vision. He also discovered and described the auditory tube, suggested that the brain is responsible for intelligence, and studied the ramifications of blood vessels.

Writing at about the same time, the Greek philosopher Pythagoras also suggested that the brain was the center of intelligence. He believed that the physical and emotional well-being of an individual was related to the ratio of the four humors: phlegm, yellow bile, black bile, and blood. These four humors were related to the four elements: water, fire, earth, and air, respectively, whose properties were moist, dry, cold, and hot. A healthy individual would possess a proper combination of these fluids, whereas a disproportionate ratio would be responsible for a diseased state of the body and/or mind. This belief in humors became a basic tenet of Hippocratic medicine. Unfortunately, Aristotle's writings lent credence to this line of thinking; thus, it persisted well into the Middle Ages. Aristotle, however, did make major contributions to the study of anatomy by correctly describing many organs and structures of the human body. He may also have been the first anatomist to illustrate his descriptions with drawings.

Shortly after the decline of Athens, the Greek scholars of Alexandria, especially Herophilus, pioneered in the teaching of anatomy by the use of human dissections. For his work in this field, Herophilus is considered the founder of anatomy, and his dissertations (all lost) encompassed many areas of the subject. The next four centuries saw a decline in anatomic studies until the advent of Galen, possibly the greatest physician of his age. His writings on anatomic structures were so precise and well researched that they constituted the solid bases of medicine for longer than a millennium. He believed that structure and function were closely interrelated, and his painstaking studies of the spinal cord illuminated his theories, which survived into the early 19th century. Soon after Galen, the Roman Empire collapsed and Europe entered its Dark Ages. During this period, it was the Persian physicians, chiefly Avicenna writing around 1000 AD, who were responsible for keeping the scientific perspectives of medicine and anatomy alive.

A major landmark of anatomic history occurred in 1224, when Frederick II proclaimed that to be permitted to perform surgery one must have studied anatomy by dissecting a human body. Although this edict established anatomy as a discipline unto itself, no major advance occurred for another 350 years. The next important achievement came with Leonardo da Vinci, whose brilliant anatomic illustrations added new emphasis to the functional appreciation of structure. He, more than anyone before him, was able to display the results of his dissections and simplify the complexities of the human body. Hence, the study of human anatomy returned to Europe, flourishing during the Renaissance. This enlightened period of humanistically oriented culture permitted questioning of secular dogma.

The teachings of the ancients were at last openly opposed by the Belgian physician Andreas Vesalius, who applied strict scientific discipline to his anatomic observations. He single-handedly revised the discipline of anatomy and wrote a treatise that was the forerunner of modern anatomy textbooks. Within a generation or so of Vesalius, another great anatomist, William Harvey, wrote about the blood vessels and the heart. His work, the cornerstone of the study of the structure and function of the circulatory system, revolutionized medicine, physiology, and anatomy.

The invention of the microscope around this time opened new vistas in anatomy, permitting the marvelous discoveries of Wirsung, Malpighi, Purkinje, Golgi, Cajal, and Ehrlich. Discussion of these anatomists is outside the scope of this brief historical survey, but interested readers are encouraged to refer to books dealing with the history of medicine or anatomy.

Modern anatomy textbooks approach the subject from a systemic, regional, or surgical point of view. A systemic anatomy textbook, as the name implies, treats the body as if it were organized into neat, self-contained systems, such as the skeletal, muscular, nervous, and circulatory systems, each of which is detailed in the text. Such an approach is valuable, especially in a reference textbook, because it describes each structure in a continuous fashion.

Textbooks that treat the subject in a regional manner divide the body into specific areas, such as upper extremity, lower extremity, thorax, and head and neck, and discuss the contents of each region (i.e., osteology, myology, nervous, and vascular elements). Descriptions do not exceed the boundaries of the region, regardless of the fact that many structures (e.g., vessels, nerves, and muscles) are not wholly contained within that specified area. Textbooks of surgical anatomy are based on such a regional approach, with emphasis on surgical techniques, approaches, and normal anatomic variations.

The head and neck comprise a highly specialized region of the body. The structures contained within this region are closely interrelated because they are compacted into a small, complicated area. Other regions of the body, where interrelationships are less complex, lend themselves to a systemic approach. The head and neck region does not. Consequently, the present textbook is written from a regional point of view because the authors continue to believe this approach is more likely to promote better student understanding.

The regional method synthesizes morphologic features for the reader by correlating relationships as the reader progresses through the various anatomic divisions of the head and neck. Furthermore, this approach aids not only those who have constant access to a laboratory situation but also those who do not. And, finally, this approach eliminates the need to synthesize the final product from its component parts, thus assisting the student in mastering the intricacies of this fascinating region of the body.

Anatomic Concepts

2

Key Terms

Anterior and Posterior are the anatomic terms for "front" and "back." Sometimes the terms ventral and dorsal are used to depict anterior and posterior, but these terms are usually applied to quadrupeds.

Anatomic Position is that position of the body (facing forward with palms forward) from which the position of all structures are described.

Cranial or Superior and Caudal or Inferior are terms applied to "headward" and "tailward."

Horizontal or Transverse Plane is a plane at right angles to the sagittal plane.

Medial and Lateral are terms used to describe positions relative to the midline of the body. For example, a structure located closer to the midline than another structure is described as being medial to it or, if farther away, lateral to it.

Median Plane or Midsagittal Plane is a plane through the midline of the body from anterior to posterior. Any plane that passes parallel to this plane is called a sagittal plane.

Mesial and Distal are terms that relate to tooth locations that are described from the median plane. Thus, canine teeth are mesial to premolar teeth, whereas molar teeth are distal to premolar teeth.

Proximal and Distal are positions relative to the body. For example, the elbow is proximal to the wrist, whereas the fingers are distal to the wrist.

Superficial and Deep are self-explanatory (e.g., skin is **superficial** to muscle, whereas the heart is **deep** to the lungs). Alternate terms for superficial and deep are external and internal.

The word **anatomy**, which has been derived from the Greek words **ana** and **tomē**, literally means to "cut up" or dissect. The human body, therefore, is described in an anatomy text as if it were dissected layer by layer. Because the study of anatomy is a descriptive science and the descriptions are related spatially, a student of anatomy must become familiar with the language an anatomist uses in describing these spatial relationships. Without understanding the basic vocabulary, the student would be unable to learn the subject effectively and to communicate with peer professionals.

DIVISIONS OF ANATOMY

Summary Bite. Four major categories of anatomy study include: developmental anatomy, neuroanatomy, microscopic anatomy, and macroscopic anatomy.

The science of human anatomy is generally divided into four major categories of study. **Developmental anatomy**, commonly referred to as human embryology, deals with the study of how the mature body is formed, beginning with a fertilized ovum. **Neuroanatomy** is the specialized study of the nervous system, including that of the brain and spinal cord. **Microscopic anatomy** is the division of anatomy that studies the fine details of the human body using the microscope. This division is more commonly referred to as **histology**, the study of tissues. **Macroscopic** or **gross anatomy**, on the other hand, is that division of anatomy that studies the human body with the unaided eye.

Gross Anatomy

Summary Bite. Gross anatomy is the study of the human body with the unaided eye, and it may be studied systemically or regionally.

Gross anatomy of the human body may be studied from one of two approaches. **Systemic anatomy** is the approach that describes and discusses each system separately and in its entirety (e.g., studying all of the muscles of the body that compose the muscular system before discussing the components of any other system).

Regional Anatomy

Summary Bite. Regional anatomy confines itself to a particular region of the body without extending the study outside the region.

Regional anatomy details a region of the body, such as the head and neck, studying all systems in that area as a complete, integrated unit.

The regional approach used in this text provides the student with a more comprehensive presentation of an anatomic region, thus enhancing an understanding of interrelationships between the various systems of the body.

DESCRIPTIVE ANATOMIC TERMS

Summary Bite. Human anatomic terms are spatially related to the anatomic position defined as erect with the palms facing forward.

Human anatomic structures are described spatially relative to the anatomic position, defined for the human as an erect position with the palms of the hands facing forward (Fig. 2-1). Structures on the "front" side of the body are described as being **anterior**, whereas those on the "back" of the body are termed **posterior**. Occasionally, other terms may be used for anterior and posterior, such as **ventral** in place of anterior and **dorsal** in place of posterior (Fig. 2-2). The terms ventral and dorsal are perhaps more appropriate when related to quadrupeds, although embryologists and neuroanatomists prefer these terms.

Similarly, alternate terms may be used in referring to directions aimed at the head or tail. **Cranial** or **superior** means "toward the head," whereas **caudal** or **inferior** refers to "tailward," although neuroanatomists prefer the term **rostral** for cranial or superior. The terms **superficial** and **deep** are used to describe positions relative to the surface of the body from any aspect. The ribs are superficial to the lungs but deep to the skin. Alternate terms for superficial and deep are **external** and **internal**, respectively.

Proximal and **distal** are terms generally applied to positions close to or away from the body, respectively. For example, the wrist is proximal to the finger but distal to the elbow. The teeth are described as being either **mesial** or **distal** to each other in the dental arch from the median plane of the face. For example, the canine tooth is mesial to the first premolar and distal to the lateral incisor. **Medial** and **lateral** are terms applied in relationship to the midline of the body. A structure, A, located closer to the midline than another structure, B, is therefore medial to structure B.

An anatomy student must also learn to visualize several imaginary planes passing through the body serving to divide it in one way or another. The **median plane** passes vertically through the body from

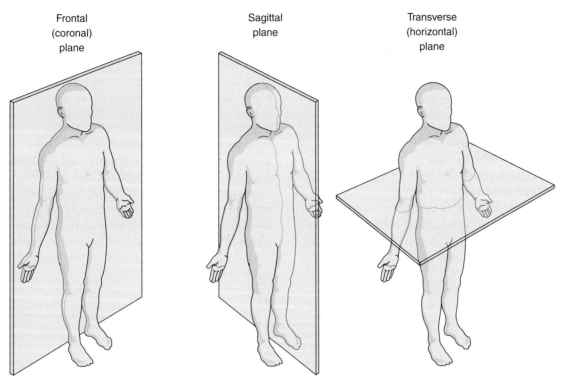

Figure 2-1. Human figure in the anatomic position (palms facing forward), illustrating frontal (coronal), sagittal, and transverse (horizontal) planes.

anterior to posterior at the midline. This plane divides the body into symmetric right and left halves, except for certain areas of the viscera. This plane may also be referred to as the **midsagittal plane**. Any plane parallel to this plane is simply a **sagittal plane**.

A plane through the body at right angles to the midsagittal plane is the **horizontal** or **transverse plane**, providing a cross section with superior and inferior parts. Another plane passes at right angles to the midsagittal plane, again in a vertical direction, and is the **frontal** or **coronal plane**, dividing the body into anterior and posterior sections (Fig. 2-3).

Although the previously described terms are applied to the entire body, they are also appropriately used in describing the structures in head and neck anatomy.

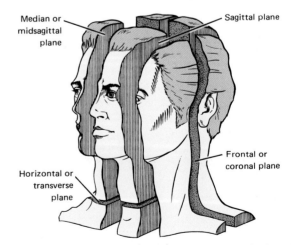

Figure 2-2. Human figure and a quadruped figure illustrating comparative planes and directional references with alternate terminology.

Figure 2-3. Planes of reference and alternate terminology in the anatomy of the head and neck.

ANATOMIC VARIATION

Summary Bite. Anatomic variation is often the rule rather than the exception and the student must learn to recognize and interpret its significance.

A student of anatomy must learn early that anatomic variation is frequently the rule rather than the exception. Structures observed in the cadaver often do not conform to the descriptions found in anatomy textbooks. The major structures might not vary so much but, as the finer details are studied, variations clearly emerge. For example, a student would not expect great variation in the number of bones present in a cadaver, and the variation is not great. However, the individual processes on the bones and their relationships are not at all constant from one individual to another. Similarly, muscles might display slightly different origins, insertions, and tendons. Nerves might not arise from the segment as described. Variations in blood supply are common; thus, a particular region might be supplied from an entirely different source than that described.

It is important that the student learn to recognize anatomic variations as they exist, whether or not they are described. Furthermore, the student must learn to interpret logically the significance of these variations and perhaps to extrapolate their effects on the living individual. Mastering this diagnostic technique helps enable the professional to make rational decisions regarding anatomic variations observed in clinical practice.

Body Systems

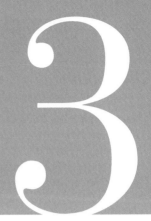

Key Terms

Autonomic Nervous System is an involuntary (visceral) motor system serving smooth muscles, cardiac muscles, and glands.

Cardiovascular System is composed of the heart, arteries, capillaries, veins, and the blood. The two-pump heart circulates blood through the pulmonary circuit to oxygenate the blood and to rid it of carbon dioxide, and it pumps the oxygen-rich blood in the systemic circuit to the remainder of the body. Additionally, the cardiovascular system transports water, hormones, and nutritive materials and exchanges these for waste and carbon dioxide, which it will deliver for elimination. Most of these exchanges take place in the capillary beds within the tissues.

Endochondral Bone Formation is a method of bone development where bone forms on a cartilage model which it eventually replaces.

Enteric Nervous System is the third division of the autonomic system, located wholly within the wall of the alimentary canal; it functions in regulating the process of digestion. The enteric nervous system is composed of about the same number of neurons as are present in the spinal cord. Although the sympathetic and parasympathetic nervous systems exercise a modulating effect on the enteric nervous system, it can function on its own if the connections are severed.

Integument includes the skin, hair, nails, and glands.

Intramembranous Bone Formation is a method of bone development where the bone forms within the surrounding mesenchyme.

Muscle usually spans across a joint from a bony origin on one side of the joint to insert upon a bone making up the other side of the joint. Contraction of the muscle, which is controlled by nerve stimulation, will alter the angle of the joint. Some muscles, such as those of the facial expression, originate and insert in connective tissue proper rather than bone.

Parasympathetic Nervous System is a division of the autonomic nervous system composed of a two-neuron chain originating in either the brain or sacral spinal cord and synapsing with the second neuron within an autonomic ganglion. This second neuron innervates the effector organs (smooth muscle,

cardiac muscle, and glands). The parasympathetic nervous system is "calming" as it returns the body to a homeostatic state.

Skeleton is composed of bone whose articular ends are usually covered with cartilage to absorb shock and reduce friction. The skeleton is made up of a series of bones comprising the axial skeleton and others comprising the appendicular skeleton.

Sympathetic Nervous System is a division of the autonomic nervous system composed of a two-neuron chain originating in the thoracic and first two or three lumbar spinal cord segments and synapsing with the second neuron within an autonomic ganglion. This second neuron innervates the effector organs (smooth muscle, cardiac muscle, and glands). The sympathetic system provides for the "fight or flight" response.

Human beings, just as all other animals, are composed of a complex aggregate of specialized **cells**. These cells—the building blocks of all living things—have become specialized to perform certain functions, a "division of labor."

CELLULAR ORGANIZATION

⮩ **Summary Bite.** Cells are organized into tissues, organs, and organ systems based on their specializations relative to structure and function.

Because structure and function are interrelated, it is possible to group these cells and the material they export into the extracellular spaces into functional classifications based on morphologic features. Similar specialized cells organized to perform a specific role are grouped into **tissues**. Thus, the cell classifications of epithelium, connective tissue, muscle, and nerve represent all of the specializations relative to structure and function.

Tissues fabricated together and performing in unison to accomplish a particular function make up an **organ**. Organs acting together to accomplish specific functionary roles are referred to as **organ systems**. Thus, the body possesses a myriad of cells organized into tissues and organs performing together as the integumentary, skeletal, muscular, circulatory, endocrine, digestive, respiratory, excretory, reproductive, and nervous systems.

Although it is not the purpose of this text to detail the systems of the body, it is nevertheless essential that students possess a satisfactory knowledge of the systems encountered in the head and neck. By learning or reviewing a brief overview of each

of these systems, students will reach a common starting point for studying the anatomy of the head and neck.

INTEGUMENTARY SYSTEM

⮩ **Summary Bite.** The integumentary system is composed of the skin and its derivatives, including the hair, nails, and glands.

The integument, or skin, includes its derivatives—the hair, nails, and glands. It functions to protect the underlying structures against intrusion from the outside and from loss from within. Furthermore, it serves as a sensory receptor, a body temperature regulator, and an organ of secretion and excretion.

Skin

⮩ **Summary Bite.** The skin covers the body except where it becomes continuous with the mucous membranes at the orifices of the body. It possesses many specializations in different regions of the body.

The skin forms a pliable covering over the body and becomes continuous with mucous membranes at the orifices of the body, as at the anus, urethra, vagina, nares, and the oral cavity. The skin is thickest over the back, the palm of the hand, and the sole of the foot, where it is about 6 mm thick. The thinnest skin, which overlies the tympanic membrane and the eyelid, is about 0.5 mm thick. In most areas of the body the skin is loosely attached to the underlying structures, thus permitting it to be easily displaced. It is, however, firmly attached to the periosteum of the tibia, to cartilage of the ear, and over joints of the fingers and the palm of the hand.

Skin color is primarily controlled by three factors: blood, carotene, and melanin. Variation in color is related to degree of vascularity, oxygen content of blood, skin thickness, and profuseness of pigmentation. Under certain conditions, physiologic changes may produce a transient increase in pigmentation, as evidenced in the tanning process from exposure to sunlight. The external genital areas, the axilla, and the areola of the mammary gland display constantly deeper pigmentation.

Skin possesses fine furrows or creases extending in various directions across its surface. These furrows tend to divide the surface into polygonal areas. Some of these areas are large, whereas others (e.g, on the back of the hand) are small. Epidermal ridges and sulci (furrows) on the fingers, palms, and soles are organized in a specialized fashion of whorls and curves peculiar to each individual. This particular uniqueness provides the basis for fingerprint identification. Epidermal ridges provide friction against slippage in walking and in grasping. Ducts of sweat glands open on the summits of the ridges, whereas in areas covered with hair, the shafts emerge at points of intersection of the furrows. Typically, the secretions of the sebaceous glands empty in the furrows also.

Structure

Summary Bite. Skin is composed of the epidermis, which is made up of the avascular epidermis, a stratified squamous keratinized epithelium, as well as the underlying connective tissue, known as the dermis, which houses blood vessels, nerve endings, connective tissue, sebaceous and sweat glands, hair follicles, and smooth muscles.

Skin is composed of two layers: the **epidermis**, or surface layer, and the underlying **dermis**. The epidermis is without blood vessels but is penetrated by sensory nerve endings. In general, the epidermis is only about 1 mm thick and is composed of several layers of stratified squamous epithelial cells. Histologists have subdivided these layers into five distinct groups based on morphologic features and function. The deepest layer, the **stratum basale** (formerly known as the **stratum germinativum**), overlies the dermis and is primarily responsible for producing all of the epidermal cells above it, which are being shed constantly. As these cells mature, they produce **keratohyalin**, which is eventually transformed into keratin in the superficial layers. The most superficial layer, the **stratum corneum**, is composed of dead cells and keratin and forms a horny layer whose thickness is related to the trauma it experiences.

The dermis underlying the epidermis possesses the blood supply, lymphatic channels, and nerve endings. It also contains sebaceous and sweat glands, hair follicles, and the smooth muscles of the skin. The interface of the epidermis and dermis is thrown into interdigitations of **epidermal ridges** and **dermal ridges (dermal papillae)**, which serve to secure the two layers (Fig. 3-1).

The dermis is composed of two basic layers—a superficial papillary layer and the deeper reticular layer—containing collagenous and elastic fibers, which account for its strength and elasticity. The deepest layer of the dermis sits on a subcutaneous connective tissue layer. The interface of these two layers is somewhat interdigitated so that when the layers are separated from each other the dermal side appears to exhibit a dimpled appearance similar to an orange peel. These dimples are sites of entry for nerves and blood vessels into the skin from the subcutaneous connective tissue.

The subcutaneous connective tissue (**hypodermis**) is a loose, fibrous connective tissue containing fat and some elastic fibers. It may be termed **loose areolar tissue** or **superficial fascia**. Some areas of the body possess large deposits of fat in this layer and are designated **panniculus adiposus**. Certain other areas, notably the eyelids, penis, and scrotum, as well as the nipple and areola of the mammary gland, are devoid of subcutaneous fat. Embedded in this layer are the roots of the hair follicles, blood vessels, secretory portions of the sweat glands, and nerves with special sensory endings for pressure. Overlying some joints, the hypodermis contains **bursae**, which are fluid-filled sacs that provide lubrication for movement of the skin as the joint is flexed. Many mammals, such as the horse, possess voluntary muscles in the hypodermis that permit flinching of the skin. Muscles of this nature, originating in the hypodermis and inserting in the dermis, are present in the scalp, face, and neck. Here they are grouped in humans as the **muscles of facial expression**. Involuntary (smooth) muscles are also represented in this layer, muscles such as the dartos muscle of the scrotum and the muscles of the nipple and areola of the mammary gland.

Hair

Summary Bite. Hair is found in nearly all places on the body except the palms, the soles, and a few other places. If hair is straight, its cross-sectional shape is round; if hair is curly, its cross section is flattened.

Hair is found on nearly all parts of the body with the exception of the palms, the soles, the dorsum

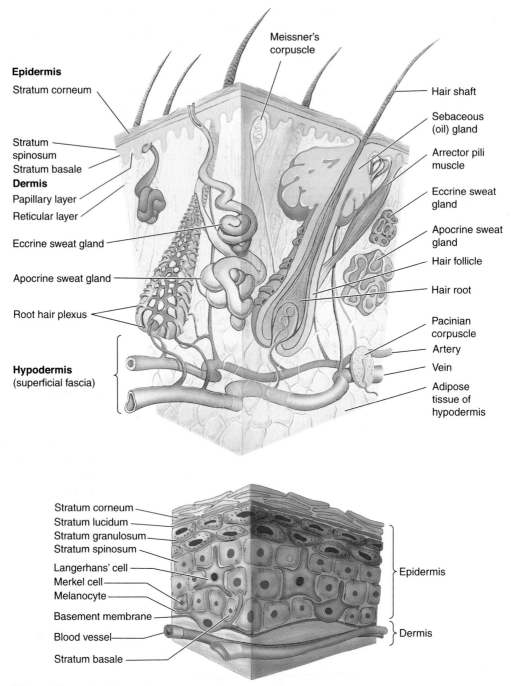

Figure 3-1. Skin structure. Observe the interface between the highly cellular epidermis and the underlying dermis where hair follicles, smooth muscles, and sebaceous and sweat glands originate, but reside mostly in the deeper layer of the dermis and the hypodermis, alongside vascular and nerve elements.

of the terminal digits, the nipples, the umbilicus, and the skin portion of the genitalia. Hair is also absent in areas of skin that are transitional to mucous membrane, such as the lips and nares. The cross section of hair may be round, causing it to be straight, or it may be flattened, producing curly hair. The eyelashes, hair of the pubic region, and hair in the beard are very thick, whereas in other areas of the body it may be so thin that it may go unnoticed. Hair on the scalp may remain for up to four years, whereas the eyelashes may survive only for a few months.

Hair is a product of the epidermis, whose deeper cells invade the dermis and form a hair follicle from which the nonliving hair develops. The dermis responds by forming a papilla to nourish the regenerative cells of the follicle. Thereafter, the hair grows surfaceward, finally exiting the skin. The free part of the hair is called the **shaft** and that within the follicle is the **root**. Color is imparted to the hair by melanin and red pigment in the hair cells.

Each hair has in association with it one or more sebaceous glands, whose ducts open into the neck of the hair follicle. Involuntary muscle fibers (**arrector pili**) arise in the dermis and attach to the hair follicle, serving to erect the hair, squeezing out the secretions of the sebaceous glands and producing "goose bumps" on the flesh (Fig. 3-1).

Nails

Summary Bite. Nails are composed of highly keratinized epithelial cells that form nail plates at the distal ends of the terminal digits.

The nails, which grow approximately 1 mm per week, are modifications of epidermal cell layers on the terminal digits. It should be noted that toe nails grow at a slower rate. The vascular nail bed, formed by the lower germinal layer of the epidermis and the dermis, on which lies the translucent nail plate, imparts a pinkish hue to the nail. The visible part of the nail is the body and the hidden portion behind the nail wall is the root. The nail is formed in the proximal part near the whitened lunula, which may be covered by eponychium (cuticle). The epidermis is thickened under the distal portion of the nail, forming the hyponychium.

Glands

Summary Bite. Glands of the skin include sweat glands, sebaceous glands, and the mammary glands (modified sweat glands).

Glands of the skin include the sebaceous glands, the sweat glands, and the mammary glands (the last will not be discussed in this text because they are remote to the head and neck). The sebaceous glands have been described in their association with hair follicles, but there are nonfunctional sebaceous glands, known as Fordyce granules, located in regions of the body devoid of hair, namely, the lips, the corners of the mouth, and sometimes within the oral cavity. In addition, these glands may be found in most areas of the genitalia as well as the areola and nipple. The secretory cells are constantly destroyed and become part of the oily secretion **sebum**, which protects the skin and hair from undue drying.

Sweat glands are widely distributed, being absent only from the lips, parts of the ear, the skin of the nipple, and some skin areas of the genitalia. Sweat glands are most dense over the palms and soles. The clear, noncellular fluid produced by the sweat glands regulates body temperature as it evaporates from the surface of the skin, cooling it (Fig. 3-1).

MUSCULAR SYSTEM

Summary Bite. The muscular system is composed of specialized cells that have the capacity to contract, which permits movement. There are three types of muscles: skeletal, cardiac, and smooth.

Cells specialized to function in contraction on stimulation comprise the muscles of the body. Skeletal muscles are usually attached from bone to bone, across a joint. On contraction, muscles change the angle of the joint, producing motion. In this way, muscles acting in concert, effect movement. Such motion may be under conscious control (**voluntary**) or not under conscious control (**involuntary**). Muscles that affect smiling, walking, writing, and so on are voluntary muscles, whereas those used in altering the diameter of blood vessels or controlling the bowel are in the involuntary category.

The body has three types of muscles: skeletal, cardiac, and smooth. The first two are striated and the last is not. Skeletal muscle is under voluntary control, whereas cardiac and smooth muscles are involuntary.

Structure

Summary Bite. The contractile elements are the myofibrils composed of actin and myosin, whose organization makes the skeletal and cardiac muscle cells appear striated, whereas smooth muscle cells do not exhibit striations.

Microscopically, the muscle cell is referred to as a **muscle fiber**. The cytoplasm of skeletal and cardiac muscle cells contains many contractile elements called **myofibrils**, which are composed of actin and myosin. The fibril arrangement in these muscles is such that the muscle fiber appears to be cross-banded in alternate light and dark striations. This appearance is responsible for the name **striated muscle**. Skeletal muscle fibers are long, cylindrical, multinucleated cells whose nuclei are located peripherally (Fig. 3-2).

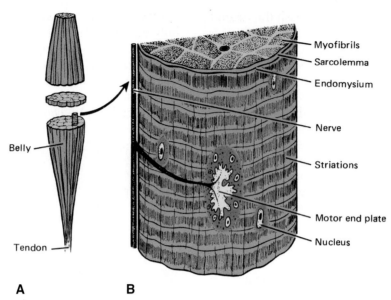

A   B

Figure 3-2. Skeletal muscle. **(A)** Belly of muscle shown with fascicles in cross section. **(B)** A detailed section of a single muscle fiber.

Smooth and **cardiac muscle** cells, in contrast, each possess only one centrally located nucleus. Microscopic evaluation reveals no striations within the cytoplasm of smooth muscle cells.

Smooth Muscle

Summary Bite. Smooth muscle is involuntary, nonstriated, and contains a central nucleus. It is the contractile element in blood vessels and forms the walls of the viscera.

Smooth muscle is a nonstriated, fusiform muscle containing a centrally placed nucleus. This involuntary muscle is the contractile element in vessel walls and forms the walls of the viscera, where it forms longitudinal and circular layers reinforcing the hollow viscera. Contractions of these layers in the gastrointestinal (GI) tract are responsible for peristalsis. Each hair of the skin possesses a smooth muscle attached at its base. Contractions of these muscles causes "gooseflesh." Because smooth muscle is involuntary, it is innervated by the autonomic nervous system.

Cardiac Muscle

Summary Bite. Cardiac muscle is found in the heart. It is striated and branched and joins to form intercalated discs. Each cell posses a centrally placed nucleus.

Cardiac muscle is found mostly in the muscular pump, the heart. Cardiac muscle fibers are striated in a fashion similar to skeletal muscle cells, but each cell possesses only one centrally located nucleus. Features unique to cardiac muscle are its branching and its anastomosing, or joining together, of the cells, and its transversely oriented **intercalated discs**, located at the junction of any two fibers. This muscle type is unique in that it possesses an ability to modify its contractive actions by altering the wave of impulses received from the nervous system.

Skeletal Muscle

Summary Bite. Skeletal muscle is the most abundant muscle. Skeletal muscle is voluntary and highly striated. The cells are very large and multinucleated. Skeletal muscle is responsible for body movements.

Skeletal muscle is by far the most abundant muscle in the body. In fact, it comprises about 40% of the total body weight. Skeletal muscle size varies from the large muscles of the leg to the very small stapedius muscle (only about 2 mm long), which is attached to the tiny stapes bone of the middle ear cavity.

Each skeletal muscle fiber is encased in a thin connective tissue covering, the **endomysium**. A **muscle fascicle**, composed of a group of muscle fibers, is bundled into a separate connective tissue sheath, the **perimysium**. The entire muscle, composed of many fasciculi, is wrapped in yet another connective tissue sheath, termed the **epimysium** or **deep fascia**.

Attachment

Summary Bite. The connective tissue coverings of muscle fibers attach to bone via tendons. A flattened attachment such as is present on the skull is termed aponeurosis. Bursae form around the attachment of some tendons, providing lubrication, reduction of frictional forces, and protection.

At the attachment to bone, the endomysium, along with the epimysium and perimysium, merge to form the tendon, a dense, regular, collagenous connective tissue, silvery white in color. Tendons are extremely strong and at the their attachment site on bone the periosteum is absent. In certain regions of the body, such as in the muscles of the scalp, attachment is by an **aponeurosis**, a broad, flat, sheetlike structure, instead of a tendon.

Some attachments are provided with **bursae**, which lubricate the tendon as it passes over bone. Often a **synovial sheath** encloses a tendon, forming a tubular sac that is capable of secreting a **synovial fluid**, which functions to reduce friction. Friction is also reduced by the epimysium, the deep fascia of the body. Because the deep fascia encloses muscles and bone in a continuous manner, it also serves to contain the spread of infection.

Tendinous attachments to bone are usually described as the **origin** and **insertion** of the muscle. Generally, the muscle is described as arising from the origin, possessing a fleshy belly (the contractive portion), and inserting at the insertion site. The origin is usually the more proximal and/or fixed area, with the insertion being the more distal or movable area. Movement is usually described relative to the muscle insertion position moving toward the origin while the body is in the anatomic position. It must be stressed that these are not inviolate rules but, rather, are arbitrarily used by anatomists as aids in describing function. These rules are especially difficult to apply in the head and neck; thus, learning muscle functions in this region of the body is painstaking.

Although the previous description of bone-to-bone origin and insertion is the usual occurrence, the muscles of facial expression do not follow this rule. Generally, these muscles arise from bone or fascia and insert into the skin of the face. On contraction, they produce movements of the skin that we recognize as facial expressions.

Form

Summary Bite. Muscle size, form, and fiber arrangement is indicative of its power and direction of the movement it produces across a joint.

Examining a muscle's size, form, and fiber arrangement in relation to its insertion into the tendon will indicate the relative strength of the muscle as well as the direction of its force. Muscle fibers that approach the tendon in an oblique fashion afford more power. Muscles whose anatomy takes this form are **pennate**. Fibers entering a tendon at two oblique angles, as do the veins of a feather, are said to be **bipennate**. Multiples of this architectural arrangement produce **multipennate** muscles, which exhibit the greatest strength.

Action

Summary Bite. Terms employed to describe muscle action are not easily applied to all movements. However, most are intuitive, such as flexion and extension across a joint and adductors and abductors moving things toward or away from the midline. Actions about the head and neck are protrusion, retraction, elevation, rotation, and depression.

Muscle action is described according to the movement effected in the part in motion from the anatomic position (this basic reference position was shown in Fig. 2-1). Although individual actions are often difficult to separate given the complexities of a variable motion—as, for example, in mandibular movement—they are expressed in a few anatomic terms. **Flexion** is described as motion that reduces the angle of a joint, whereas **extension** increases the joint angle. Making a fist uses the flexor muscles; opening a closed fist uses the extensor muscles. **Adduction** and **abduction** describe motion toward and away from the body centerline, respectively. Terms describing movements of the head and neck—**protrusion**, **retraction**, **elevation**, **rotation**, and **depression**—are self-explanatory.

Several other terms are used to describe various other motions created by the action of a muscle; however, because these are of no concern to the study of the head and neck, their discussion will be omitted here. Often, names assigned to muscles reflect the architecture of the muscle, its form or shape, its attachments and action, or, in some cases, a combination of these features. However, seldom does a muscle function independently. Indeed, movements are so complex that muscles must function in a cooperative and integrated manner to accomplish a total desired movement. To recognize this complexity, anatomists have created additional terms that indicate how a muscle functions in producing a total movement. Muscles may be **prime movers** or **synergists**, which assist a prime mover. Certain other muscles, such as the strap muscles attached to the hyoid bone, serve as

fixators, so that other actions may be initiated by yet other muscles. **Antagonists** function in such a manner that the action they develop is in opposition to the desired function of yet other muscles (**agonists**). In addition to aiding in the production of smooth movement, antagonists protect the musculoskeletal system from damaging itself, as might occur through a violent movement.

Nerve Control

Summary Bite. Voluntary muscle contraction is controlled by nerves that interact with the muscle fiber at the motor end plate stimulating the muscle fiber to contract. Other nerve fibers enter the muscle to relay sensory and proprioceptive information back to the central nervous system.

Voluntary muscles must receive nerve stimulation to contract. The number of nerve fibers in a muscle depends on the muscle's size and the degree of control required of the muscle. The extrinsic muscles of the eye, for instance, are well endowed with nerve fibers, whereas the muscles of the back possess fewer nerve endings. As the nerve fiber approaches the muscle, it branches to innervate many muscle fibers. The **motor end plate** is that part of the muscle fiber's cell membrane where the nerve fiber forms a synapse with the muscle cell and the impulse is transmitted (Fig. 3-2). In addition to this nerve fiber, which serves a motor function, other fibers enter the muscle, which will conduct sensations of pain and proprioception from the muscle and surrounding connective tissue back to the central nervous system (CNS). These nerves provide sensory data to the CNS so the motor function may be reprogrammed either voluntarily or involuntarily, as might be necessary for the individual to take protective measures.

When a muscle fiber is stimulated, it contracts maximally according to the "law of all or none." It holds, then, that fine movements are accomplished by stimulating fewer nerve fibers, resulting in activation of only a portion of the total muscle fibers at a given time.

Energy requirements necessary for the work performed by the muscles demand a rich vascular supply. It is a general rule throughout the entire body that nerves and blood vessels travel together as **neurovascular bundles**, are named alike, and enter the muscle together. Larger muscles, requiring additional vascularization, may have additional arteries entering their surfaces without associated nerves. In such cases, the artery usually arises from a nearby vascular trunk. Whereas nerve supply to a muscle is specific, vascular supply might not be; therefore, vascular supply is provided by region.

SKELETAL SYSTEM

Summary Bite. Bone and cartilage are specialized connective tissues that make up the skeletal system. As a system they perform many functions, including protection, attachment for muscles, leverage, mineral storage, and blood formation.

The elements of the skeletal system—bone, cartilage, and the joints—are composed of intercellular materials and cells specialized in performing certain functions for the body. Functions unique to this system include support, protection, providing attachment for muscles, leverage, mineral storage, and blood formation.

Support is derived from the mineral salts that are deposited in the matrix and fibers secreted by the cells of the system. Through this process, the skeletal system provides form and a framework on which all of the remaining systems of the body are supported and held together.

Protection is afforded to the soft tissues of the body, including the viscera, lungs, and brain, by encasing them in partially enclosed structures, such as the rib cage and pelvis, or in an enclosed chamber, the skull.

The skeletal system also provides sites of attachment for skeletal muscles along the bones and across the joints. The various parts of the skeletal system then can be used as levers for the production of motion as a result of muscle contraction. In addition to their function in providing leverage, bones become calcified by mineral deposits during development and growth and, therefore, serve as reservoirs for mineral storage. The predominant minerals stored are calcium, magnesium, and phosphate.

A final major function of the skeletal system is blood cell formation. The interiors of most bones, including the epiphyses of long bones, flat, irregular, and short bones, house bone **marrow**, whose specialized cells have the capacity of differentiating and maturing into circulating blood cells. Although the liver and spleen are active in blood cell production prenatally, they cease this function prior to birth; thus, after birth, bone marrow becomes the principal site of blood cell production.

Skeleton

Summary Bite. The bony skeleton is composed of 206 bones divided into an axial and an appendicular skeleton.

The skeletal system, composed of 206 bones, is divided into the **axial skeleton** and the **appendicular skeleton** according to the following distribution:

Bone	Number
Axial Skeleton	
Skull	28
Hyoid	1
Vertebral Column	26
Ribs and Sternum	25
Subtotal	80
Appendicular Skeleton	
Upper Limbs	64
Lower Limbs	62
Subtotal	126
Total	206

This number is not constant because slight variations can exist among individuals. Many bones do not fuse together until after infancy; therefore, infants possess more bones than adults. Occasionally, some skull bones, which develop as bilateral halves, do not fuse in the midline, thus remaining doubled. The frontal bone is one example of this phenomenon, in some cases remaining divided into two separate bones at the **metopic suture** instead of fusing at the midline.

Accessory bones might also develop in bones possessing multiple ossification centers that fail to unite. This condition gives rise to **Wormian bones**, often observed in the larger flat bones of the skull. **Sesamoid bones** develop within tendons either for additional leverage, as in the patella (kneecap), or as a means of reducing friction at the joint. Several of these bones may be present, but again the number varies among individuals.

The **axial skeleton** comprises the bones making up the longitudinal axis and protects the spinal cord, brain, and vital organs. It also supports the head and neck, along with the trunk and its appendages. A major part of this portion of the skeleton is the **skull**, composed of many bones more or less tightly sutured together forming the cranial vault to protect the brain, as well as bones forming the face. The mandible and bony ossicles of the ear are bones that are separate from the skull proper, but they are still considered part of the skull. Although the hyoid bone does not articulate with the skull, it is occasionally listed as part of the skull because of its functional association.

The **vertebral column** is the major foundation of the skeleton and protects the spinal cord. Attached to the vertebral column are the ribs, which enclose and protect the lungs and heart and attach anteriorly to the medial, anteriorly placed sternum. The five fused sacral vertebrae and four coccyx form part of the pelvis, serving to protect the pelvic viscera. These last nine constitute the remaining components of the axial skeleton.

The **appendicular skeleton**, composed of some 126 bones, makes up the remaining skeletal system. The bones of the **superior extremity** include those of the hand, arm, and pectoral girdle. The pectoral girdle attaches the bones of the superior extremity to the axial skeleton. The **inferior extremity** includes the bones forming the foot and leg and the pelvic girdle. Here the pelvic girdle attaches the extremity to the axial skeleton.

Bone Classification

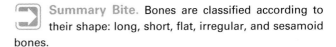 Summary Bite. Bones are classified according to their shape: long, short, flat, irregular, and sesamoid bones.

Bones may be classified on the basis of their general shape. These shapes include **long bones**, as found in the arms and legs, **short bones**, as in the wrist and ankle, **flat bones**, like those forming the skull, and **irregular bones**, such as the vertebrae. **Sesamoid** bones are also described as a separate category.

Bone is a composite of cells and organic matrix secreted by bone cells with deposited inorganic salts crystallized within the matrix. This complex organization produces a lightweight structure with a great tensile strength and the ability to withstand compression. The tubular design of long bones, consisting of a thin layer of compact bone external to spongy bone with its trabeculae, increases the structural strength of the bone. The articular ends of bones usually covered by the articular cartilage are designated as **condyles** or **heads**. The shaft of the bone may possess several characteristic landmarks indicating much information. Terms used to describe these features include **smooth areas**, indicating a periosteum cover only; elevations, in the form of **lines**, **crests**, **ridges**, **processes**, **tubercles**, **tuberosities**, and **spines**, indicating points of attachments; depressions, such as **pits**, **foveae**, and **fossae**, indicating intervals between elevations or sites where a structure may be housed; **grooves** and **sulci**, indicating linear depressions housing particular structures; **foramina** and **notches**, indicating openings or holes; and **canals** or **meatuses**, indicating passageways or tunnels.

Joints

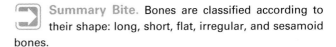 Summary Bite. Joints are formed when two or more bones come together. They may be classified as fibrous, cartilaginous, or synovial, depending on the make-up of the union components.

Two or more bones coming together form a joint. Sometimes the union is such that movement is prevented, whereas in other instances movement is the function of the joint. Joints can be classified as **fibrous**, **cartilaginous**, or **synovial**, depending on the structural articulations of the opposing bones (Fig. 3-3).

Fibrous joints include two types: **syndesmoses** and **sutures**. The syndesmosis joint permits only slight movement between the two bones, which are separated by a layer of fibrous connective tissue. The interosseous membrane between the radius and the ulna is an example. Sutures are joints like those between the flat bones of the skull. Here the individual bones interdigitate tightly along serrated edges, rendering them almost immovable. The fibrous tissue between these bones is continuous with the periosteum.

Some believe that gentle manipulative techniques on the cranial sutures may be used to treat a myriad of health problems. However, it is now suggested that this concept is no longer accepted. **Cartilaginous joints** are represented by **synchondroses** and **symphyses**. Opposing bony surfaces of this group are united by cartilage. A synchrondrosis is a temporary joint that will eventually be ossified into a bony component. The epiphyseal plate on the ends of the growing long bones is an example of this type of joint. A symphysis is a cartilage joint between two bones. It is located in the midline and is interposed between the fusion of the bones, as in the mandibular symphysis and the pubic symphysis.

Synovial joints, the most abundant type in the body, afford the greatest degree of joint movement. The articular surfaces of the bones are covered by hyaline cartilage. The entire joint is in turn covered by ligaments forming an articular capsule, which is lined by synovial membrane. Occasionally, the joint is separated by an **articular disk (meniscus)**. This meniscus is continuous with the capsule peripherally, but its articular surfaces are not covered with synovial membrane. A variety of synovial joints exist in the body, each permitting only a particular type of movement. These movements are categorized using six different terms. Because most of these terms are not associated with the joints of the head and neck, they will be defined as discussion of individual joints requires.

Articulations of the synovial joint are usually of a gliding or sliding character. The joint contains synovial fluid, which acts as a lubricant and also supplies nutrients to the avascular articular cartilage. Synovial joints are richly supplied with sensory nerve endings, principally of the proprioceptive variety, as well as with pain and stretch receptors. Articular capsules and ligaments are highly vascularized, forming capillary networks over the synovial membranes (Fig. 3-4).

Bone Development

Summary Bite. Bone formation may occur in either of two ways: intramembranous bone formation or endochondral bone formation.

During embryogenesis and postnatal growth, bone may develop in one of two ways. It may be formed directly in mesenchyme, in which case the mode is intramembranous. Most of the flat bones of the skull are formed in this manner. The other method of bone formation involves bone being elaborated on and replacing a cartilage template. This is endochondral bone formation and represents the manner in which long bones and most other bones of the body are formed.

Intramembranous Bone Formation

Summary Bite. Intramembranous bone formation begins in a highly vascularized region where mesenchymal cells develop into bone-forming cells.

Intramembranous bone formation begins as the area destined to become bone becomes highly vascularized and the mesenchymal cells develop into **osteoblasts**. These bone-forming cells then begin secreting collagen and a matrix composed of mucoproteins, constituting the **osteoid**. These osteoblasts possess long cell processes that communicate with other osteoblasts and nearby blood vessels. At this stage, the osteoid is a rubbery, tough, somewhat elastic material as yet uncalcified.

Mineral ions of calcium and phosphate, circulating in the blood, begin to diffuse into osteoid tissue and are deposited on the surfaces of collagen fibers as fine crystals. This imparts a hardness and rigidity to the osteoid in the process of becoming bone. Osteoblasts (cells that were responsible for secreting the matrix) become trapped in **lacunae** and are now renamed **osteocytes**.

Endochondral Bone Formation

Summary Bite. Endochondrial bone formation takes place as bone cells invade and replace a cartilaginous template.

Endochondral bone formation begins after a cartilage template has been formed in an area destined to become bone. The hyaline cartilage miniaturized model, which continues to grow while at the same time being replaced by bone, originally develops in mesenchyme in a fashion similar to that of intramembranous bone. Condensation of mesenchymal cells is followed by differentiation into **chondroblasts**, which secrete a

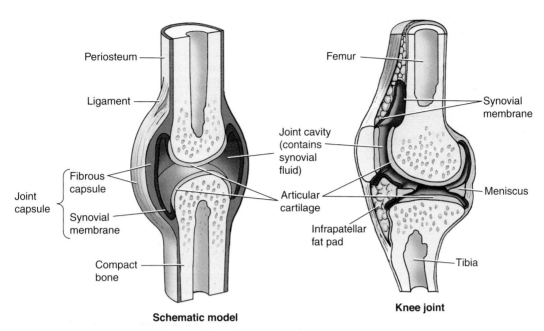

Schematic model   **Knee joint**

A **Synovial joint**

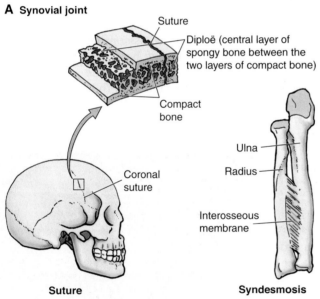

Suture   **Syndesmosis**

B **Fibrous joints**

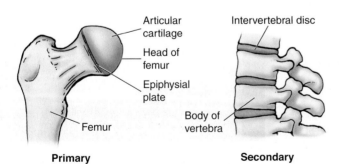

Primary   **Secondary**

C **Cartilaginous joints**

Figure 3-3. Joint types. **(A)** Synovial joint. **(B)** Fibrous joint. **(C)** Cartilagenous joints.

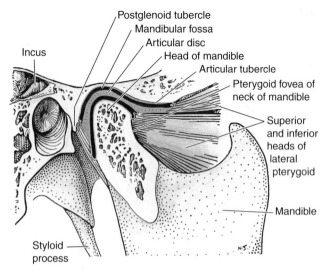

Sagittal section

Figure 3-4. Temporomandibular joint. A portion of the condyle has been cut away, revealing the disc and joint cavity.

viscous polysaccharide matrix interspersed with collagen fibers. The chondroblasts eventually become entrapped in a lacuna within the matrix and are then renamed chondrocytes. Because the matrix might not become calcified soon after formation, if at all, chondrocytes might continue to divide within the lacuna, indicative of **interstitial growth**. Later, the entrapped cells become quiescent, ceasing to produce matrix. Once these cells stop secretion, the only method of enlarging the cartilage model is by **appositional growth** at the periphery by cells differentiated from the perichondrium.

Because of the nature of the cartilage matrix, it does not become infiltrated by blood vessels. Nutrients reach the cells by diffusion only; therefore, chondrocyte metabolism is low compared with that of osteocytes in bone. This low metabolic rate accounts for the slow repair of cartilage.

During endochondral bone formation, the perichondrium of the cartilage model becomes vascularized at mid-diaphysis (shaft), causing the chondrogenic cells to become osteoprogenitor cells, which proliferate to form osteoblasts—cells that elaborate bone in this region. Eventually a **periosteal bud**, composed of mesenchymal cells, osteoprogenitor cells, hemopoietic cells, and blood vessels, invade the model and the cartilage begins to calcify. Simultaneously, osteoprogenitor cells differentiate into **osteoblasts** and start elaborating bony tissue on the calcified cartilage. Then **chondroclasts (phagocytic cells)** begin to destroy the calcified cartilage–calcified bone complex and new bone is elaborated in the remaining space, thus developing a **primary ossification center**. This process spreads outward from the center and, in the case of a

long bone, for example, it may take many years to complete.

The bony structure continues to elongate at its **epiphyses** (ends) by cartilaginous growth. The center of the **diaphysis** of the long bone is composed of **cancellous bone**, which is finally remodeled to withstand stresses on it. Later, much of it is replaced with **red bone marrow** composed of specialized stem cells that give rise to blood cells. The wall of the shaft is composed of very hard and strong **compact bone** to which muscles are attached via tendons (Fig. 3-5).

The architecture of the bone is in a constant state of change in response to the mechanical stresses placed on it. The mandible and maxillae, for example, are constantly being restructured to meet the changing stresses imposed by growth as well as by tooth eruption, movement, wear, and loss. This constant simultaneous growth and remodeling process is achieved by resorbing bone from certain areas and depositing new bone in other areas. The cells associated with the process of resorption are the **osteoclasts**, whereas the osteoblasts responsible for depositing new bone are derived from the osteoprogenitor cells of the **periosteum** covering the bone or the **endosteum** lining the medullary cavity. This is the process that permits the orthodontist to move teeth because tension stimulates

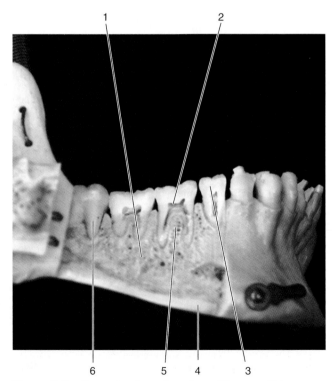

Figure 3-5. Bone structure. A section of the mandible reveals the cancellous bone located interior to the very hard, compact bone located on the surface. (1) Spongy bone; (2) Pulp cavity; (3) Premolar; (4) Compact bone; (5) Bony trabeculae; (6) Molar root.

new bone formation, whereas pressure activates resorption (**Wolff's Law**).

Cartilage

Summary Bite. Hyaline cartilage is at the growing ends of bone and the template for endochondral bone formation; fibrocartilage is in the intervertebral discs; and elastic cartilage is in the ear, auditory tube, epiglottis, and larynx.

Any discussion of bone requires the mention of the articulating cartilages that serve as connective tissue at the joints. Cartilage is a supporting tissue that possesses a firm but somewhat pliable anatomy, permitting it to withstand compression and great stresses at the joints.

Cartilage also serves as the template for endochondral bone formation and functions in long bone growth, as previously discussed. Although cartilage is formed in a fashion similar to bone, it is poorly vascularized and innervated. Three types are recognized: **hyaline**, **fibrous**, and **elastic**. Hyaline cartilage is the type found in the cartilage template of long bones and at their growing ends. Hyaline cartilage is located also at the joints as articulating cartilage and may be found also in the tracheal rings and larynx. Fibrocartilage is present in the intervertebral discs, in the pubic symphysis, and in the mandibular symphysis. Elastic cartilage occurs in the external ear, the auditory tube, the epiglottis, and some components of the larynx.

CIRCULATORY SYSTEM

Summary Bite. The circulatory system is composed of two parts: the cardiovascular system and the lymphatic vascular system.

The circulatory system is composed of two parts working in unison to maintain the internal environment. The heart, arteries, veins, capillaries, and blood comprise the cardiovascular system, whereas the lymph nodes, spleen, tonsils, thymus, lymph, and lymphatic vessels make up the lymphatic system.

Cardiovascular System

Summary Bite. The cardiovascular system is composed of the heart, arteries, veins, capillaries, and blood.

The cardiovascular system functions to provide transportation of oxygen, water, nutritive materials, and hormones to the tissues of the body in exchange for carbon dioxide and wastes that will be further transported to excretory organs for elimination from the body.

Blood, the fluid tissue of the cardiovascular system, is composed of cells and plasma. The cells are **erythrocytes (red blood cells)** and **leukocytes (white blood cells)**. Erythrocytes, which are manufactured in red bone marrow, transport oxygen and carbon dioxide gases to and from the body tissues, respectively. Leukocytes, also manufactured in the bone marrow, are diverse in origin and function. Agranular leukocytes, which include **lymphocytes** and **monocytes**, originate in red bone marrow and lymphatic tissues. They function in the defense of the body and are especially well represented in the immune system. Granular leukocytes include **eosinophils**, **neutrophils**, and **basophils**. These cells are generally assigned the functions of protecting the body from outside invasion and combating infection. **Blood platelets**, formed elements also found in the blood, assist in coagulating the blood. The **plasma** (liquid portion of the blood) is composed of water, proteins, enzymes, and salts as well as the products of digestion and excretion. This fluid leaks out of the capillary walls, becoming the extracellular fluid (tissue fluid) bathing the cells with its contents and picking up wastes before its return to the circulatory system via either venous or lymph capillaries.

The heart, arteries, veins, and capillaries comprise the closed system for the transportation function of the cardiovascular system. The heart is a double pump in that it serves two circuits for blood flow that are completely separated from each other in a normal healthy adult heart. The **pulmonary circuit**, located in the right side of the heart, receives venous (deoxygenated) blood in the right atrium from the body via the **superior and inferior venae cavae** and from the walls of the heart via the **coronary sinus**. During muscular contraction, the pooled blood is pumped from the right atrium through the **right atrioventricular (tricuspid) valve** into the **right ventricle**. Blood in the ventricle is then pumped out the **pulmonary trunk**, which divides into **right and left pulmonary arteries** transporting the blood to the lungs for oxygenation and some excretion (Fig. 3-6).

Oxygenated blood returns from the lungs in the **pulmonary veins** to enter the left side of the heart in the **left atrium**. The blood is now in the **systemic circuit**, where it is pumped through the **left atrioventricular (bicuspid)** valve into the enlarged, very muscular **left ventricle**. From here, the blood will be pumped out of the **aorta** to be distributed by arteries throughout the entire body (Fig. 3-6).

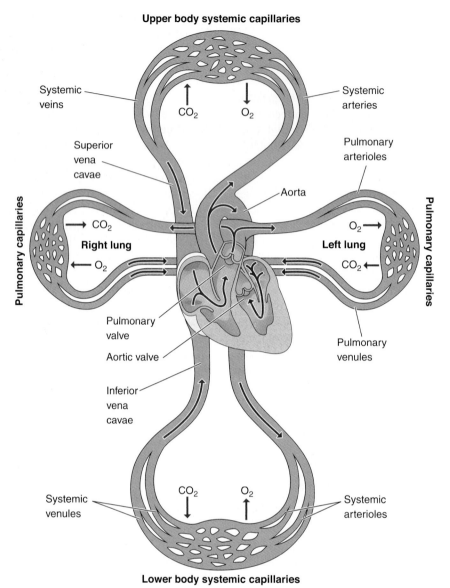

Upper body systemic capillaries

Systemic veins

Systemic arteries

Superior vena cavae

Pulmonary arterioles

Aorta

CO_2 O_2

Pulmonary capillaries

CO_2

Right lung

O_2

O_2

Left lung

CO_2

Pulmonary capillaries

Pulmonary valve

Aortic valve

Pulmonary venules

Inferior vena cavae

Systemic venules

CO_2 O_2

Systemic arterioles

Lower body systemic capillaries

Figure 3-6. Schematic representation of the cardiovascular system.

The **arteries** branch like a tree, becoming smaller and smaller, with each branching leading away from the heart. The blood flows away from the heart from large arteries to small arteries to **arterioles** and **metarterioles** and finally to **capillaries** with a bore large enough only to permit red blood cells to traverse one or two at a time (Fig. 3-7). In the **capillary bed**, gases and nutrients are exchanged for wastes, whereas hormones and enzymes are delivered for body maintenance. Muscles in the walls of the vessels control the blood flow to the periphery, thus aiding in the control and management of body temperature and oxygen requirements.

The cardiovascular system is under control of the nervous system. The rate and force of the heartbeat is modulated by the autonomic nervous system through the specialized cells within the heart musculature. These specialized cells have the innate capacity to perpetuate the rate of heartbeat, but the rate has to be modified by nerve impulses arising from the autonomic nervous system. The blood vessels, particularly the arteries, are also under control of the autonomic nervous system. Nerve impulses to the muscular walls of the arteries elicit either dilation or contraction of the vessel lumen, thereby increasing or decreasing the rate of flow.

Specialized sensory mechanisms to monitor blood pressure and oxygen and carbon dioxide tension within the bloodstream are located in the carotid arteries within the neck. The **carotid sinus**, located at the beginning of the internal carotid artery, responds to changes in blood pressure. The

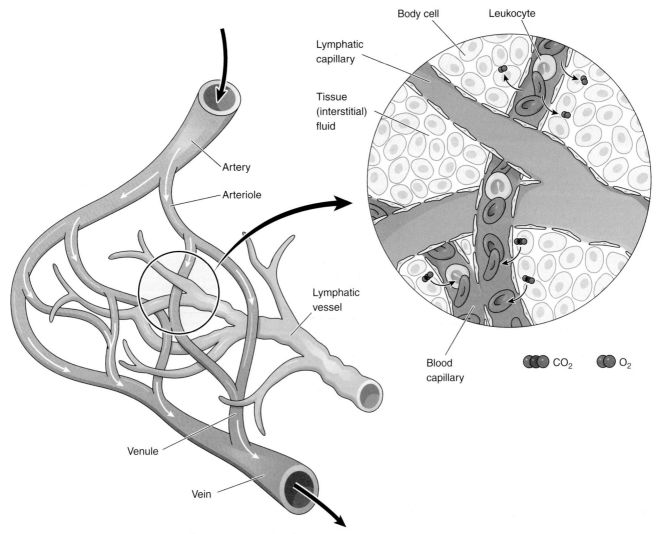

Figure 3-7. Diagram illustrating the capillary bed where tissue fluids leave the blood vessels to bathe the tissues before being taken into the lymphatic capillary.

carotid body, located at the bifurcation of the common carotid artery, is a chemoreceptor sensitive to changes in oxygen and carbon dioxide tension as well as hydrogen ion concentration within the blood. When stimulated, both of these specialized receptors, served by cranial nerves, evoke an autonomic response aimed at returning the system to homeostasis (Fig. 3-8).

Lymphatic System

Summary Bite. The lymphatic system is composed of the lymph nodes, spleen, tonsils, thymus, lymph, and lymph vessels.

The lymphatic system begins as an extensive system of capillary beds collecting the lymph (extracellular fluid) from the tissues (Fig. 3-7). The capillaries empty into larger lymphatic vessels, and eventually the lymphatic vessels empty their contents into the bloodstream in the large veins at the base of the neck. Between the capillary beds and the point of entry into the bloodstream, the lymph passes through one or usually several **lymph nodes**, which act as filters. Here, lymphocytes reside in **lymphoid nodules** and in the paracortex and are propagated for circulation in the bloodstream to sites for combating foreign intrusion. Lymph capillaries within the small intestine, called **lacteals**, receive fatty products of digestion which are eventually transported to the bloodstream via the **thoracic duct**.

In addition to the lymph nodes, the lymphatic system also includes the spleen, thymus, and tonsils, which are responsible for other lymphatic functions such as the filtering of blood and the maintenance of immunocompetence.

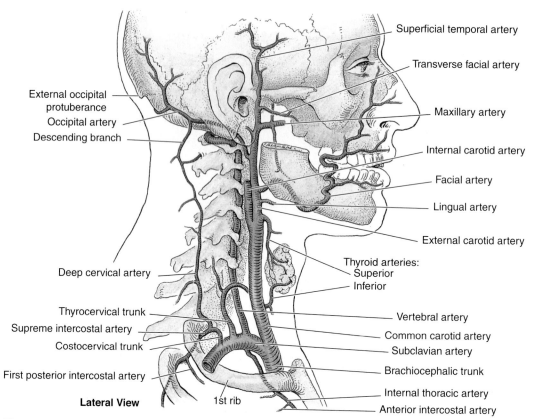

Figure 3-8. Schematic diagram of the carotid artery and the distribution of its vessels in the neck and head.

NERVOUS SYSTEM

Summary Bite. The nervous system is divided into the peripheral nervous system (PNS) and the central nervous system (CNS). The PNS is composed of 12 pairs of cranial nerves and 31 pairs of spinal nerves. The CNS is composed of the brain and spinal cord.

The nervous system is a complex organization of tissue, ramifying throughout the body, functioning to collect information from within and from outside the environment of the body. The nervous system sorts this information, then reacts to perceived challenges imposed on it. Included within the functions of this system is the process of cognitive faculties occurring in the highest centers of the brain.

The nervous system is divided morphologically, for descriptive purposes, into two divisions: the peripheral nervous system (PNS) and the central nervous system (CNS). The **PNS** comprises 12 pairs of cranial nerves emanating from the brain and 31 pairs of spinal nerves originating from the spinal cord. The

CNS is composed of the brain and the spinal cord (Fig. 3-9).

Structure

Summary Bite. The nervous system is made up of neurons (impulse-conducting cells) and neuroglial cells that support the neurons.

The tissue of this system is made up of specialized cells, **neurons**, which conduct impulses, and **neuroglial** cells, which serve in a supporting capacity.

A neuron, the basic structural unit of the system, possesses the ability to perceive stimuli (**irritability**) and to transmit physiochemical impulses along its processes (**conduction**) to effector organs and/or other neurons. The neuron is composed of a **cell body** (soma, perikaryon) and its processes. The cell body contains the nucleus and cytoplasm containing **Nissl bodies** (rough endoplasmic reticulum), which may be made visible by light microscopy through the use of special stains. Neuron cell bodies are located either in a **ganglion**, if outside the CNS, or in **nuclei**, if within the CNS. Radiating from the cell body are

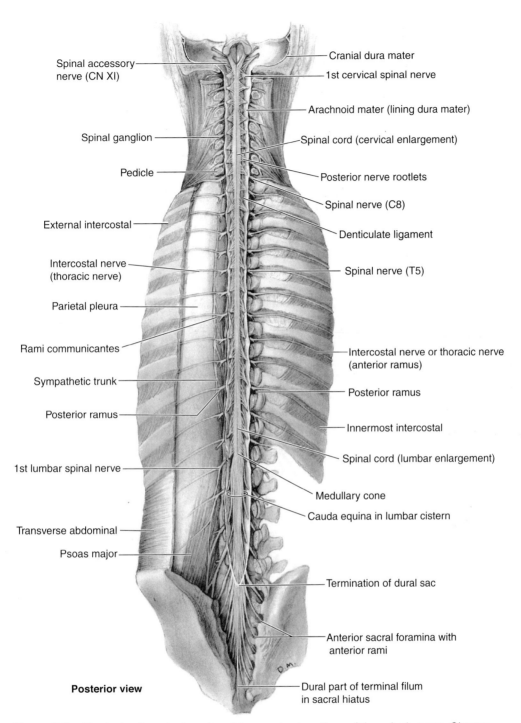

Spinal accessory nerve (CN XI)

Cranial dura mater

1st cervical spinal nerve

Arachnoid mater (lining dura mater)

Spinal ganglion

Spinal cord (cervical enlargement)

Pedicle

Posterior nerve rootlets

Spinal nerve (C8)

External intercostal

Denticulate ligament

Intercostal nerve (thoracic nerve)

Spinal nerve (T5)

Parietal pleura

Rami communicantes

Intercostal nerve or thoracic nerve (anterior ramus)

Sympathetic trunk

Posterior ramus

Posterior ramus

Innermost intercostal

Spinal cord (lumbar enlargement)

1st lumbar spinal nerve

Medullary cone

Cauda equina in lumbar cistern

Transverse abdominal

Psoas major

Termination of dural sac

Anterior sacral foramina with anterior rami

Posterior view

Dural part of terminal filum in sacral hiatus

Figure 3-9. The brain, the spinal cord, and the proximal portions of the spinal nerves. Observe the nerve plexus in the neck.

freely branching processes called **dendrites**, which transmit impulses toward the cell body, and a singular **axon**, which transmits impulses away from the perikaryon. The axon emanates from the cell body at a bulge called the **axon hillock**. The arrangement of processes around the cell body might vary from that described here and are thus supplied with descriptive terms (Fig. 3-10).

Axons may or may not possess a fatty **myelin sheath** covering composed of the wrapping of Schwann cell plasmalemma (in the PNS) or oligodendroglia cell membrane (in the CNS). These

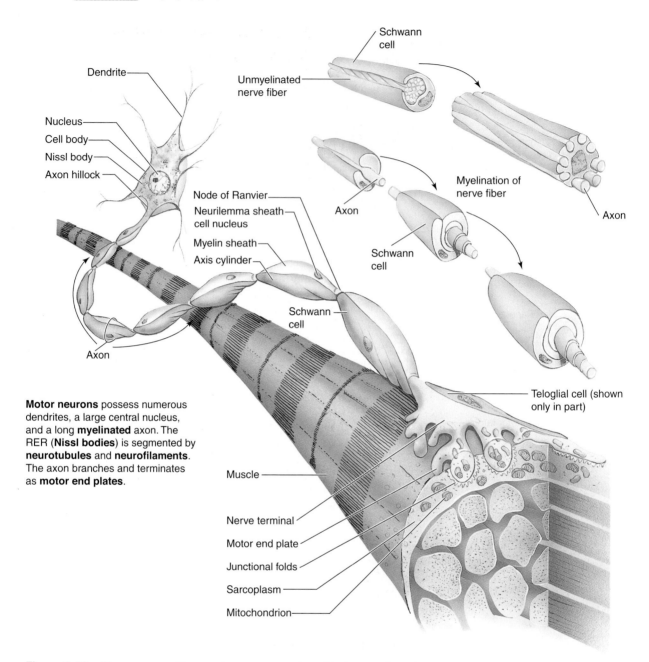

Dendrite

Nucleus
Cell body
Nissl body
Axon hillock

Node of Ranvier
Neurilemma sheath
cell nucleus
Myelin sheath
Axis cylinder

Schwann
cell

Axon

Schwann
cell

Unmyelinated
nerve fiber

Myelination of
nerve fiber

Axon

Schwann
cell

Axon

Teloglial cell (shown
only in part)

Motor neurons possess numerous
dendrites, a large central nucleus,
and a long **myelinated** axon. The
RER (**Nissl bodies**) is segmented by
neurotubules and **neurofilaments**.
The axon branches and terminates
as **motor end plates**.

Muscle

Nerve terminal

Motor end plate

Junctional folds

Sarcoplasm

Mitochondrion

Figure 3-10. Motor neuron. Observe the axon synapsing with the muscle at the motor end plate.

myelin sheaths are of variable thickness and completely surround the **axis cylinder**, except at regular
intervals along the axon. These intervals, called the
nodes of Ranvier, impart a linked-sausage appearance to the axon. Myelinated or unmyelinated axons
are covered by a **neurilemma sheath** composed of
Schwann cells (in the PNS) or oligodendroglia (in the
CNS). The speed of conduction of an impulse along
a nerve fiber is related to the absence or presence
and the thickness of the myelin sheath (Fig. 3-10).

Functional Components

Summary Bite. Neurons are either of a sensory
(afferent) function, an intercalated (connecting) function, or a motor (efferent) function.

See Chapter 18 for a more thorough discussion.
Neurons are categorized functionally as sensory,
intercalated (connecting), or motor. Sensory (afferent) and motor (efferent) functions are each further

subcategorized to facilitate description of a neuron's specific function. **General somatic afferent** refers to sensory function (modality) perceived from the body and transmitted to the spinal cord or brain. Sensations such as pain, temperature, and touch to the skin are perceived by neurons in this category. Also in this category is sensation from muscles, tendons, and joints, referred to as "proprioception." **General visceral afferent** is the sensory modality received from within the viscera (glands, organs, and membranes). **General somatic efferent**, a motor component, serves to provide innervation to all of the skeletal muscles of somatic origin, whereas **general visceral efferent** stimulation provides motor innervation to smooth muscles, cardiac muscles, and glands.

Sensory and motor functions within the head are carried by the cranial nerves. Certain muscle groups and the sense organs for hearing, smell, taste, and sight make this group "special." The senses of sight and hearing are transmitted by **special somatic afferent** sensory neurons, whereas taste and smell are transmitted by **special visceral afferent** sensory fibers. Similarly, the motor component to the "special" muscles (branchiomeric origin) is the **special visceral efferent**. Because no "special" category exists for glandular secretomotor function in the head, the **general visceral efferent** component remains for the glands, smooth muscles, and mucous membranes of this region. Note that certain of the cranial nerves carry **general visceral afferent** sensory components from the viscera of the head as well.

Peripheral Nervous System

Summary Bite. The PNS represents those nerve fibers that receive stimuli from the interior or exterior of the body (i.e., sight and hearing) and transmit it to the CNS for processing. The PNS also delivers motor function from the CNS to the periphery.

Sensory neurons originating peripherally (e.g., in skin) may possess nerve endings specialized for receiving various stimuli, such as cold, hot, touch, and pressure. Nerve endings transmitting pain, on the other hand, are free and without specializations. Dendrites of the spinal nerves are connected to their cell bodies located in the **dorsal root ganglion**, which is just outside the spinal cord. The axons pass from the ganglion via the **dorsal root** into the **dorsal horn** (sensory) of the spinal cord. Here they may terminate, enter the white matter of the cord to ascend or descend before synapsing on connecting neurons in the spinal cord, or ascend to conscious levels in the brain (Fig. 3-11).

Cell bodies of spinal motor neurons are located in the **ventral horn** (motor) of the spinal cord. Their axons traverse the **ventral root** on leaving the spinal cord. Just beyond the dorsal root ganglion area, the sensory and motor roots unite, forming a spinal nerve that thus carries both sensory and motor components (Fig. 3-11). Motor fibers destined for muscle will continue on to **synapse** at the **motor end plate**, a specialized ending between the nerve and the muscle (Fig. 3-10).

Sensory nerve endings located, for example, in the patellar ligament of the knee do not have their

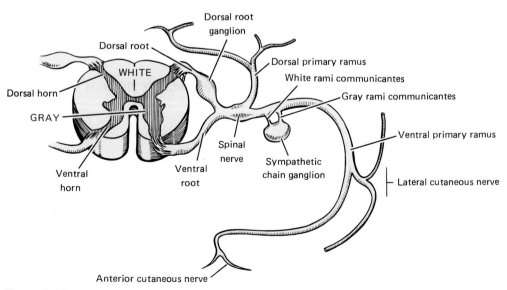
Figure 3-11. Typical thoracic spinal cord segment and spinal nerve.

terminals in the dorsal horn but, instead, terminate directly on motor neurons in the ventral horn of the spinal cord, thus effecting a **reflex arc** that bypasses connecting neurons. Rapid opening of the mouth as a result of painful stimuli from biting down on a piece of bone while chewing is an example of a reflex arc in the fifth cranial nerve.

Central Nervous System

Summary Bite. The central nervous system is composed of the brain and spinal cord.

The central nervous system is represented by the brain, which is housed with the skull, and the spinal cord, which is housed within the vertebral canal surrounded by the divisions of the vertebrae. The brain and spinal cord are responsible for analysis, integration, and response for the body via sensory input and motor output.

Coverings

Summary Bite. The CNS possesses three separate meninges that encase it: dura mater, arachnoid, and the pia mater.

The CNS is composed of the brain and the spinal cord (see Chapter 17). Each is delicately covered by several layers of meninges and is protected by bone—either the skull around the brain or the bony vertebral column that surrounds the spinal cord.

The meninges covering the brain and spinal cord are continuous and completely enclose the CNS. Three separate layers make up the meninges: a tough outer layer, the **dura mater**; an inner delicate layer closely applied to the brain and the spinal cord and their vessels, the **pia mater**; and an intermediate layer, the **arachnoid**, which is closely applied to the dura. Only a potential space exists between the dura and arachnoid, known as the **subdural space**. The **subarachnoid space**, located between the arachnoid and pia layers, contains the cerebrospinal fluid that functions in bathing and further protecting the CNS.

Autonomic System

Summary Bite. The autonomic nervous system, by definition, is a motor system controlling the viscera, cardiac and smooth muscle, and glands. It is subdivided into the enteric, sympathetic, and parasympathetic systems.

The **autonomic (involuntary, visceral) nervous system** exerts control over the viscera of the body, serving

cardiac muscle, smooth muscle, and/or glands. By definition, the autonomic nervous system is purely motor in function. Its manner of functioning is different from that previously described in that innervation is accomplished via a two-neuron chain between the CNS and the effector organ (smooth muscle, cardiac muscle, and glands). The cell body of the first neuron in the chain is located in the CNS (brain or spinal cord), whereas the cell body of the second neuron is located in one of the autonomic ganglia, all of which lie outside the CNS (Figs. 3-11 and 3-12).

The autonomic system is subdivided into the enteric, sympathetic, and parasympathetic systems. The enteric nervous system is located in the wall of the digestive system and functions in the autonomic control of the digestive system. It is influenced by the other two components of the autonomic system. The enteric nervous system is not associated with the head and neck and, therefore, will not be discussed in this textbook.

Sympathetic Nervous System

Summary Bite. The sympathetic nervous system is that system which puts the body ready for action ("fight or flight").

The **sympathetic system** generally prepares the body for action—as in the "fight or flight" response—by increasing heart rate, respiration, blood pressure, and blood flow to the skeletal muscles; dilating the pupils; and generally "shutting down" visceral activity. Neurons of the sympathetic system originate in the intermediolateral cell column of the spinal cord in the thoracic and upper lumbar segments (T1 to L2–L3). Thus, they are often referred to as the **thoracolumbar outflow** of visceral efferent fibers (Fig. 3-13A).

Parasympathetic Nervous System

Summary Bite. The parasympathetic nervous system serves to "calm" the body, returning it to a homeostatic state.

Parasympathetic innervation, conversely, functions to calm the body by decreasing heart rate, respiration, and blood pressure; constricting the pupils; and increasing visceral activity. Both systems innervate many organs of the body where their antagonistic actions serve to balance functioning to maintain homeostasis.

Neurons of the parasympathetic system originate either in the brain in certain nuclei of cranial

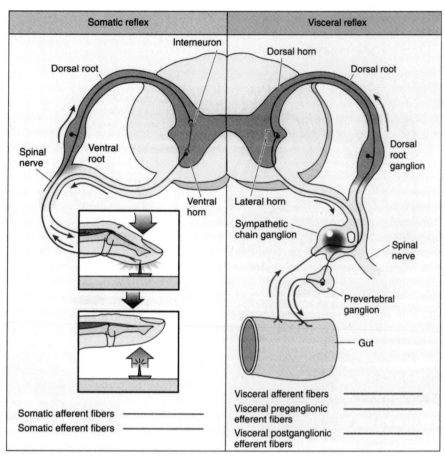

Figure 3-12. Schematic representation comparing the somatic and visceral nervous systems.

nerves III, VII, IX, and X (**cranial outflow**) or in the sacral spinal cord from the intermediolateral cell column of spinal nerves S2–S4 (**sacral outflow**). Together, this system is known as the craniosacral outflow (Fig. 3-13B).

The cell body of the first neuron within the two-neuron chain of the autonomic system is located within the visceral efferent column of the CNS. The axon of this neuron will synapse on the cell body of the second neuron in the chain, located in one of the autonomic ganglia; thus, this axon is **preganglionic**. The axon of the second neuron is **postganglionic** and extends to the effector organ. The sympathetic system is served by the autonomic ganglia located along most of the spinal segments. These ganglia are known as the **sympathetic chain ganglia (paravertebral ganglia)** and are connected to each other by the **sympathetic trunk** and the several **collateral ganglia (preaortic ganglia)** along the major abdominal blood vessels (Figs. 3-11 and 3-13A). Ganglia of the parasympathetic system are located close to the structures innervated and are called **terminal ganglia**, four of which are in the head, whereas others,

the **enteric ganglia**, are located within the wall of the alimentary canal (Fig. 3-13B).

Preganglionic sympathetic fibers reach the chain ganglia via the **white rami communicantes**, a connection between the spinal nerve and the ganglion transmitting the myelinated fibers. The postganglionic fiber may enter the spinal nerve via the **gray rami communicantes** directly or after ascending or descending in the sympathetic trunk. Preganglionic fibers synapse only one time; therefore, those destined to synapse in the collateral ganglia do not synapse in the chain ganglia (Figs. 3-11 and 3-13A).

Preganglionic parasympathetic neurons of the cranial outflow originate in cranial nerves III, VII, IX, and X only and may be distributed to the terminal ganglion via the cranial nerve of origin or by the named preganglionic fiber. Postganglionic fibers are distributed by other nerves serving the organ (Fig. 3-13B).

Acetylcholine is the neurotransmitter of both preganglionic sympathetic and parasympathetic neurons and postganglionic parasympathetic neurons. However, **noradrenaline** is the primary neurotransmitter of postganglionic sympathetic neurons

Parietal distribution | Visceral distribution

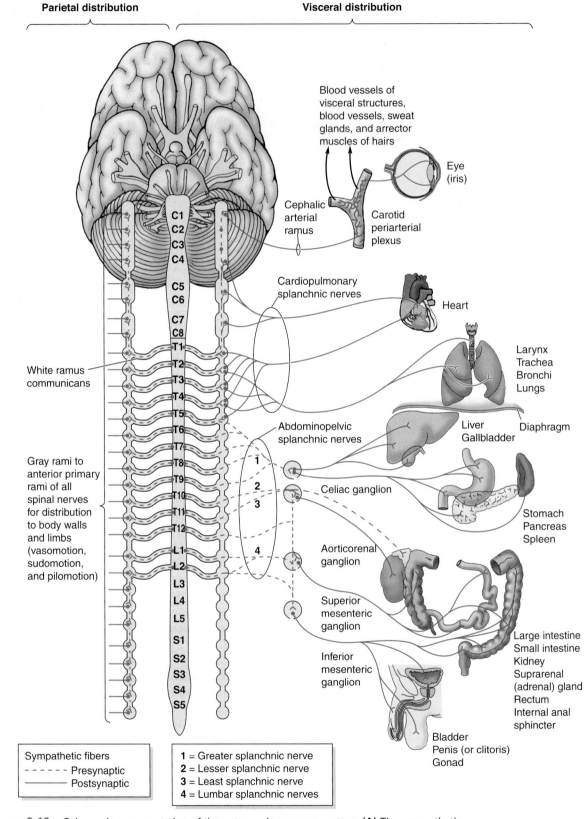

Figure 3-13. Schematic representation of the autonomic nervous system. **(A)** The sympathetic nervous system. *(continued)*

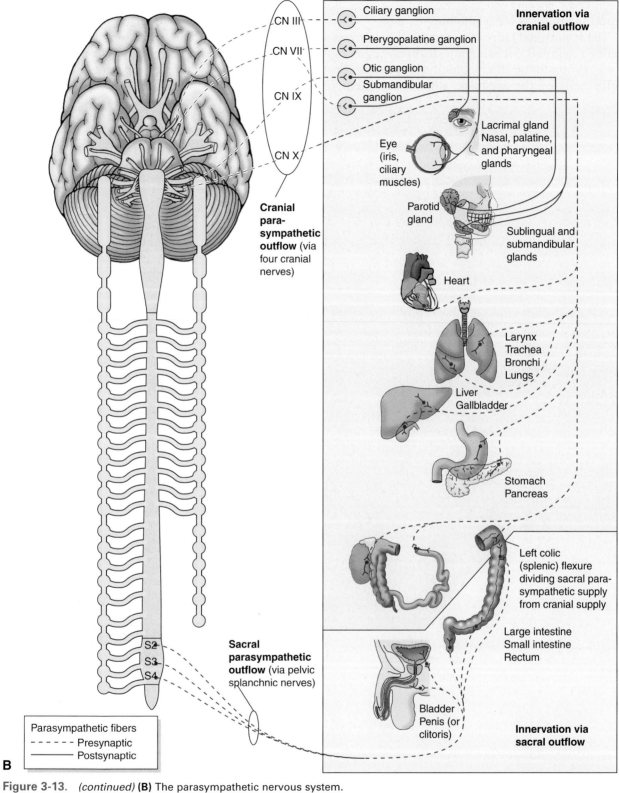

Figure 3-13. *(continued)* **(B)** The parasympathetic nervous system.

except those serving sweat glands. In this case, the neurotransmitter is acetylcholine.

The suprarenal (adrenal) medulla functions as a modified sympathetic ganglion. It receives preganglionic sympathetic fibers which synapse on chromaffin cells of the medulla, stimulating them to produce catecholamines, which give rise to epinephrine and norepinephrine, which are released into the bloodstream. The epinephrine produced here prepares the body for "fight or flight" during stress or fear. The norepinephrine produced here is short-lived.

The Oral Cavity, Palate, and Pharynx

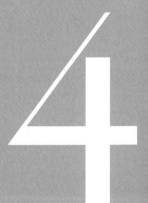

Key Terms

Lips are the highly vascular fleshy structures that guard the entrance to the oral cavity. The dry, red vermilion zone gives way to a wet epithelium lining the vestibule.

Oral Cavity Proper is that part of the oral cavity lying within the space created by the dental arches and their surrounding gingiva of each jaw. It is bounded superiorly by the palate and inferiorly by the muscular tongue.

Palate forms the roof of the oral cavity proper and consists of an anterior-placed bony palate and the posterior soft palate.

Pharynx is a mucous-lined tube attached to the base of the cranium coursing inferiorly to become continuous with the esophagus. It serves as an airway to the larynx and as a passageway for food and drink to the esophagus.

Teeth are arranged on both the maxillary and mandibular arches and articulate with the teeth on the opposing arch during occlusion. While they are in occlusion the oral cavity proper and the vestibule are separated. The deciduous dentition possesses 20 teeth, which is later replaced by the permanent dentition possessing a complement of 32 teeth.

Tongue forms the floor of the oral cavity proper and consists of the body, the freely moving portion, and the base which is attached to the hyoid bone.

Vestibule is that portion inside the oral cavity lying between the dental arches and the cheeks laterally and the lips anteriorly.

This chapter provides an overview of the anatomy of the oral cavity as it would be observed in an oral examination. In addition, some pertinent clinical aspects of the variations in normal anatomy of the oral cavity are addressed where appropriate. Subsequent chapters detail regional dissections pertinent to a thorough understanding of the anatomic structures of the head and neck.

The oral cavity (mouth) is the entry portal of the digestive system. It is bounded anteriorly by the **lips** and posteriorly by the **oropharyngeal isthmus (isthmus faucium)**, a more or less circular aperture that guards the entrance to the pharynx. The oral cavity is lined with mucous membrane composed of stratified squamous epithelium and an underlying dense, irregular, collagenous connective tissue that houses minor salivary glands. For purposes of description, the oral cavity is subdivided into two major regions: the outer **vestibule** and the inner **oral cavity proper**.

LIPS

Summary Bite. The highly vascular fleshy lips guard the entrance to the mouth. The red vermilion zone gives way to mucus membrane leading into the oral cavity.

The lips are two fleshy, mobile structures guarding the entrance to the mouth. They are covered externally with skin that overlies muscle, glands, and connective tissue. Internally they are lined with a mucous membrane. The red portion of the lips, whose coloration is caused by a rich vascular bed visible through the thin epithelium, is termed the **vermilion zone**. Because it is not a wet membrane, it must be kept moistened with the tongue to prevent drying. The skin and vermilion zone join at the **vermilion border**.

The superior lip is bounded laterally by the **nasolabial groove** extending from the **ala (wing)** of the nose to a short distance lateral to the corner of the mouth. A slight shallow, vertical depression in the midline from the nose to the vermilion border is the **philtrum (Cupid's bow)**, and just inferior to this depression is the **labial tubercle**, a fleshy bump of varying size in the vermilion zone (Fig. 4-1). The inferior lip is separated from the chin by the **labiomental groove**.

The two lips are connected laterally by the **labial commissures**, which are thin folds of tissue that are easily viewed when the mouth is slightly opened. Occasionally a slight depression is noted in the center of the labial commissure, known as the **commissural**

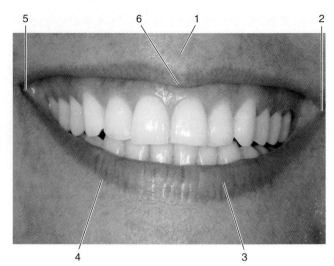

Figure 4-1. Anatomy of the lips and adjacent area. (1) Philtrum; (2) Commissural lip pit; (3) Vermilion zone; (4) Vermilion border; (5) Labial commissure; (6) Labial tubercle.

lip pit. The **oral fissure (rima of the mouth)** is the zone between the superior and inferior lips, which may be opened or, when the two lips are in contact with each other, closed.

The lips develop from several sources, including the median nasal (intermaxillary segment), maxillary, and mandibular processes. Many of the structures just described are fusion remnants of these embryologic origins and often become more pronounced with advancing age. A more detailed description of the development and congenital deformities of the lips is presented in Chapter 5.

VESTIBULE

Summary Bite. The vestibule is the space between the lips and the cheeks external to the teeth in occlusion.

The vestibule is the cleft or space between the lips and cheeks externally and the teeth and gingiva of the dental arches internally when the teeth are in occlusion. The vestibule communicates with the exterior through the oral fissure of the lips and with the oral cavity proper via the interdental spaces and the interval posterior to the last molar teeth in each dental arch (Fig. 4-2).

Laterally, the vestibule is referred to as the **buccal vestibule**, whereas anteriorly, in the region of the lips, it is termed the **labial vestibule**. The **mucobuccal** and/or **mucolabial folds (fornix)** represent the location point at which the regionally named vestibular mucosa turns to become the alveolar mucosa. Located

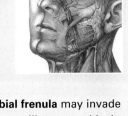

Clinical Considerations

Lips

Cleft lip, often associated with cleft alveolar and primary palate, is the result of a developmental defect and occurs in approximately 1 in 1,000 births. The terminology and severity of this and associated defects in the palate are discussed in detail in Chapter 5.

Congenital commissural lip pits may be observed infrequently at the angle of the mouth in the commissure. These are remnants of development and are not clinically significant (Fig. 4-1). The mouth from corner to corner normally spans between the first premolar teeth.

As the mouth is opened the oral fissure becomes an oval to circular aperture.

Abnormally large superior labial frenula may invade the interdental space between the maxillary central incisors, thus causing a large diastema. This may be relieved by severing the frenula (frenectomy). If after a reasonable time the diastema persists, orthodontic treatment may be necessary.

---

in the superior labial vestibule is the **incisive fossa** represented by a shallow depression superior to the incisor teeth.

The bulge extending into the labial vestibule from the alveolar ridge over the root of the superior canine tooth is the **canine eminence**, whereas the shallow depression just lateral to it is the **canine fossa** (Fig. 4-3).

Protruding into the roof of the buccal vestibule in the vicinity of the first molar is the zygomatic process of the maxilla. This structure may easily be palpated. The nearly vertical anterior border of the masseter muscle may also be palpated in the posterior buccal

vestibule because it extends from the angle of the mandible to the zygomatic arch.

The region of the maxilla posterior to the zygomatic process and superior to the last molar is the **maxillary tuberosity**. This is an important area anatomically because it serves as an injection site for anesthesia of the posterior superior alveolar nerve.

The parotid gland empties its salivary secretions into the buccal vestibule at a small orifice opposite the second maxillary molar. This opening, which appears elevated in the mucosa, is the **parotid papilla (Stenson duct)**. Several other small minor salivary glands that are regionally named—for example, the

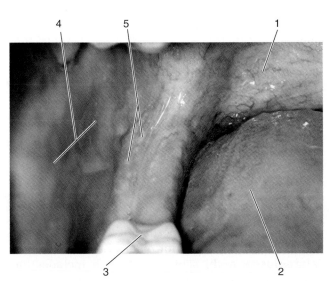

Figure 4-2. Buccal vestibule illustrating buccal mucosa and Fordyce granules. (1) Palate; (2) Tongue; (3) Molar; (4) Buccal vestibule; (5) Fordyce granules.

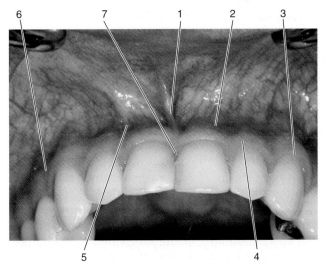

Figure 4-3. Superior labial vestibule indicating regionally named gingiva covering anatomic regions of maxillae. (1) Superior labial frenulum; (2) Mucogingival junction; (3) Marginal gingiva; (4) Attached gingiva; (5) Alveolar mucosa; (6) Canine fossa.

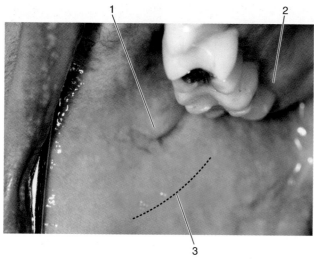

Figure 4-4. Buccal vestibule with opening of parotid duct opposite the second maxillary molar. Accessory buccal glands open onto the mucosa of the vestibule. (1) Parotid papilla; (2) Lingual gingiva; (3) Accessory buccal glands.

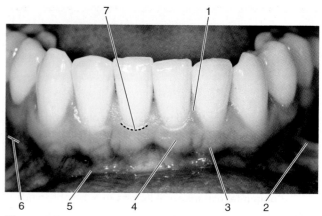

Figure 4-5. The lower jaw, including the regional areas of the mucosa and gingiva. The free gingival groove represents the area above the dotted line. (1) Interdental papilla; (2) Labial frenulum; (3) Mucogingival junction; (4) Attached gingiva; (5) Mucolabial fold; (6) Canine eminence; (7) Free gingival groove.

buccal glands and **labial glands**—also open into the vestibule via microscopic openings (Figs. 4-2 and 4-4).

In most individuals, small yellow spots may be observed in the buccal mucosa lateral to the corner of the lips. These are **Fordyce granules**, composed of defunct sebaceous glands that became trapped in the mucosa during development (Fig. 4-2).

Extra reflections of labial mucosa appear as folds of tissue in the midline attaching the superior and inferior lips to the gingiva. These are the **labial frenula** (sing. frenulum), where the superior labial frenulum is the most prominent (Fig. 4-3). Often, additional frenula may be observed in the labial and buccal vestibules.

Occasionally, the superior labial frenulum is so broadly attached that it interferes with normal eruption of the central incisors, thereby producing a diastema. Correction of this condition usually requires surgical removal of the frenulum between the central incisors to permit the teeth to return to the normal position.

The **gingiva (gum)** is covered by the **gingival mucosa**, which folds back on itself to form a free edge, known as the **gingival margin**, which surrounds the inferior margin of the clinical crowns of the teeth. The vestibular gingiva in this region becomes continuous with the gingiva of the oral cavity proper.

The **interdental papilla** lies between the teeth in the interdental spaces, and the **retromolar papilla** is that specialized area of the gingiva distal to the last molars in both dental arches. The coronal-most aspect of the interdental papilla of the molar region usually possesses a concavity known as the **col**.

Gingival mucosa is pale pink and stippled in good oral health. The **alveolar mucosa** overlies the alveolar

processes of both the maxillary and mandibular arches. Its red hue is caused by the visibility of its vascularity through the nonkeratinized epithelium of its mucosa. Where the alveolar mucosa blends into the remaining vestibular mucosa is not easily distinguished. However, a rather sharp, scalloped line, the **mucogingival junction**, separates the gingival mucosa from the alveolar mucosa (Figs. 4-3 and 4-5).

ORAL CAVITY PROPER

Summary Bite. The oral cavity proper is that part of the oral cavity lying internal to the dental arches of each jaw and their surrounding gingiva. It is bounded superiorly by the palate and inferiorly by the muscular tongue.

The oral cavity proper lies internal to the dental arches and their contained dentition and gingiva. It is bounded superiorly by the palate and inferiorly by the muscular tongue and reflections of the mucous membrane extending from the mandibular gingiva in the **sublingual sulcus (groove)** to the base of the tongue. Anterolaterally, it is bounded by the lingual surfaces of the teeth, lingual gingiva, and lingual alveolar mucosa.

The posterior boundary of the oral cavity proper is formed by the vertical portion of the soft palate superiorly and by the **anterior pillar of the fauces (the palatoglossal arch)**. This arch, which includes the palatoglossus muscle and overlying oral mucosa, extends from the soft palate to the sides of the base of the tongue (Fig. 4-6).

Clinical Considerations

Vestibule

A fold of mucosa in the posterior-most boundary of the vestibule connecting the maxillary and mandibular alveolar regions covers the **pterygomandibular raphe**. The raphe is a tendinous inscription between the buccinator and superior constrictor muscles that is attached to the pterygoid hamulus and the area of the **retromolar triangle** of the mandible (Fig. C4-1).

The superior labial frenulum frequently possesses a tag of tissue located on its anterior surface approximately midway between its attachments at the lip and gingiva. This tissue lends an irregular surface to the frenulum. This small mass is nonpathologic and may be regarded as a hyperplastic anomaly. The region of the buccal mucosa adjacent to the mandibular retromolar papilla contains an aggregation of accessory buccal glands that results in a prominence in the mucosa. This, along with the retromolar papilla, is often referred to incorrectly as the **retromolar pad**.

Occasionally, a white line, the **linea alba**, may be observed on the buccal mucosa representing that area of the mucosa in close proximity to the occlusal surfaces when the jaws are in the closed position (Fig. C4-2).

The space of the vestibule is somewhat reduced when the mouth is opened by the forward movement of the coronoid process of the mandible as its condyle moves forward and downward. This may interfere with dental radiographic procedures in the maxillary molar area and in preparing study models and making maxillary dentures.

The masseter muscle also impinges on the vestibular space as the mouth is closed and teeth are clenched. The anterior edge of this muscle may be palpated in the clenched position by inserting a finger in the buccal vestibule. The presence of this muscle must be taken into account when fitting a mandibular prosthesis.

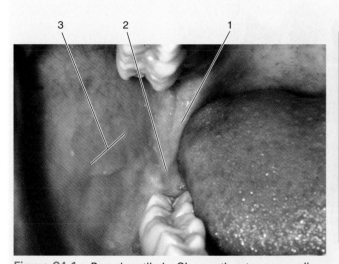

Figure C4-1. Buccal vestibule. Observe the pterygomandibular raphe and the retromandibular triangle. (1) Pterygomandibular raphe; (2) Retromolar pad; (3) Buccal vestibule.

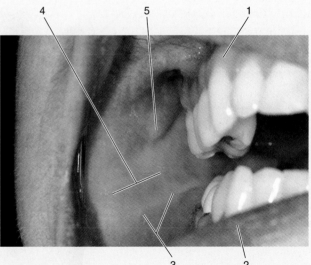

Figure C4-2. Buccal vestibule. Observe the linea alba and the parotid papilla. (1) Attached gingiva; (2) Lower lip; (3) Linea alba; (4) Buccal vestibule; (5) Parotid papilla.

Communication of the oral cavity proper with the vestibule has been discussed previously; now its communication with the pharynx will be described.

The oral cavity communicates with the oral pharynx via the **oropharyngeal isthmus**, the **fauces**. This aperture is bounded by the soft palate superiorly, by the surface of the posterior one third of the tongue inferiorly, and by the palatoglossal arch laterally. Anything posterior to these named structures lies in the pharynx. For example, the palatine tonsil lies in a tonsillar crypt between the palatoglossal and palatopharyngeal arches. Thus, the palatine tonsil

4 5 6 1 2 3

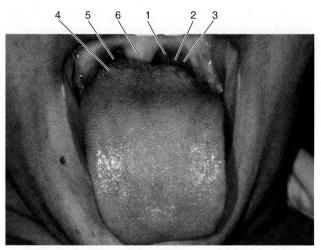

Figure 4-6. The body of the tongue and the anatomy of the anterior and posterior pillars of the fauces. (1) Pharynx; (2) Palatopharyngeal arch; (3) Tonsilar fossa; (4) Posterior 1/3 of tongue; (5) Lingual tonsil; (6) Uvula.

is considered to be in the pharynx because its position is posterior to the palatoglossal arch (Figs. 4-6 and 4-7).

TONGUE

 Summary Bite. The tongue, lying in the floor of the oral cavity proper, is divided into a body and the base.

The tongue, a muscular organ, is divided for descriptive purposes into the body, which lies relatively free in the oral cavity, and the base, which is fixed to the hyoid bone. The base spans the oral cavity and pharynx. The dorsum of the body possesses the **median sulcus**, a shallow groove superficially dividing the tongue longitudinally in the midline into right and left halves.

The surface mucosa exhibits specialized zones demarcating the remnants of the embryologic origin of the tongue. The **sulcus terminalis** may be observed as a posteriorly directed, V-shaped shallow groove separating the anterior two thirds (or body) from the posterior one third (base) of the tongue. The terminal sulcus is the developmental dividing line.

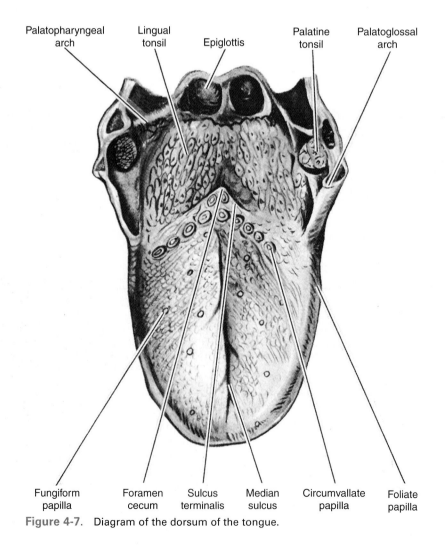

Palatopharyngeal arch   Lingual tonsil   Epiglottis   Palatine tonsil   Palatoglossal arch

Fungiform papilla   Foramen cecum   Sulcus terminalis   Median sulcus   Circumvallate papilla   Foliate papilla

Figure 4-7. Diagram of the dorsum of the tongue.

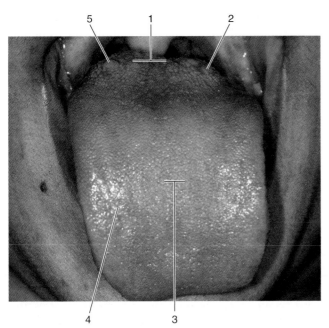

Figure 4-8. Dorsum of the tongue illustrating fungiform papillae and circumvallate papillae of its base. (1) Base of tongue; (2) Circumvallate papilla; (3) Body of tongue; (4) Fungiform papilla; (5) Lingual tonsil.

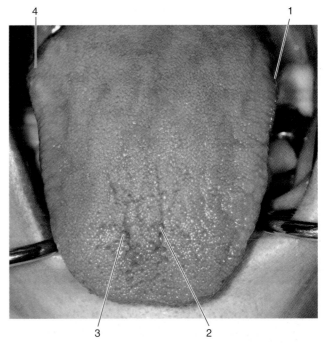

Figure 4-9. Dorsal surface of the tongue illustrating the papillae associated with its body. (1) Foliate papilla (left side); (2) Filiform papilla; (3) Fungiform papilla; (4) Foliate papilla (right side).

That is, anything anterior to it is in the oral cavity, whereas anything posterior to it is in the pharynx. The posterior one third and base will be described here because they may be observed when the tongue is protruded, as in an oral examination (Fig. 4-8).

Lying alongside but anterior to the terminal sulcus is a row of 8 to 10 mushroom-shaped **circumvallate papillae (vallate papillae)**. These structures possess taste buds and receive the ducts of the serous **glands of von Ebner**, one of the few named groups of minor accessory salivary glands. The remaining mucosal surface of the dorsum of the anterior two thirds of the tongue possesses specialized projections, known as lingual papillae. The most numerous are the **filiform papillae** and, interspersed among them are the mushroom-shaped **fungiform papillae**; the former present a rough surface and they present no taste buds, whereas the latter display a few taste buds on their dorsal surface (Fig. 4-8).

On the posterolateral aspect of the anterior two thirds of the tongue are vertical furrows known as the **foliate papillae**; their taste buds degenerate after the first couple of years of life (Fig. 4-9). Located in the midline, just posterior to the apex of the sulcus, is the **foramen cecum**, a shallow, pitlike depression that is a remnant of the developmental **thyroglossal duct** (see Chapter 5). The rest of the dorsal surface of the posterior one third of the tongue exhibits irregular bulges in its mucosa representing the **lingual tonsils**.

The mucosa of the ventral surface of the tongue is smooth and without surface papillae. The medially placed **lingual frenulum** attaches the anterior two thirds of the tongue to the floor of the mouth (Fig. 4-10).

On either side of the frenulum, extending almost to the tip of the tongue, surface bulges may be observed representing the underlying **glands of Blandin-Nuhn**, another group of the named, minor accessory salivary glands. These glands are mixed, producing both serous and mucus saliva, which empty into the oral cavity via several minute pores.

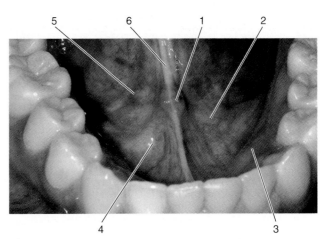

Figure 4-10. Anterior floor of the mouth. Observe the sublingual fold overlying the sublingual gland. (1) Lingual caruncle; (2) Sublingual sulcus; (3) Mandibular torus; (4) Sublingual fold; (5) Sublingual vein; (6) Lingual frenum.

The bilateral **deep lingual veins** may be observed through the nearly transparent mucosa on either side of the frenulum coursing just deep to the mucosa along the tongue's inferior surface from the tip to the deep regions in the floor of the mouth, where the vein disappears from view.

Lateral to the vein is a fringed fold of mucous membrane, the **plica fimbriata** (Fig. 4-9), which often exhibits tissue tags from its free edge. Ducts of the glands of Blandin-Nuhn open into the oral cavity through the fringes of the plica fimbriata. Just above the floor of the mouth on either side of the lingual frenulum is an elevation of the mucous membrane (**plica sublingualis**) overlying the bulging **sublingual glands** (Fig. 4-10).

On closer examination one may observe several small openings along the surface of the plica sublingualis representing the **small sublingual ducts (ducts of Rivinus)**. In addition, a large **sublingual duct (duct of Bartholin)** from the sublingual gland joins the **submandibular duct (Wharton duct)** just before its entry into the oral cavity for the delivery of saliva from the submandibular gland. The Wharton duct empties at the **sublingual caruncula**, an enlarged (Fig. 4-11) papilla adjacent to the lingual frenulum. **Incisive glands**, a small group of minor accessory salivary glands, may also be found on the floor of the oral cavity on either side of the lingual frenulum just posterior to the mandibular incisors.

A more thorough discussion of the development, structure, vascularization, innervation, and function of the tongue is presented in Chapter 15.

PALATE

Summary Bite. The palate forms the roof of the oral cavity and is composed of the anterior hard palate and the posterior soft palate.

The **palate**, representing the roof of the oral cavity, is divided into the **hard palate**, comprising the anterior two thirds, and the **soft palate**, comprising the remaining posterior one third (Fig. 4-12). Mucoperiosteum covers part of the bony skeleton of the hard palate, whereas mucous membrane covers the muscular soft palate. Anterolaterally, the palatal mucosa blends into the alveolar and gingival mucosae surrounding the lingual surface of the maxillary teeth.

Posteriorly, the palate blends into the anterior and posterior pillars of the fauces laterally. The free posterior border of the soft palate terminates in the inferiorly directed **uvula**, located in the midline. The **palatine velum** is that area of the soft palate represented by the superiorly placed posterior free margin and the laterally placed pillars of the fauces (Fig. 4-13).

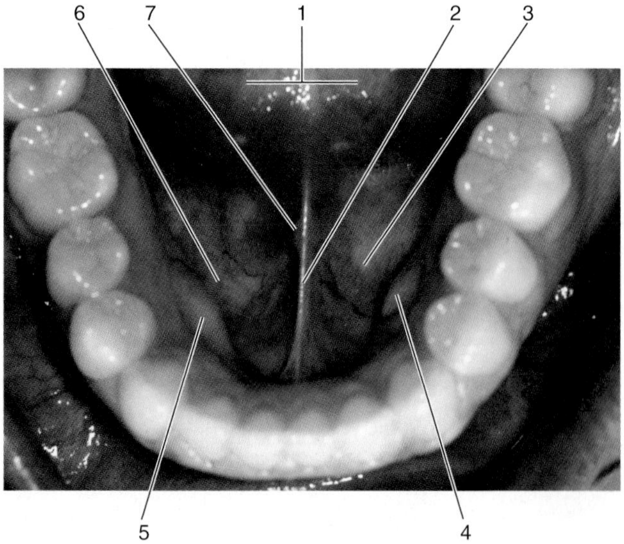

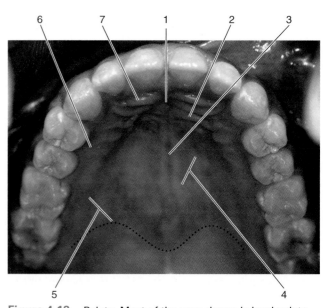

Figure 4-11. Floor of the mouth. Observe the sublingual caruncula indicating opening of the submandibular duct at the base of the lingual frenulum. Of special interest are the mandibular tori. (1) Tongue (ventral surface); (2) Lingual frenum; (3) Sublingual fold; (4) Mandibular torus (left side); (5) Mandibular torus (right side); (6) Sublingual sulcus; (7) Lingual caruncle.

Figure 4-12. Palate. Most of the area shown is hard palate with its rugae and incisive papilla. The most posterior aspect behind the dotted line covers the palatine bone. Anterior aspect is fatty, giving way to a glandular region posteriorly. (1) Incisive papilla; (2) Palatine rugae (left side); (3) Median palatine raphe; (4) Anterior hard palate (fatty region); (5) Posterior hard palate (glandular region); (6) Palatal gingiva; (7) Palatine rugae (right side).

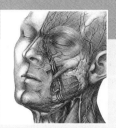

Clinical Considerations

Tongue

Normally, the tongue varies considerably in size and surface presentation, and this variation is often the result of developmental abnormalities. Some of the more common inconsequential anomalies are **microglossia** (small tongue), **macroglossia** (large tongue), **fissured tongue** (excessive fissures in dorsum) (Fig. C4-3A), **median**

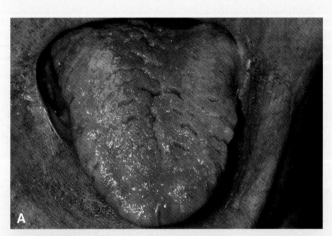

rhomboid glossitis (an area devoid of lingual papilla), and **crenated tongue** (indentations along the margins pressing on the teeth in occlusion) (Fig. C4-3B).

Other anomalies exist, particularly in the lingual papilla, which manifest themselves in many ways, each of which has been supplied with a descriptive term. Space does not permit their descriptions here. Textbooks in oral diagnosis should contain this information.

If the lingual frenulum is attached to the tip of the tongue too far anteriorly, a condition known as **ankyloglossia (tongue-tied)** exists. This condition limits speech because of the immobility of the tongue. Ankyloglossia may be surgically corrected by clipping the frenulum (frenectomy) to shorten its extent.

The thyroglossal duct normally atrophies during fetal life. Incomplete atrophy leads to formation of a midline cyst or accessory thyroid in the vicinity of the foramen cecum. Depending on the size of this **lingual thyroid**, other structures in the vicinity may be obliterated and/or hidden from view.

Floor of Mouth

The floor of the oral cavity proper frequently possesses bony swellings along the lingual surface of the mandible known as **mandibular tori** (Fig. 4-11). Additional **bony exostoses** may be present on the buccal surface of the mandible in the vicinity of the alveolar processes. The tori present radiographic opacity, whereas the buccal exostoses seldom demonstrate radiographic change. Neither of the two conditions presents problems, except in denture construction when they must be removed surgically. Difficulty may be encountered in placing films for dental radiographs and in preparing study models.

A **retrocuspid papilla**, a small papule, may often be observed on the lingual gingiva adjacent to the mandibular cuspid. Such a papilla is not clinically significant.

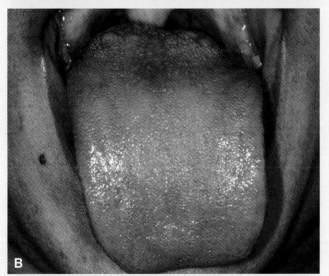

Figure C4-3. Tongue forms. **(A)** Fissured tongue. Note the deep furrows on the surface. This represents a congenital anomaly rather than a pathologic condition. **(B)** Large tongue. Observe the slight scalloped region along the lateral border apparently indicating the lingual aspect of the occlusal arch.

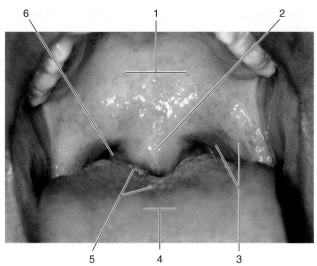

Figure 4-13. Soft palate illustrating the uvula and palatoglossal and palatopharyngeal folds. (1) Soft palate; (2) Uvula; (3) Palatopharyngeal/Palatoglossal arches; (4) Body of tongue; (5) Circumvallate papilla; (6) Lingual tonsil.

The mucoperiosteum displays some specializations in its surface, especially anteriorly. A median **palatine raphe**, the developmental fusion of the palatine shelves, may be observed on the hard palate.

Located in the midline of the palate, immediately behind the central incisors, lies a small, oval-shaped surface prominence termed the **incisive papilla** (Fig. 4-12). This structure covers the oral opening of the incisive canal through which the nasopalatine nerves and nasopalatine arteries are transmitted to the anterior palate. It is an important landmark for anesthesia of the anterior palate. Posterior to this region is a series of transverse folds that appear to radiate from the incisive papilla. These folds are the **palatine rugae**, which are vestigial in humans but may serve accessory masticating and special sensory functions in some lower animals.

Lateral to this area of the palate and beneath the covering mucosa is the **fatty region**. Moving posteriorly, the fatty region is replaced by a **glandular region**, housing the mucous, minor palatine glands extending into the soft palate. Near the midline and just posterior to the hard palate is the **palatine fovea**, a small depression or pit that receives the ducts of some of the **palatine glands** of the hard and soft palates (Fig. 4-12).

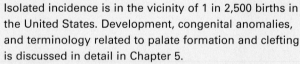

Clinical Considerations

Palate

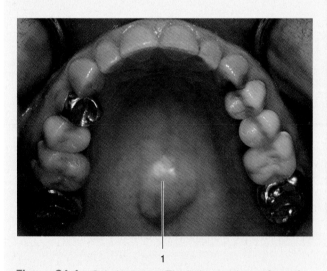

Figure C4-4. Palatine torus. The bulge on the surface of the palate is a bony exostoses and does not represent a pathologic condition. It may be necessary to remove it before preparing a denture. (1) Palatine torus.

The developmental defect of greatest concern to the dental profession is the cleft palate.

Isolated incidence is in the vicinity of 1 in 2,500 births in the United States. Development, congenital anomalies, and terminology related to palate formation and clefting is discussed in detail in Chapter 5.

The normal shape of the palate is classically described as vaultlike, but this varies in individuals from narrow to wide, flat or high, and so on. Frequently, one may observe a midline bulge in the palate resulting from excess bone growth. This is termed **palatine torus** and presents no problem except during denture construction, at which time it must be removed surgically (Fig. C4-4).

Whenever anesthetic injections are to be administered in the palate they should be given, if possible, in an area away from the mucoperiosteum. If an injection must be given in the area covered by mucoperiosteum (hard palate), care must be exercised and the injection must be given slowly to prevent tearing of the collagenous bundles away from the bone.

The palate is formed by the fusion of the intermaxillary segment with the two lateral palatine processes of the maxillae. This fusion is initiated early in development and serves to separate the common oronasal cavity into separate nasal and oral cavities, thus limiting their communication only through the pharynx. A more thorough account of development and congenital anomalies associated with the palate is presented in Chapter 5.

TEETH

Summary Bite. Teeth are arranged on the maxillary and mandibular arches. They articulate with their counterpart on the opposing arch and during occlusion, and when they do that they separate the oral cavity proper from the vestibule.

The teeth are arranged in a row on both the **maxillary** and the **mandibular dental arches**. They form a boundary between the vestibule and the oral cavity proper. As discussed previously, the gingiva of the vestibule and the oral cavity proper become continuous in the interdental spaces.

The **permanent teeth** are named similarly on each side and in the two arches. There are two **incisors**, one **canine (cuspid)**, two **premolars (bicuspid)**, and three **molars**; thus, eight teeth are in each quadrant of the jaw, for a total complement of 32 teeth. This is the normal complement of teeth found in a mature adult. The third molar, **wisdom tooth**, is often slow to erupt and may not present itself in the oral cavity. Occasionally it is congenitally absent, thereby reducing the total complement of teeth (Figs. 4-14 and 4-15).

Deciduous teeth, as the name implies, are those that are eventually shed or replaced. Thus they represent the complement of teeth present in childhood. Each quadrant contains the following deciduous teeth: two incisors, one canine, and two molars. The molars occupy the same position as will the permanent premolars; thus, there are five deciduous teeth in each quadrant for a total of 20 teeth (Fig. 4-16).

The two dentitions, deciduous and permanent, may be expressed in a dental formula as in the following diagrams:

Deciduous

	M	C	I	I	C	M	
Maxilla	2	1	2	2	1	2	= 20
Mandible	2	1	2	2	1	2	

Permanent

	M	P	C	I	I	C	P	M	
Maxilla	3	2	1	2	2	1	2	3	= 32
Mandible	3	2	1	2	2	1	2	3	

The teeth develop from substances elaborated by certain layers of the primitive oral ectoderm and certain specialized cells of the ectomesenchyme. As the teeth develop, the **alveolar processes** of the maxilla and mandible form the bony socket surrounding it. The tooth is anchored in its **alveolus** by a calcified tissue, the **cementum**, and a soft tissue, the **periodontal ligament**. The clinical crown of the tooth is that part exposed in the oral cavity, whereas the root lies in the bony alveolus, out of view. **Enamel** overlies **dentin** in the crown, where it terminates just below the gingival line at the **neck**. The dentin in the root is overlaid by the cementum, which anchors the tooth to the bone via the periodontal ligaments. The central core of the tooth is composed of the soft-tissue pulp containing blood vessels, nerves, and lymphatics that reach the area through the apical foramen at the tip of the root (Figs. 4-17 and 4-18).

The tooth has an **occlusal surface** that contacts the same surface of its counterpart on the opposing dental arch on closure of the mouth. **Buccal surface** and **lingual surface** refer to the vestibular surface and the oral cavity proper surface, respectively. The **incisal edge** is the cutting edge of the anterior teeth. The premolars and molars possess **cusps** (raised knobs on the occlusal surface). Also, because embryologically the teeth form from the midline laterally, the surface that most closely approximates the midline is considered to be the **mesial** aspect; that which is in the opposite direction is the **distal** aspect (Fig. 4-14).

Odontogenesis

Odontogenesis, the development of teeth, begins in the middle of the sixth week of gestation (Fig. 4-18). Although a continuous process, it is arbitrarily subdivided into various stages. These are the bud, cap, and bell stages, followed by apposition, root formation, and eruption.

The basal layer of the ectodermally derived presumptive **oral epithelium** of the stomadeum undergoes proliferation, both on the maxillary and mandibular arches, along the region of the future dental arches, forming a horseshoe-shaped band of ectodermal tissue, the **dental lamina**, surrounded by neural crest-derived ectomesenchyme.

The epithelially derived cells are separated from the underlying and surrounding connective tissue

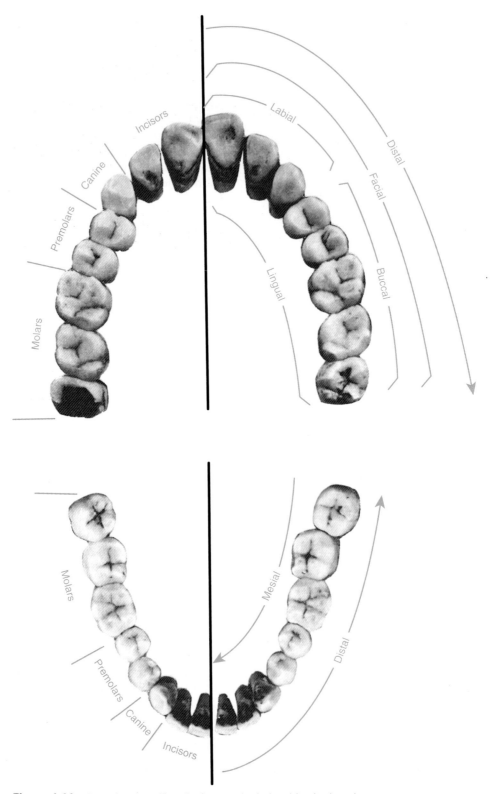

Figure 4-14. Dental arches. Terminology and relationships in dental anatomy.

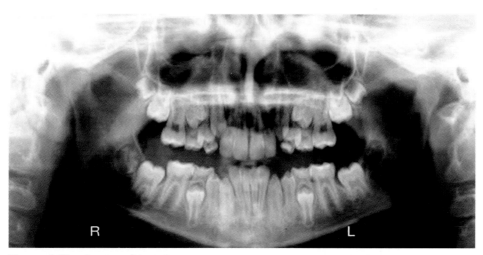

Figure 4-15. Panographic radiograph of the jaws.

elements by a thin acellular layer, the **basement membrane**.

Bud Stage

Along with the formation of the dental lamina, 10 round epithelial structures, each referred to as a **bud**, develop at the distal aspect of the dental lamina of each arch. These correspond to the 10 deciduous teeth of each dental arch, and they signify the **bud stage** of tooth development.

Each bud is separated from the ectomesenchyme by a basement membrane. Ectomesenchymal cells congregate deep to the bud, forming a cluster of cells, which is the initiation of the condensation of the ectomesenchyme. The remaining ectomesenchymal cells are arranged in a more or less haphazardly uniform fashion.

Cap Stage

Cells of the inferior aspect of each tooth bud proliferate, forming a larger, more expanded structure, the **cap**. The cap is said to be composed of an epithelially derived **enamel organ**, which is separated by the basement membrane, from a condensation of ectomesenchymal cells, known as the **dental papilla**.

Enamel Organ

The cells in the core of the enamel organ are known as the **stellate reticulum**. It is completely enveloped by the two regions of a single layer of epithelial cells, the squamous to low–cuboidal-shaped **outer enamel epithelium (OEE)** and the cuboidal to low–columnar-shaped **inner enamel epithelium (IEE)**. They contact each other at the rim-shaped **cervical loop**, which represents the presumptive cervix of the future tooth. Some cells of the stellate reticulum form a group of flattened cells, known as the **enamel knot (Ahren knot)**.

The **dental papilla**, the future pulp of the tooth, fills the concavity of the enamel organ. It is composed of a vascularized embryonic connective tissue whose mesenchymal cells are derived from neural crest.

The **dental follicle (dental sac)** is a membranous structure that surrounds the tooth germ. It will give rise to the periodontal ligament, cementum, and alveolus.

The **succedaneous lamina**, a cordlike epithelial band, arises from each enamel organ and will give rise to the enamel organ of that permanent tooth which will replace the deciduous tooth presently being formed. This permanent tooth germ will also go through the same stages of odontogenesis, but at a later date than its deciduous counterpart.

Bell Stage

Mitotic activity of the enamel organ enlarges this structure and forms a new cell layer, the **stratum intermedium**. The enlarged structure resembles a bell, hence the **bell stage** of tooth development. The cell layers of the inner enamel epithelium elongate and become tall, columnar cells. Because of this histologic change, the bell stage is said to be the stage of **histodifferentiation**.

Additionally, the entire bell-shaped enamel organ changes its morphology to form the template for the future tooth; therefore, the bell stage is also said to be the stage of **morphodifferentiation**.

Enamel Knot

The process of morphodifferentiation is responsible for the establishment of the template of the presumptive tooth, that is, the enamel organ will assume the

Deciduous dentition

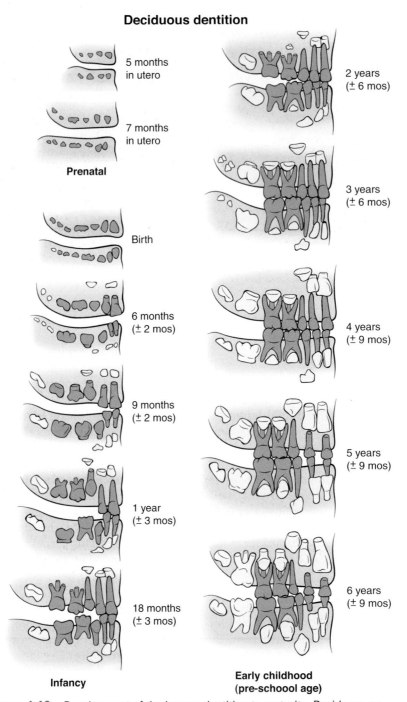

Figure 4-16. Development of the human dentition to maturity. Deciduous or primary teeth are darker in the illustration. *(continued)*

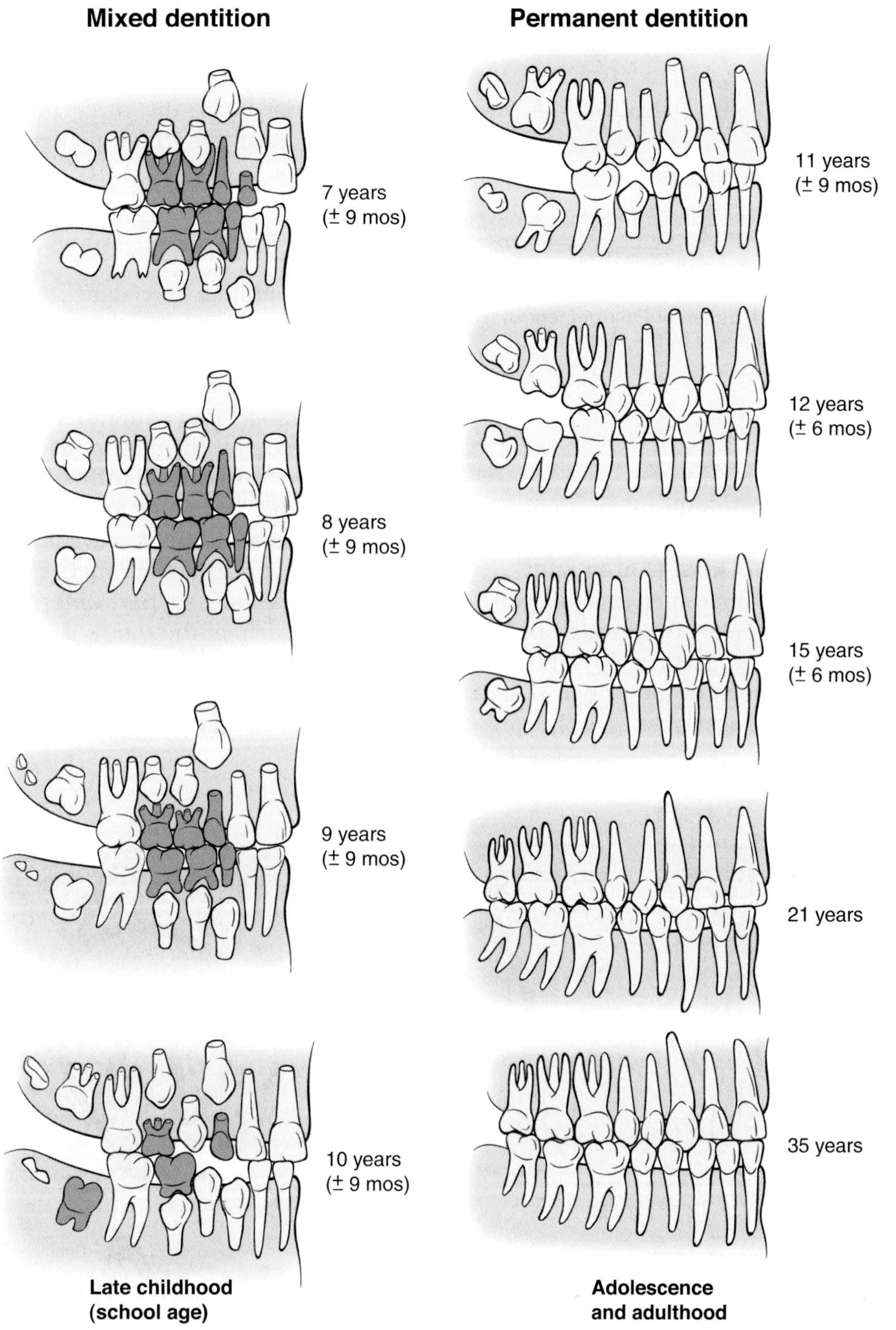

Mixed dentition

Permanent dentition

7 years
(± 9 mos)

8 years
(± 9 mos)

9 years
(± 9 mos)

10 years
(± 9 mos)

11 years
(± 9 mos)

12 years
(± 6 mos)

15 years
(± 6 mos)

21 years

35 years

**Late childhood
(school age)**

**Adolescence
and adulthood**

Figure 4-16. *(Continued)*

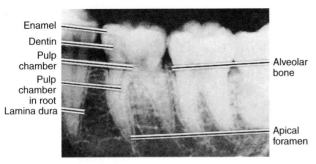

Enamel

Dentin

Pulp chamber

Pulp chamber in root

Lamina dura

Alveolar bone

Apical foramen

Figure 4-17. Radiographs of the teeth. Enlargement of a molar tooth illustrating the anatomy of the tooth and the alveolus.

shape of an incisiform, caniniform, or molariform tooth. It has been recently discovered that this event is controlled by the **enamel knot (Ahren knot)**.

It appears that the ectomesenchymal cells of the dental papilla induce the cells of the enamel knot to begin to express signaling molecules, thus transforming the enamel knot into one of the principal signaling centers of tooth morphogenesis.

Origin of the Permanent Molars

The posterior regions of the upper and lower dental laminae elongate and each newly elongated region forms three buds, the three **permanent molars** of each quadrant, for which no deciduous counterparts exist. Therefore, these 12 permanent molars are referred to as **accessional teeth**.

Apposition

The tall, columnar cells of the dental papilla, the **pre-odontoblasts**, begin to elaborate a collagen-rich substance known as dentin matrix, and these cells are now referred to as **odontoblasts**.

The initial layer of dentin matrix is different from the remainder of the dentin matrix of the tooth and is referred to as **mantle dentin**.

In response to the formation of mantle dentin, the preameloblasts become ameloblasts and secrete the first layer of enamel matrix. Since this very first layer of enamel matrix differs from most of the enamel matrix of the tooth, it is referred to as **aprismatic enamel matrix**. Thus, the dentinoenamel junction has just been established in a very small region of the developing tooth germ.

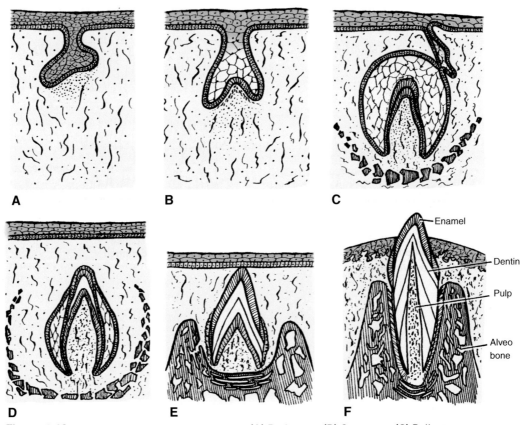

A

B

C

Enamel

Dentin

Pulp

Alveo bone

D

E

F

Figure 4-18. Tooth development in the human. **(A)** Bud stage. **(B)** Cap stage. **(C)** Bell stage. **(D)** Appositional stage. **(E)** Beginning of eruption. **(F)** Eruption into the oral cavity.

Odontoblasts retreat on a daily basis, and they apparently move approximately 4 to 8 μm per day. During this motion they elaborate dentin matrix. As aprismatic enamel matrix is being formed, the ameloblasts retreat (as did the odontoblasts) but in the opposite direction.

As they move away from the odontoblasts, each forms a short, blunt **Tomes process** and manufactures enamel matrix around this process. As the enamel matrix is secreted, the ameloblast withdraws its Tomes process, leaving a space in the enamel matrix, known as **rod space**, which quickly becomes filled with enamel matrix, and a small block of enamel matrix is known as a **rod segment**. Every day, each ameloblast manufactures a single rod segment; these rod segments are placed on top of one another, forming an **enamel rod (enamel prism)**. Because of these rod segments, the enamel formed is known as **prismatic enamel**.

Root Formation

Root formation begins when dentinogenesis and amelogenesis approach the cervical loop. Possibly influenced by the presence of enamel and dentin near the cervical loop, this structure begins to undergo mitosis and grows in an apical direction as an epithelial cylinder that surrounds the dental papilla. This epithelial cylinder, the **Hertwig epithelial root sheath**, is composed of two layers of cells, an outer and an inner layer, derived from the outer enamel epithelium and the inner enamel epithelium, respectively.

Because of the absence of a stellate reticulum and stratum intermedium, the inner layer of the Hertwig epithelial root sheath will not form enamel. However, these cells will provide signaling molecules that will cause the peripheral layer of cells of the dental papilla to differentiate into odontoblasts and elaborate dentin matrix. These cells will also form, on the surface of mantle dentin, an enamel-like **hyaline layer of Hopewell-Smith**, a substance that facilitates the adherence of cementum to the radicular dentin.

Radicular Dentinogenesis

Radicular dentin formation is similar to coronal dentin formation in that there is a layer of mantle dentin matrix formed first. The bulk of radicular dentin, known as circumpulpal dentin, is manufactured similarly to its coronal counterpart.

Cell Rests of Malassez

Subsequent to the formation of the hyaline layer of Hopewell-Smith, the Hertwig epithelial root sheath (which was composed of two continuous layers of epithelial cells) begins to undergo partial degeneration.

It becomes a network of epithelial cords surrounding the root of the tooth, and is called the **rest cells of Malassez**.

Cementoblasts

Ectomesenchymal cells, derived from the dental follicle, pass through the discontinuities among the network of epithelial cords and, proceeding between the newly formed dentin and the now incomplete inner layer of the Hertwig epithelial root sheath, differentiate into **cementoblasts**. The cementoblasts manufacture **cementum matrix**, which mineralizes to become **cementum**.

Detailed information regarding developmental processes, as well as information on the complex anatomy and function of the individual teeth, is available in texts of oral histology, embryology, and dental anatomy.

PHARYNX

Summary Bite. The muscular pharynx is a mucosal lined tube attached to the base of the cranium, coursing inferiorly to become continuous with the esophagus. It serves as an airway to the larynx and as a passageway for food and drink to the esophagus.

The **pharynx** is a muscular tube lined with mucous membrane. It extends in an inferior direction from the base of the cranium to the level of the sixth cervical vertebra, where it becomes continuous with the esophagus. The pharynx possesses several attachments along its length; therefore, its mobility is somewhat restricted.

The pharynx lies behind the nasal cavity, oral cavity, and larynx. Although its posterior wall presents a continuous surface, superiorly its anterior wall is interrupted by the choanae of the nasal cavity and the isthmus of the oral cavity. Thus, the pharnyx serves to conduct air to the larynx from the nasal and oral cavities as well as food to the esophagus from the mouth.

The muscular wall of the pharynx is composed of three overlapping muscles, originating from several anatomic structures in their vicinity and all inserting into a longitudinal line, the **posterior median raphe**, in the dorsal wall of the pharynx.

The three muscles are the **superior pharyngeal**, **middle pharyngeal**, and **inferior pharyngeal constrictors**, each named for its relative location. Each muscle possesses fibers that ascend and descend from their origin to be inserted into the raphe. This fanned-out arrangement provides for a strong but

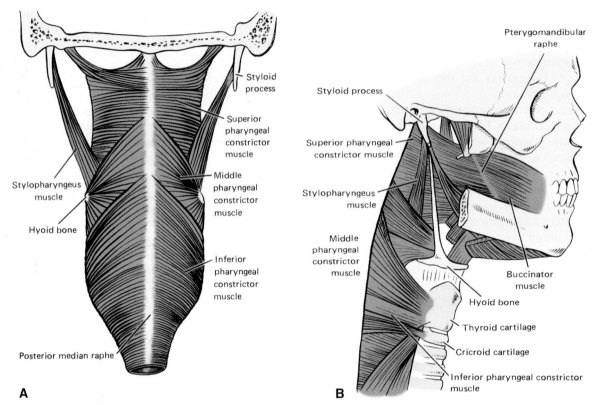

Figure 4-19. Muscles of the pharynx. **(A)** Posterior view illustrating the posterior median raphe. **(B)** Lateral view demonstrating fiber directions.

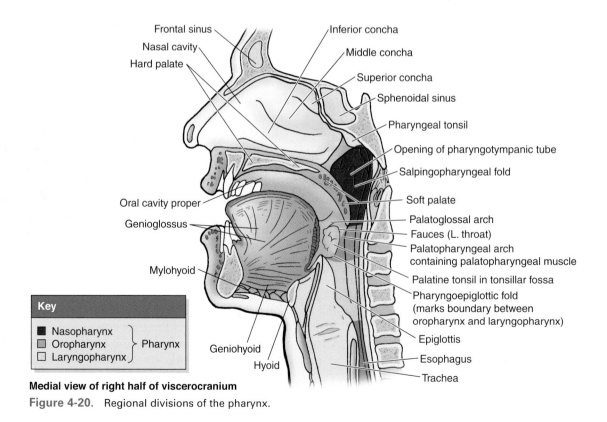

Medial view of right half of viscerocranium

Figure 4-20. Regional divisions of the pharynx.

flexible multilayered wall whose muscle fibers course in a direction oblique to each other (Fig. 4-19).

The pharynx, for purposes of description, is divided into three anatomic regions: the **nasopharynx**, **oropharynx**, and **laryngeal pharynx** (Fig. 4-20). The most superior portion, the nasopharynx, begins at the superior attachment to the sphenoid and occipital bones and ends at the soft palate. This is the widest part of the pharynx and is in communication with the nasal cavity via the choanae and with the middle ear cavity via the **auditory tube (Eustachian tube)**. A fold of mucous membrane, in the area of the auditory tube, covers the **salpingopharyngeus muscle**, which blends into the pharyngeal wall. In the **pharyngeal recess**, behind the lip of the auditory tube, is the **pharyngeal tonsil** (Fig. 4-20).

During swallowing, the nasopharynx is sealed off from the oral cavity by the elevation of the soft palate superiorly and posteriorly against the posterior and lateral walls of the pharynx. This may be observed during an oral examination by having the patient open the mouth, protrude the tongue, and say "ah." This causes the palate to be elevated and permits observation of the oropharynx extending from the palate to the larynx.

The lateral wall of the pharynx is formed by the **palatopharyngeal fold** covering the palatopharyngeus muscle. This fold, arising from the soft palate, is also called the **posterior pillar of the fauces**, whereas the fold anterior to this, the **palatoglossal fold**, is also called the **anterior pillar of the fauces**. This fold is not a part of the lateral wall of the pharynx; rather, it is the fold that covers the palatoglossal muscle, one of the extrinsic muscles of the tongue

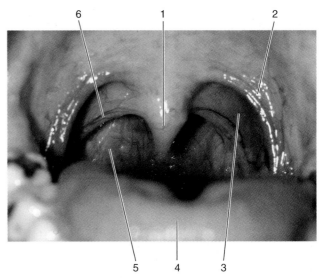

Figure 4-21. The shared anatomy of the oral cavity/oral pharynx with the tonsilar sinus separating the oral cavity from the oral pharynx. (1) Uvula; (2) Palatoglossal arch; (3) Palatine tonsil fossa; (4) Body of tongue; (5) Oropharyngeal wall; (6) Palatopharyngeal arch.

(Fig. 4-21). Note that the sinus between the two folds houses the palatine tonsil.

Anteriorly, the base of the dorsum of the tongue lies in the pharynx. Inferiorly, the epiglottis projects into the oral pharynx behind the tongue, separated by two small pouches (**valleculae**) located on either side of the epiglottis (Fig. 4-7).

A more thorough discussion of the pharynx is found in regional descriptions that follow in Chapter 16.

Clinical Considerations

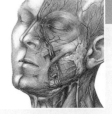

Oropharynx

Small clumps of lymphoid tissue surround the entry into the deep portions of the digestive tract at the oropharynx. This **lymphatic ring of Waldeyer** is well developed in the child and regresses with advancing age.

It is possible to view the posterior nasal choanae, the auditory tubes, and the larynx during an oral examination by illuminating the oropharynx and using a dental mirror.

On examination of the oropharynx, a ridge of tissue on the posterior pharyngeal wall may be observed on a plane with the soft palate. This ridge, known as the **Passavant bar**, represents the contact zone between the pharynx and the palate when it is elevated for sealing off the nasopharynx from the oropharynx.

Embryology of the Head and Neck

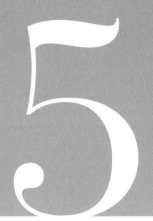

Key Terms

Cleft Lip results when the maxillary process and the intermaxillary segment fail to fuse with one another. This may be observed as a notching of the lip to a unilateral cleft lip that may reveal the unfused maxillary process and the intermaxillary segment. More severe malformations may result in a bilateral cleft lip with neither of the maxillary processes fused with the intermaxillary segment.

Cleft Palate results from failure of the lateral palatine shelves to fuse in the midline (or with the intermaxillary segment), thus

failing to separate the oronasal cavity into a nasal cavity superior to the palate and an oral cavity inferior to the palate.

Foramen Cecum is the small pit at the apex of the V-shaped terminal sulcus separating the anterior two thirds of the tongue (body) from the posterior one third (base) of the tongue. The primordium of the thyroid gland, derived from the pharyngeal wall at the foramen cecum, migrates into the neck to be positioned ventral and inferior to the thyroid cartilage.

Muscles of Facial Expression are specialized muscles about the face that arise from the hypodermis or bone and insert into the dermis of the face, neck, or scalp. Coordinated contractions of these muscles, especially about the mouth, nose, and eyes, convey emotions in humans. This group of muscles arises from the second pharyngeal arch and is innervated by the facial nerve (cranial nerve VII), the nerve of second arch.

Muscles of Mastication are the four bilateral pairs of muscles developed from the mandibular arch that are attached to the mandible and whose contractions supply the forces for mastication. These muscles are innervated by the mandibular division of the trigeminal nerve (cranial nerve V).

Pharyngeal Arches are the five bars of condensed mesenchymal tissue interposed between the successive pairs of the pharyngeal pouches and grooves (clefts). Each pharyngeal arch gives rise to bone, cartilage, vascular, muscle, and nerve components.

Pharyngeal Grooves form concurrently around the stomodeal neck area on the lateral surface of the embryo where they approximate, but do not contact, the corresponding pharyngeal pouches.

Pharyngeal Pouches are the five pairs of endodermally lined out-pouchings of the pharyngeal gut that develop just posterior to the ruptured buccopharyngeal membrane and invade the laterally positioned mesenchyme.

Primary Palate (Premaxilla) develops from the intermaxillary segment (formed by the fused median nasal swellings) as it grows down from the nose to form the nasal septum, columella, philtrum of the upper lip, labial tubercle, and into the mouth where anterior teeth supporting structures and gingiva develop. The primary palate is that triangular portion of the hard palate that is located behind the four incisor teeth and is bounded by imaginary lines drawn from the space between the lateral incisors and canine teeth of either side and extending to the incisive foramen.

Stomatognathic System includes the muscles of mastication and the structures within the mouth for ingesting and masticating food. This system also forms sounds produced by the larynx into speech for communication.

Stomodeum is the primitive mouth cavity in the human embryo. This shallow space is lined with ectoderm and is separated from the cephalic end of the pharyngeal gut by the buccopharyngeal membrane.

The Rathke Pouch develops in the oral ectoderm of the roof of the primitive oral cavity just anterior to the buccopharyngeal membrane. This evaginating pouch comes in contact with a pouch developing from the floor of the diencephalon. These two structures give rise to the pituitary gland.

THE HEAD AND NECK

The head and neck comprise the most complicated portion of the human anatomy. The complex bony skull houses the brain, which is the control and coordination center for all body functions. Connected to the brain are the special sense organs of taste, hearing, smell, and sight. These organs perceive stimuli from the environment and transmit these sensations to the brain via the cranial nerves. Located in the head is the **stomatognathic system**, including the muscles of mastication and the structures within the mouth for ingesting and masticating food. This system also forms sounds produced by the larynx into speech for communication. In addition, the face possesses a special system of muscles, the muscles of facial expression, whose coordinated contractions about the mouth, nose, and eyes convey our emotions. And finally, the nose serves as the point of entry to the respiratory system and olfaction and incidentally as an entranceway for disease.

Indeed, no other region of the body is so complex or performs so many complicated functions as the head and neck. Because of its intricate nature, the compactness of the region, the ramifications of anomalies and congenital defects, and the disease manifestations arising in the head and neck, perhaps no other region of the body is served by so many specialized areas of medicine and surgery.

HEAD AND NECK DEVELOPMENT

Summary Bite. Understanding developmental processes in the head and neck is necessary for comprehending nerve–muscle relationships in normal patients as well as in those with congenital defects to arrive at the proper diagnosis and treatment.

An understanding of the developmental processes that form the head and neck ultimately helps students assimilate and remember the vast amount of information necessary to master the study of head and neck anatomy. For example, understanding nerve–muscle relationships in development and subsequent muscle migrations away from their embryonic origin is of particular importance in the head and neck as it relates to adult morphology and as an explanation of congenital defects. Understanding these elements of development helps one arrive at sound reasoning for diagnosis and management of congenital defects about the head and neck as well as for treatment modalities of many disease manifestations.

Descriptive Language for Head and Neck Development

Summary Bite. Terms that are applied in describing human development sometimes have been incorrectly carried over from descriptions of development in lower animals.

Language used in describing the developmental anatomy of the head and neck may be particularly confusing to students who have not yet studied embryology. Early development within vertebrate animals is similar; indeed, to the untrained eye it would be difficult to distinguish an early human embryo from many of those of lower animals. For this reason, much of the terminology used in embryology is generally applied to all vertebrates, creating some confusion to the untrained individual in the specific study of human development.

The term **branchia**, for example, literally means "gill"; consequently, it is the term used to describe the embryologic development of gills in fish. This term is sometimes used in describing the embryologic formation of the head and neck in human beings. Obviously, humans do not possess gills; however, the term is not used without reason. Many of the head and neck structures in humans are homologues of gill structures in the primitive vertebrates. The equivalent term used in descriptions of human head and neck development is **pharyngeal**. This term, although not completely accurate, will be used in this text. The terms **groove** and **cleft** may also be used interchangeably, but this should not create misunderstanding.

Genetic and Molecular Aspects of Development

Summary Bite. Related genes on all chromosomes control patterning, thus either facilitating or inhibiting normal development.

A group of related genes located in the chromosomes of all cells are responsible for **patterning**, a term used to define the spatial relationship of specific predetermined periods of development. These genes are turned on or off as a result of intracellular and extracellular phenomena that cause them to be either activated or suppressed, thus facilitating or impeding the normal sequence of development.

Homeobox Genes

Summary Bite. Homeobox genes code for transcriptional factors that turn on a cascade of genes responsible for regulating segmentation and axis formation. These genes control the "window of opportunity" for normal development.

A specific group of highly conserved genes, known as **homeobox genes**, code for the synthesis of transcriptional factors—proteins that bind to and regulate the expression of other genes. Thus, these homeobox genes as well as certain growth factors

are essential for the temporal sequencing of developmental events. For example, certain genes can be switched on only after being activated by the synthesized products (i.e., proteins) coded from other genes. By the same token, these same genes might not be activated if certain other genes have been activated before them. This implies that there is a "window of opportunity" in development when certain events must take place, indicating that most events in embryologic development are sequential and that each event must take place neither before nor after the period of opportunity written in the DNA code. Hence, these homeobox genes are responsible for establishing a temporospatial pattern of developmental events as occurs in segmentation and axis formation. When this does not progress properly, development does not proceed normally, resulting in anomalies, congenital defects, and, if severe enough, death to the developing embryo.

Signaling Cells and Target Cells

Summary Bite. Signaling cells produce growth factors, signaling molecules, or ligands bound for other cells which have receptors for these molecules on their surface; these cells are known as target cells. Such cell-to-cell interaction triggers a sequence of developmental events.

During development, cells must interact with each other, either indirectly by receptor-mediated binding of the product of a particular cell or directly by cellular contact between the cells. Accordingly, there are **signaling cells** and **target cells** in all developmental processes. The products of these signaling cells are referred to as **growth factors**, **signaling molecules**, or **ligands**, which reach target cells via body fluids.

Target cells possess receptor molecules on their plasmalemma that will bind only signaling molecules produced by the signaling cell, which fit together like a lock and key. When the cellular interaction is physical cell-to-cell contact, the cells must be able to recognize each other by the binding of their corresponding ligand–receptor molecules. Once this has been accomplished, the signaling cell interacts with the target cell, triggering a series of sequential events influencing a single gene or a group of genes. This may result in releasing new signaling molecules; altering the activities of the target cell; causing the target cell to differentiate into another cell type; causing proliferation of the target cell; or causing the target cell to undergo apoptosis and die.

The process whereby the signaling cell causes the target cell to differentiate into another cell type is called **induction**. Each event in development possesses

Clinical Considerations

Abnormal Development of the Head and Neck

Abnormalities in the embryologic development of the head and neck lead to a great variety of malformations with varying degrees of severity. The head and neck develop under the control of autosomal and sex-linked inheritance, modulated by the great influence of environmental factors.

The interdependence of events and the sequencing of development during this rather short embryonic period, perhaps before the woman is even aware of her pregnancy, contributes to the possibility of malformation.

a specific induction period (window of opportunity) that precludes the actual development. The most severe congenital defects occur from interference during induction rather than during actual growth and development. For example, a particular teratogen may cause cleft palate in a developing fetus when introduced during the actual formation of the palate, yet may have no effect at all when introduced at a later date when the palatal shelves have approximated but have not as yet fused with each other.

PHARYNGEAL ARCH, GROOVE, AND POUCH DEVELOPMENT

Summary Bite. During early development at the cephalic end of the embryo, a series of pharyngeal arches with grooves between them may be observed on the external surface. These surround the development of out-pocketing of the pharyngeal gut just caudal to the buccopharyngeal membrane.

In the human embryo, the **stomodeum** or primitive mouth cavity, a shallow depression lined with ectoderm, is separated from the cephalic end of the pharyngeal gut by the **buccopharyngeal membrane**, which ruptures during the fourth week of gestation (Fig. 5-1).

Just anterior to the buccopharyngeal membrane, a midline diverticulum known as the **Rathke pouch** develops in the oral ectoderm of the roof of the primitive oral cavity. This evaginating pouch comes in contact with a pouch developing from the floor of the diencephalon. Further development of these two opposed structures gives rise to the **pituitary gland**.

During the fourth and fifth weeks of gestation, as the buccopharyngeal membrane is degenerating, communication is established between the future

oral cavity and the pharynx. Concomitant with this event, out-pouchings of the pharyngeal gut develop just posterior to the ruptured buccopharyngeal membrane, forming five pairs of **pharyngeal pouches** that invade the mesenchyme laterally. Although it was once thought that the neural crest cells of the pharyngeal arches were responsible for patterning skeletal components of the arches, it is now clear that the endodermal lining of the pharyngeal pouches regulates this patterning.

Concurrent with the formation of the pouches in the pharyngeal wall, four pairs of grooves develop around the stomodeal neck area on the lateral surface of the embryo. These **pharyngeal grooves (branchial grooves)** invade the underlying mesenchyme approximating, but not contacting, their corresponding pharyngeal pouches. Invasion by the pouches and the grooves produces a condensation of mesenchymal

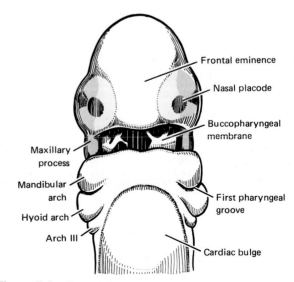

Figure 5-1. Frontal view of an embryo at 4 to 5 weeks of age. Observe the branchial arch formation and the ruptured buccopharyngeal membrane.

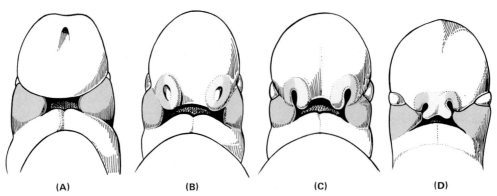

Figure 5-2. Developing face. **(A)** Fourth week. **(B)** Fourth to fifth week. **(C)** Fifth to sixth week. **(D)** Sixth to seventh week. Note how the nose develops and the eyes appear more anteriorly placed, illustrating the nasolacrimal groove.

tissue interposed between successive pairs of pouches and grooves (clefts). These five bars of condensed mesenchymal tissue are the **pharyngeal (branchial) arches** (see Figs. 5-2, 5-3, and 5-4).

The mesenchymal cells forming much of the ventral regions of the developing pharyngeal arches are derived from neural crest cells originating from the vicinity of the midbrain region and the rhombomeres. During early pharyngeal arch formation, these cells express homeobox gene (**Hox** gene) products indicative of the region of their origin.

Continued development and growth of the arches results in their fusion in the anterior midline. Each arch will develop its own bone, cartilage, vascular, muscular, and nerve components. The arches form sequentially from rostral to caudal, with the first arch being most highly developed and the last arch being poorly developed. The first and second arches are named "mandibular" and "hyoid" arches, respectively, whereas the remaining three are unnamed. The discussion of pharyngeal arch derivatives that follows is summarized in Table 5-1.

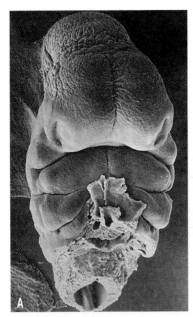

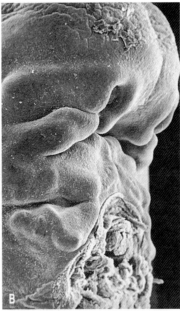

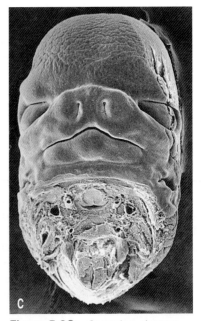

Figure 5-3A. Scanning electron micrograph of a stage 15 (8.0-mm) human embryo in frontal view. Observe the maxillary processes, mandibular process, hyoid and third pharyngeal arch processes, and nasal pits. ×52.

Figure 5-3B. Scanning electron micrograph of a stage 17 (11.7-mm) human embryo in lateral view. Observe the nasal pits, median and lateral nasal processes, maxillary processes, mandibular process, and hyoid arch. ×57.

Figure 5-3C. Scanning electron micrograph of the face of a stage 18 (17.5-mm) human embryo in frontal view. Observe the fused processes making up the nose, the maxillary processes, and the mandibular processes delineating the mouth. ×14.

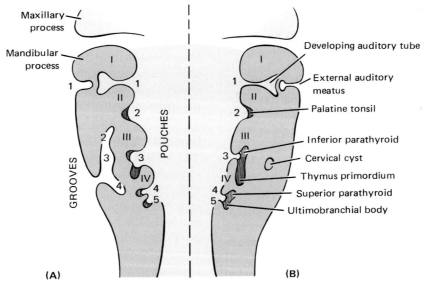

Figure 5-4. Early development of the pharyngeal grooves and pouches. **(A)** Early development. **(B)** Later development. Observe the second arch overgrowing the second, third, and fourth grooves leaving a cervical cyst in drawing **B**. Note the diverticula of pouches three and four as each develops dorsal and ventral prolongations.

Table 5-1 Pharyngeal Arch Derivatives and Their Innervation

Arch	Skeletal	Ligaments	Muscle	Nerve
I Mandibular	Meckel's cartilage Maxillae Mandible Malleus Incus	Sphenomandibular Anterior ligament of malleus	Muscles of mastication (temporalis, masseter, medial and lateral pterygoids) Tensor veli palatini Tensor tympani Digastric (anterior belly) Mylohyoid	Cranial nerve V (trigeminal) mandibular div.
II Hyoid	Reichert's cartilage Hyoid (part) Lesser cornu Body, upper part Styloid process	Stylohyoid	Muscles of facial expression (platysma, buccinator, frontalis, occipitalis, auricular, orbicularis, oculi, oris) Stapedius Digastric (posterior belly) Stylohyoid	Cranial nerve VII (facial)
III	Hyoid (part) Greater cornu Body, lower part		Stylopharyngeus Cricothyroid Pharyngeal constrictors[a]	Cranial nerve IX (glossopharyngeal) Cranial nerve X (vagus) External branch of superior laryngeal nerve[b]
IV } VI	Thyroid cartilage Laryngeal cartilages (cricoid, arytenoid, corniculate, cuneiform)		Intrinsic laryngeal muscles— except cricothyroid	Pharyngeal plexus[c] Cranial nerve X (vagus) Recurrent laryngeal nerve[b]

[a]The origin of some of the muscles of the pharynx is as yet unclear. The pharyngeal constrictors may in fact receive innervation from more than one source.
[b]Although this named branch of the vagus nerve is traditionally described as the motor innervation to the identified laryngeal muscles, it is important to remember that the motor fibers of the vagus nerve, at least in this region, are actually motor fibers contributed to the vagus nerve from the cranial portion of the accessory nerve (cranial nerve XI).
[c]Several of the pharyngeal and associated muscles of the soft palate are innervated by branches of the pharyngeal plexus—a complex of the nerves located on the posterior aspects of the pharynx consisting of contributions from cranial nerves IX and X (IX is sensory, whereas X is motor, although these motor fibers are contributed from XI). Fibers from the superior cervical ganglion also contribute to the pharyngeal plexus, serving vasomotor functions.

Derivatives of the Pharyngeal Arches

Summary Bite. Five pharyngeal arches develop in the human. The first two are named, whereas the remainder are known by Roman numerals only. They are the mandibular arch (I), hyoid arch (II), arch III, arch IV, and arch VI. Arch V is missing in humans. Each arch has skeletal, cartilage, and ligament components, and specific associated muscles, and its derivatives are innervated by a specific cranial nerve.

Mandibular Arch (I)

The first pharyngeal arch, the **mandibular arch**, is located between the stomodeum and the first pharyngeal groove. This arch divides early in its development into two unequal portions, the dorsally positioned **maxillary process** lying close to the eye and the ventrally placed **mandibular process** (Figs. 5-1, 5-2, 5-3, and 5-4). **Meckel cartilage**, the cartilage of this arch, develops in this arch, forming a primitive support. Later, Meckel cartilage regresses and forms two of the bony ossicles, the incus and malleus of the middle ear dorsally, whereas ventrally the cartilage becomes incorporated into the mandibular symphysis. However, it should be noted that most of the mandible develops by intramembranous bone formation rather than by endochondral formation on Meckel cartilage. Skeletal derivatives of this arch, arising from the maxillary process, also include the premaxilla, maxilla, zygoma, and part of the temporal.

The perichondrium of Meckel cartilage will become the sphenomandibular ligament and the anterior ligament of the malleus.

The muscles of mastication (masseter, temporalis, medial, and lateral pterygoids) and some muscles accessory to mastication, including the mylohyoid muscle and the anterior belly of the digastric muscle as well as the tensor tympani and tensor veli palatini muscles, develop within this arch. The cranial nerve providing innervation to the structures originating from this arch is the trigeminal nerve (cranial nerve V).

Mandibular arch development depends on **endothelin-1**, an epidermally derived signaling molecule that facilitates an interaction between the ectomesenchymal cells and the epithelial cells of the arch. The presence of this signaling molecule is necessary for development of structures formed from the mandibular arch.

Hyoid Arch (II)

The second pharyngeal arch, the **hyoid arch**, develops immediately behind the mandibular arch and is separated from it by the first pharyngeal groove. This arch assists in forming the anterior neck (Figs. 5-1, 5-3, 5-4, and 5-5). The cartilage of the arch, **Reichert cartilage**, gives rise to the styloid process of the temporal bone, the stylohyoid ligament, the lesser cornu, and part of the body of the hyoid bone and the third bony ossicle of the middle ear, the stapes.

The muscle mass developed within this arch migrates over the superficial face and neck, forming the muscles of facial expression. Other muscles derived from the second pharyngeal arch include the stapedius, attached to the stapes; the stylohyoid, attached to the styloid process; and the posterior belly of the digastric, attached to the hyoid bone anteriorly. Innervation to the structures derived from this arch is supplied by the facial nerve (cranial nerve VII).

HoxA-2, one of the homeobox genes, is the signaling gene of structures developed in the second pharyngeal arch. It is interesting to note that if HoxA-2 gene products are not present, first pharyngeal arch derivatives develop in the hyoid arch. Apparently, first pharyngeal arch derivatives are the default derivatives and HoxA-2 products modify the developmental process.

Third Pharyngeal Arch (III)

The unnamed third pharyngeal arch develops posterior to the hyoid arch just behind the second pharyngeal groove (Figs. 5-1, 5-3, 5-4, and 5-5). The greater cornu, the remainder of the hyoid bone, and one muscle, the stylopharyngeus, originate from this arch. This

Clinical Considerations

First Arch Defects

Defects of the first arch are the most common and of greatest significance because many structures develop from it. Because of the many possible defects, the term **first arch syndrome** is generally applied to anomalies from this arch. This term is applied to first arch malformations because they are often observed as multiple defects.

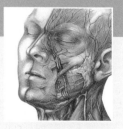

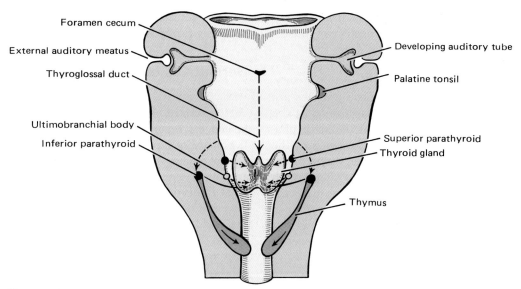

Figure 5-5. Late development of pharyngeal grooves and pouches illustrating migration of the thymus primordial and parathyroids on the dorsal side of the thyroid gland.

muscle is innervated by the nerve of this arch, the glossopharyngeal nerve (cranial nerve IX).

Fourth and Sixth Pharyngeal Arches (IV and VI)

The fourth pharyngeal arch develops posterior to the third pharyngeal arch and is separated from it by the third pharyngeal groove (Figs. 5-4 and 5-5). Technically, from the standpoint of comparative embryology, a fifth pharyngeal arch does not develop in humans, but a rudimentary sixth pharyngeal arch does. Unnamed cartilages of the fourth and sixth pharyngeal arches fuse to form the thyroid and cricoid cartilages as well as the arytenoid, cuneiform, and corniculate cartilages of the larynx. Muscles developing in the fourth pharyngeal arch include the three pharyngeal constrictor (superior, middle, and inferior) muscles and the cricothyroid muscle.

Controversy exists concerning the arch of origin of some of the pharyngeal muscles. The developmental origin of the muscles of the pharynx and soft palate has been difficult to elucidate because overlap of innervation occurs via a complex of cranial nerves and sympathetic fibers. This complex, termed the **pharyngeal plexus**, serves many of the muscles and mucous membranes of the fourth and sixth pharyngeal arch derivatives. This plexus, located on the posterior pharyngeal wall, consists of pharyngeal branches provided by the glossopharyngeal and vagus nerves, as well as branches from the superior cervical sympathetic ganglion. Glossopharyngeal contributions to the pharyngeal plexus are sensory, whereas the vagal branches are motor. However, these vagal motor branches are believed to consist mainly of fibers from the cranial portion of the accessory nerve (cranial nerve XI), contributed to the vagus before it exits the skull. The sympathetic fibers of the pharyngeal plexus are vasomotor. Although many of the structures developed in the fourth pharyngeal arch are innervated by fibers from the pharyngeal plexus, the principal named nerve of this arch is the external branch of the superior laryngeal branch of the vagus nerve (cranial nerve X). This nerve provides exclusive innervation to

Clinical Considerations

Preauricular Pits

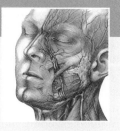

Preauricular pits may be observed in the external ear. They are usually inconsequential and result from incomplete covering of the sulci between the nodes of the first and second arch as they develop into the pinna of the ear.

the cricothyroid muscle and contributes to the innervation of the inferior pharyngeal constrictor muscle (see Chapter 16).

Muscles developing in the sixth pharyngeal arch include all of the intrinsic muscles of the larynx. Except for the cricothyroid, all of these muscles are innervated by the recurrent laryngeal branch of the vagus (cranial nerve X), the nerve of the sixth pharyngeal arch. The recurrent laryngeal branch of the vagus nerve also contributes to the innervation of the inferior pharyngeal constrictor muscle along with input from the pharyngeal plexus and the external branch of the superior laryngeal nerve, a branch of the vagus nerve. It should be remembered, however, that the motor fibers distributed by the vagus nerve at this point are probably derived from the accessory nerve (cranial nerve XI).

The pharyngeal musculature as well as the muscles of the soft palate, with the exceptions of the tensor veli palatini, which is innervated by the trigeminal nerve, and the stylopharyngeus, which is innervated by the glossopharyngeal nerve, present an embryologic enigma in that the entire muscle mass is innervated by the pharyngeal plexus and/or by named branches of the vagus nerve (cranial nerve X). Although the pharyngeal muscles and soft palate muscles (except those listed previously) are innervated by the nerve of the fourth pharyngeal arch, their precise origin in humans is as yet unclear. A detailed discussion of the contributions of each cranial nerve to the pharyngeal plexus appears in Chapter 18.

First Pharyngeal Groove

The first pharyngeal groove, separating the mandibular and hyoid arches, continues to invade the mesenchyme opposite the evaginating first pharyngeal pouch (Figs. 5-1, 5-2, 5-3, 5-4, and 5-5). The groove gives rise to the external auditory meatus and the external ectodermal lining of the tympanic membrane (eardrum). Mesenchymal proliferations from the dorsal aspects of the first and second pharyngeal arches provide the tissues that later fuse and develop into the auricle (external ear).

Mesenchymal tissues at the anterior tips of the second pharyngeal arch develop a sudden growth spurt when forming the anterior neck, causing overgrowth of the neck region and obliterating the remaining pharyngeal grooves (Figs. 5-4 and 5-5). Because these covered pharyngeal grooves are lined with ectoderm, they may remain as cervical sinuses and might later develop into cervical cysts. The impetus for this growth spurt is provided by the signaling molecules bone morphogenic protein BMP-7, sonic hedgehog, and fibroblast growth factor-8 produced by the overlying ectodermal cells. These signaling molecules target the mesenchymal cells of the hyoid arch, inducing proliferation and growth of these tissues.

Derivatives of the Pharyngeal Pouches

Summary Bite. Pharyngeal pouches are outpocketed portions of the pharyngeal foregut just behind the ruptured buccopharyngeal membrane. These five pharyngeal pouches, lined by endoderm, give rise to several organs.

First Pharyngeal Pouch

The first pharyngeal pouch, an endodermal-lined, outpocketed portion of the pharyngeal wall located between the first and second arch mesoderm, evaginates into an elongated tubotympanic recess giving rise to the tympanic cavity and the mastoid antrum, which remains connected to the pharynx as the auditory tube (Figs. 5-4 and 5-5). The endodermal lining participates in the formation of the eardrum. Thus, the closing plate between the first pharyngeal groove and the first pharyngeal pouch is the tympanic membrane, covered on its external surface by ectoderm derived from the groove and on its internal surface by endoderm derived from the pouch. Interposed between these two coverings are a few strands of mesenchymal tissue.

Second Pharyngeal Pouch

The second pharyngeal pouch remains as the tonsillar fossa between the pillars of the fauces (Figs. 5-4 and 5-5). Later, the crypts of the fossa are invaded by lymphoid tissue, which becomes organized into the palatine tonsils.

Third Pharyngeal Pouch

The third pharyngeal pouch forms two diverticula, a dorsal one whose endoderm differentiates into the definitive inferior parathyroid tissue and a ventral one that develops into thymus primordium which then fuses with its counterpart of the opposite side, forming the thymus gland (Figs. 5-4 and 5-5). These primordia become detached from the wall and begin to migrate caudally. The thymus comes to lie in the superior thoracic cavity, whereas the parathyroid primordia migrating with it will occupy the inferior pole of the posterior surface of the thyroid gland—hence its name, **inferior parathyroid**.

Fourth Pharyngeal Pouch

The fourth pharyngeal pouch, in a manner similar to the third, develops a dorsal and a ventral diverticulum. Developing from the dorsal diverticulum is the superior parathyroid, which eventually rests on the superior pole of the dorsal surface of the thyroid gland (Figs. 5-4 and 5-5). The ventral portion soon disap-

Clinical Considerations

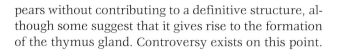

Cysts and Fistulas

As the second arch overgrows the third and fourth arches to cover the neck, the grooves are normally buried and become obliterated. **Cervical cysts** develop if obliteration does not occur, thus connecting the surface of the neck with the pharynx via the **branchial fistula**. These cysts are usually found in the neck on a line just anterior to the sternocleidomastoid muscle. Often these are not evident during childhood but may become apparent later as they enlarge. Surgery is necessary to repair the defect.

Pouch Defects

Sometimes the thymic primordia does not fuse with each other or do not descend into the chest cavity, leaving thymic tissue behind in cords along its path. This may cause ectopic placement of the parathyroid tissue from its normal location on the dorsal aspect of the thyroid. Occasionally, supernumerary parathyroid glands

develop or, infrequently, parathyroid development does not occur.

Thyroid

The epithelium destined to become the definitive thyroid tissue, which leaves a depression on the tongue (the foramen cecum), sometimes also leaves a remnant along its migration path, called the **thyroglossal duct**, along which cysts and sinuses may develop. Should these ever become infected, they may enlarge and open onto the midline of the neck, requiring corrective surgery. Rarely, the thyroid primordium fails to descend, thus forming a **lingual thyroid** at the base of the tongue. **Aberrant** or **accessory thyroid**, which may or may not be functional, may be found anywhere along the usual descent route.

---

pears without contributing to a definitive structure, although some suggest that it gives rise to the formation of the thymus gland. Controversy exists on this point.

Fifth Pharyngeal Pouch
This pouch gives rise to the ultimobranchial body, which becomes incorporated into the substance of the thyroid gland, giving rise to the calcitonin-secreting parafollicular cells of the thyroid gland (Figs. 5-4 and 5-5).

FLOOR OF THE PHARYNX

Summary Bite. The mouth, lips, gingiva, and enamel of the teeth develop from the stomodeum and the floor of the pharynx, whereas the salivary glands arise as ectodermal buds from the first arch.

The mouth is developed from the stomodeum and from the floor of the pharynx (foregut). The lips, the gingiva, and the enamel of the teeth develop from the ectodermally lined stomodeum. The salivary glands also arise from the oral cavity as ectodermal buds derived from the lining of the first arch. The

parotid gland, the first to develop, appears between the maxillary and mandibular processes. It is followed by the submandibular gland and finally the sublingual gland in the floor of the mouth.

Tongue

The tongue begins its formation in the floor of the pharynx during the fourth week of gestation, first as a small median swelling, the **tuberculum impar**, bounded by the two larger **lateral lingual swellings** (Fig. 5-6). These structures develop in the dorsal aspects of the ventral ends of the mandibular arch. Shortly thereafter, another median swelling, the **copula** develops just posterior to the tuberculum impar. It appears that this structure develops as a result of contributions from the second, third, and fourth arches. Posterior to the copula, yet another median swelling, the epiglottic eminence, which will become the epiglottis and the posterior region of the tongue, develops from the fourth arch (Fig. 5-6). The copula and the epiglottic eminence together are known as the hypobranchial eminence.

Continued growth in the lateral lingual swellings results in overgrowth of the tuberculum impar. Forward growth of the copula and the subsequent fusing with the lateral lingual swellings forms a V on

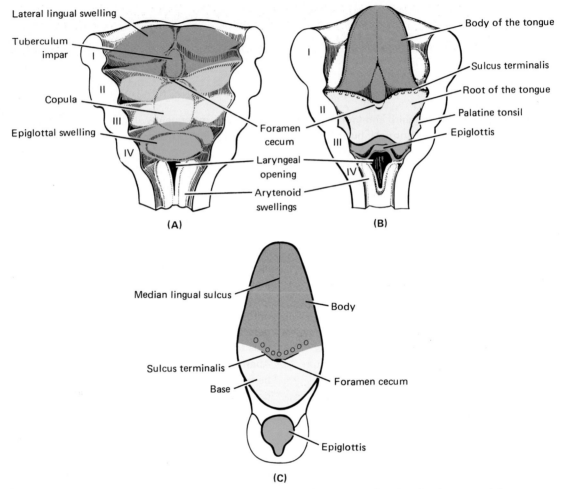

Figure 5-6. Ventral portions of the pharyngeal arches seen from above showing development of the tongue. *I* to *IV* the cut pharyngeal arches. **(A)** Five weeks (~6 mm). **(B)** Five months. Note the foramen cecum, site of the origin of the thyroid primordium. **(C)** Definitive tongue.

the tongue surface, separating, in the adult, the anterior two thirds of the tongue (body) from the posterior one third (base) of the tongue. The V-shaped groove separating the two regions is the **terminal sulcus** (Fig. 5-6). Located at the apex of the V is a small pit, the **foramen cecum**, demarcating the place where the primordium of the thyroid gland separated from the pharyngeal wall to migrate into the neck to be located ventral and inferior to the thyroid cartilage.

The tongue musculature does not arise from the pharyngeal arches. The muscle mass probably

Clinical Considerations

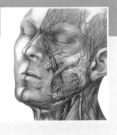

Tongue

Because the tongue develops from diverse origins, several different malformations are possible.

Ankyloglossia (tongue-tie), perhaps the most common defect, results from a shortening of the lingual frenulum, thus restricting the tip of the tongue. It occurs in 1 in 300 infants. Simply clipping the frenulum relieves this condition. An excessively large or unusually small tongue is relatively rare. **Macroglossia** is apparently the result of generalized hypertrophy of the tongue, and **microglossia** is usually associated with an underdeveloped mandibular process called **micrognathia**. Rarely, the lateral lingual swellings of the right and left sides fail to fuse, resulting in a **bifid tongue**.

Table 5-2 Derivatives of the Pharynx and the Pharyngeal Pouches

Region	Pouch I Level	Pouch II Level	Pouch III Level	Pouch IV Level	Pouch V Level
Roof		Pharyngeal tonsils			
Lateral walls	Tympanic cavity Lining of tympanum Mastoid air cells Auditory tube	Palatine tonsils and fossa	*Dorsal:* inferior parathyroid *Ventral:* thymus	*Dorsal:* superior parathyroid *Ventral:* thymus?	Ultimobranchial body—incorporated into lateral thyroid as parafollicular cells that secrete calcitonin
Floor (pharyngeal endoderm related to pharyngeal arch)	Body of tongue (anterior two thirds) Foramen cecum (remnant of rostral end of thyroglossal duct of thyroid gland)	Root of tongue (posterior one-third) Lingual tonsil	Base of tongue (in part)	Base of tongue (in part) Epiglottis	

migrates from preoccipital somites, taking with it the hypoglossal nerve (cranial nerve XII).

The multiple origin of the tongue provides the reason for its multi-innervation. The anterior two thirds, developing from the first arch ectoderm, receive sensory innervation via the trigeminal nerve and special sensation (taste) from the facial nerve. The posterior one third, developing from endoderm of arches II, III, and IV, is served by the glossopharyngeal nerve for general and special sensation, whereas the very base of the tongue is supplied by branches of the vagus nerve. The motor components to the muscles, however, are supplied by the hypoglossal nerve. (See Table 5-2 for a summary of the pharynx and its derivatives.)

FACE, NOSE, AND PALATE, DEVELOPMENT

Summary Bite. The face, nose, lips, mandible, maxillae, and the palate develop from the frontonasal prominence and the maxillary and mandibular processes as they fuse together.

Face and Nose

During the fourth week of gestation, as the maxillary and mandibular processes of the first pharyngeal arch are developing and growing anteriorly, a median bulge covering the brain enlarges and grows forward. This **frontonasal prominence**, with its two lateral thickened areas, the **nasal placodes**, develops just above the stomodeum. Later, the medial and lateral rims of the nasal placodes grow around the placode, leaving a depression, the **nasal pit**. Continued anterior growth of these rims through the fifth week causes a thinning and rupture of the epithelium covering the floor of the nasal pit. At this point, as this bucconasal membrane ruptures, a communication is established with the roof of the developing oral cavity. The lateral rims of the nasal placodes become the **lateral nasal swellings**, which will become the alae (wings) of the nose. The medial rims of the nasal placodes, known as the **median nasal swellings**, fuse together to form the **intermaxillary segment**, which will form the bulbus of the nose (Fig. 5-3B,C).

Continued growth of this intermaxillary segment anterior and inferior to the nose will give rise to the inferior aspect of the nasal septum, columella of the nose, philtrum of the upper lip, labial tubercle, and primary palate (premaxilla). The anterior teeth and their supporting structures as well as the gingiva will also develop from the intermaxillary segment (Fig. 5-7A).

During this approximately 2-week period, the maxillary swellings have moved anteriorly, meeting the intermaxillary segment and fusing with it to seal the **nasolacrimal groove**, a deep furrow running between the medial aspect of the eye and the primitive oral cavity on the face. The epithelium lining this groove separates from the surface ectoderm, finally forming the **nasolacrimal duct** (tear duct) opening into the nasal cavity (Figs. 5-3C and 5-8).

During this period, the mandibular processes have fused anteriorly, forming the mandible, thereby reducing the size of the primitive mouth. Also at this time, mesoderm of the second arch has invaded the

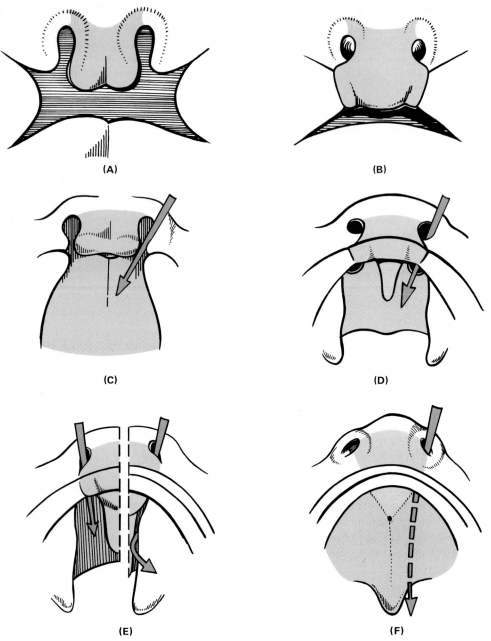

Figure 5-7. Development of the nose, mouth, and palate. **(A–B)** Formation of the nose and upper lip. **(C–F)** Formation of the philtrum, nose, and upper lip and the stages of palate formation and closure. Observe the steps of developing separate oral and nasal cavities from the early common oronasal cavity.

area, forming the muscles of facial expression over the entire face (Figs. 5-3C and 5-9).

Early development of the facial region is believed to be controlled by the migrating neural crest cells. These ectomesenchymal cells express the products of the homeobox genes, such as **MSX-1**, as well as the signaling molecules fibroblast growth factor (FGF) and sonic hedgehog (SHH). These gene products are believed to orchestrate the morphogenic events required to establish a facial anlagen. Neural crest cells

from the region of the midbrain and hindbrain migrate into the upper jaw, whereas those destined for the lower jaw and remaining arches migrate from the rhombomeres, special regions of the hindbrain.

Palate

The initial formation and continued growth of the palatal shelves appear to be under the influence of epithelial–mesenchymal interaction and growth factor,

Facial Malformations

Retinoic Acid

Retinoic acid, the acidic form of vitamin A, stimulates the expression of homeobox genes and is known to be implicated in early facial development. However, the absence as well as the excess availability of retinoic acid have been shown to result in increased incidences of severe facial malformations.

Treacher Collins Syndrome

Treacher Collins syndrome (mandibulofacial dysostosis) is a severe deformity of the face, eyes, ears, and derivatives of the mandibular arch with undeveloped zygoma bones. Although it is an autosomal dominate trait, it can be produced in laboratory animals following exposure to teratogenic doses of retinoic acid.

including transforming growth factor-α and epidermal growth factor.

As the two maxillary swellings grow anteriorly toward the midline to contribute to the formation of the upper jaw, each develops a shelflike structure that grows inferiorly to project obliquely on the side of the tongue into the sublingual sulcus (Fig. 5-10). As the tongue drops from the nasal into the oral cavity during the seventh week of development, these **lateral palatine shelves** ascend to a horizontal position above the tongue (Fig. 5-11) and fuse with each other in the midline, forming the secondary palate (Fig. 5-12). As a result of the fusion, some of the epithelial cells of the seam undergo programmed cell death, thus permitting confluence of mesenchymal tissues across the midline. However, some of the epithelial cells of the seam are transformed into mesenchymal cells under the influence of transforming growth factor-β,

whereas others migrate and become part of the epithelium lining the oral cavity.

The intermaxillary segment forms the primary palate, the triangular portion of the palate that is located behind the four incisor teeth and extends posteriorly in the midline to the incisive papilla. Fusion of the secondary palate with the primary palate separates the oronasal cavity into the nasal cavity and the oral cavity. Concomitantly, the nasal septum develops as a downgrowth within the nasal cavity and, as it fuses with the nasal aspect of the palatine shelves, it divides the nasal cavity into bilateral halves.

As the nasal wall continues to develop, diverticula form and invade the maxillae, frontal, ethmoid, and sphenoid bones, giving rise to the paranasal sinuses. (For a summary of the derivatives of facial components, see Table 5-3.)

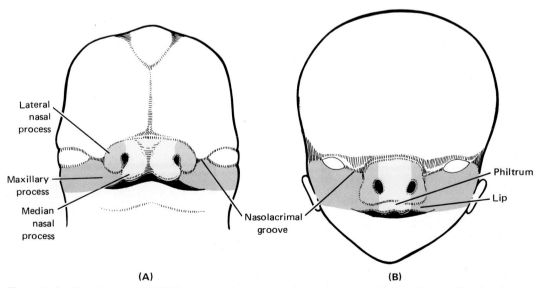

(A) **(B)**

Figure 5-8. Face formation. **(A)** The nasolacrimal groove is as yet unsealed, as are the maxillary/median nasal process seams. **(B)** The nasolacrimal groove is sealing and the upper lip and philtrum have formed.

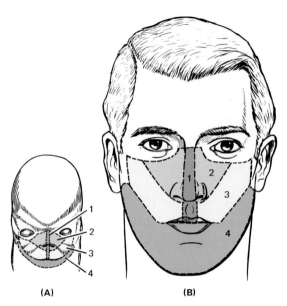

Figure 5-9. Development of the face illustrating derivatives of embryologic development. **(A)** Approximately 8 weeks of development. **(B)** Adult. (1) Median nasal process; (2) Lateral nasal process; (3) Maxillary process; (4) Mandibular process.

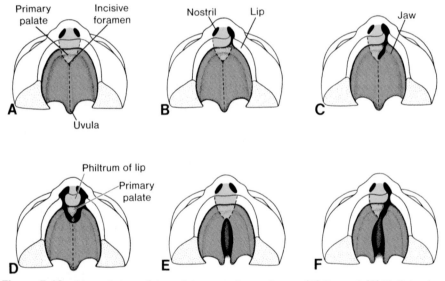

Figure 5-10. Ventral view of the palate, gum, lip, and nose. **(A)** Normal. **(B)** Unilateral cleft lip extending into the nose. **(C)** Unilateral cleft lip involving the lip and jaw extending to the incisive foramen. **(D)** Bilateral cleft involving the lip and jaw. **(E)** Isolated cleft palate. **(F)** Cleft palate combined with unilateral anterior cleft lip.

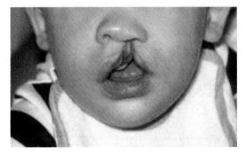

Figure 5-11. Cleft lip.

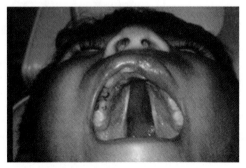

Figure 5-12. Cleft palate.

Table 5-3 Derivatives of Facial Components

Embryonic Part	Facial Derivatives	Skeletal Derivatives
Frontal process	Forehead	Frontal bone
Frontonasal process	Bridge of nose	Nasal bones
Median nasal process	Globus of nose	Ethmoid-perpendicular plate
Intermaxillary segment (fused median nasal processes)	Columella of nose Primary palate (premaxilla) Philtrum Superior labial frenulum Center portion of upper lip	Vomer
Lateral nasal process	Sides and ala of nose	
Maxillary process	Major portion of upper lip Upper cheek	Maxilla, zygoma Secondary palate
Mandibular process	Lower lip, lower cheek	Mandible

Clinical Considerations

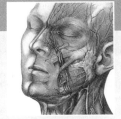

Cleft Lip and Cleft Palate

These two malformations are the most common defects observed on the face. Cleft lip occurs in about 1 of every 1,000 births in the United States, being more prevalent in boys (80%) than in girls. The incidence also seems to be related to increasing maternal age. The incidence of cleft palate is about 1 in 2,500 births. Unlike the differences noted with cleft lip, the cases observed in occurrence of cleft palate show girls (67%) to be more prone to develop the defect than boys. Some evidence points to the fact that the slower development in the female, with palatal fusion being delayed 1 week, may contribute to this condition.

Genetic and environmental factors play a large role in malformations of the lip and palate; however, space does not permit discussion of these factors here.

Cleft Lip

Cleft lip (see Fig. 5-7) may be observed only as a small notching of the lip to a **unilateral cleft lip** revealing the unfused maxillary process with the intermaxillary segment of one side. Malformation of more severe consequences results in **bilateral cleft lip** where neither of the maxillary swellings have fused with the intermaxillary segment. Extremely severe cases of bilateral cleft lip display the philtrum and the entire undifferentiated intermaxillary segment, which would have developed into the primary palate. Many cases of cleft lip present malformation of the primary palate and the anterior teeth. Rarely, the median nasal processes fail to fuse and proliferate, resulting in **median cleft lip**.

Depending on the severity of the cleft lip and the structures associated with it, surgical repair is successful, although it may require several procedures.

Cleft Palate

Posterior (secondary) cleft palate (see Fig. 5-7) results from failure of the lateral palatine processes to fuse in the midline with the intermaxillary segment, thereby permitting direct communication between the oral and nasal cavities. **Unilateral cleft palate** results when one palatal shelf does not fuse with the intermaxillary segment. When both shelves fail to fuse with each other and the median nasal septum, **bilateral cleft palate** results.

Anterior (primary) cleft palate is a consequence of fusion failure between the primary and secondary palatal processes (see Fig. 5-7). Clefts of both anterior and posterior palates result from failure of fusion between the primary palate, palatal shelves of the secondary palate, and the median nasal septum.

Varying degrees of clefting exist, the last described being most severe, and the least severe is observed simply as a bifid uvula. Factors producing cleft lip, with or without cleft palate, are distinctly different from factors producing cleft palate alone.

A team approach, involving specialists in medicine, dentistry, social work, and speech therapy, are often used to correct and rehabilitate the more serious cases of cleft palate and/or cleft lip. Although it may take several surgical and dental procedures over a number of years, along with therapy, the results are usually good.

Osteology

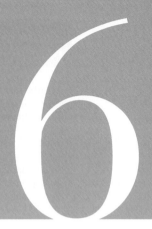

6

Key Terms

Atlas, the first cervical vertebra, is greatly modified. The body is replaced by an anterior arch whose ventral surface possesses an anterior tubercle, whereas its dorsal surface presents the **facet** for the **dens** of the axis, thus permitting rotation. Superior facets articulate with facets on the occipital bone, whereas the inferior facets articulate with facets on the axis.

Axis, the second cervical vertebra, is also modified to participate in the formation of the atlantoaxial joint. The body of the axis is modified superiorly to present a projection, the **dens**, which presents an articular facet that meets the articular facet on the internal surface of the anterior arch of the atlas, permitting the arch of the atlas to rotate about the dens of the axis.

Cervical Vertebrae are the superior seven vertebrae of the vertebral column. The superior two cervical vertebrae, the atlas and axis, support the head and permit its rotation at the atlantoaxial joint. With the exception of the 7th cervical vertebra, the transverse processes of all cervical vertebrae are pierced by the large foramen transversarium, housing the vertebral vessels and associated sympathetic plexus.

Cranium is that portion of the skull that houses the brain. Eight bones comprise the cranium, including the paired temporal and parietal bones and the unpaired ethmoid, frontal, sphenoid, and occipital bones.

Dental Arches are two in number. One is formed in the maxillae and the other is formed in the mandible. Each arch normally houses 16 teeth in the adult, which articulate with their counterparts in the opposing arch as a result of the actions of the muscles of the mandible.

Face is composed of the remaining 14 bones of the skull. These include the paired nasal, maxillae, palatine, lacrimal, zygoma, and inferior nasal conchae, and the unpaired vomer and mandible.

Hyoid Bone is a small, U-shaped bone situated horizontally in the middle of the anterior neck. It does not form a joint with another bone; rather, it is suspended by three bilateral ligaments and as many as 10 (and occasionally 11) muscles.

Mandible is the only movable bone of the skull. It is a double-jointed bone that articulates with the articular eminence of the zygomatic process of the paired temporal bones. This is made possible by several ligaments about the joints and the contractions of the muscles that act upon the mandible.

Zygomatic Arch represents most of the bony prominence of the cheek. It is formed by the zygomatic process of the temporal bone and the temporal process of the zygomatic bone. The space superior and deep to the arch is called the temporal fossa, whereas the space inferior and deep to the arch is called the infratemporal fossa. Both of these fossae are filled with three of the four muscles of mastication.

SKULL AND CERVICAL VERTEBRAE

The **skull** and **cervical vertebrae**, as well as the **hyoid bone**, comprise the bony skeletal system of the head and neck. In addition, the viscera of the neck—specifically, the larynx—contains a cartilaginous skeleton that will be discussed later. This chapter examines the skull, the cervical vertebrae, and the hyoid bone.

SKULL

Summary Bite. The bony skull is composed of 22 paired and single bones that make up the face and cranium. With the exception of the mandible, the bones of the skull are tightly attached to each other via sutures which render them immovable.

The skull, excluding the three pairs of ossicles of the ear, is composed of 22 bones, some of which are paired, whereas the others are single. Twenty-one of these bones are firmly attached to each other via **sutures** and are immovable. The only movable bone is the tooth-bearing **mandible**, which articulates with the paired **temporal bones** by a combined hinge and gliding (ginglymoarthrodial) joint, the temporomandibular joint. Articulation at this joint permits the teeth of the mandible to interact with the teeth on the opposing tooth-bearing arch, the paired maxillae, and thus function in biting, mastication, and other actions.

It is convenient to divide the skull arbitrarily into two portions, namely, the bones assisting in the formation of the face and those forming the cranium. Fourteen bones compose the face: the paired **nasal bones**, **maxillae**, **palatine bones**, **lacrimal bones**, **zygoma**, and **inferior nasal conchae**, along with the singular **vomer** and **mandible**. Eight bones comprise the cranium, the portion of the skull housing the brain: the paired **temporal** and **parietal bones** and the singular **frontal**, **sphenoid**, **ethmoid**, and **occipital bones** (Table 6-1).

Examination of the skull is normally performed first externally and then internally. Externally, it is viewed from several perspectives, namely, anterior, lateral, posterior, superior, and inferior views, whereas internally the base of the skull and the calvaria are studied.

External Aspect of the Skull

Anterior View

Summary Bite. The anterior view presents the bones of the face and the anterior portion of the calvaria.

From the anterior perspective, the skull is viewed face-on, observing all of the bones that comprise the face as well as some of the bones that form the calvaria. At first glance, the most obvious landmarks are the paired orbits separated medially and inferiorly by the anterior nasal aperture. The bony prominence of the forehead is superior to the orbits, whereas the zygomatic arch is visible lateral and inferior to the orbits. An additional obvious feature is the presence of the teeth located in the upper and lower jaws (Figs. 6-1 and 6-10).

Bearing these landmarks in mind, one may now begin a thorough examination of the anterior aspect of the skull. The forehead is formed by the squamous part of the **frontal bone**, whose posterior aspect extends to the **coronal suture**. Here, the frontal bone articulates with the right and left parietal bones, which are separated from each other by the midline **sagittal suture**. The paired **frontal eminences** are more or less prominent elevations on either side of the middle of the forehead just above the **superciliary arches**, which may be palpated in the living individual as elevations superior to the eyebrows. Between the superciliary arches is a rather smooth depressed area, the

Table 6-1 Bones of the Skull

Cranial	No.	Facial	No.	Ossicles of the Ears, No.
Ethmoid	1	Inferior concha	2	6
Frontal	1	Lacrimal	2	
Occipital	1	Mandible	1	
Parietal	2	Maxilla	2	
Sphenoid	1	Nasal	2	
Temporal	2	Palatine	2	
		Vomer	1	
		Zygoma	2	
Total	**8**		**14**	**6**

glabella. Superior to the glabella occasionally is another suture, the **metopic frontal suture**, a remnant of the postembryonic fusion between the right and left halves of the frontal bone. Inferior to the superciliary arch is the superior rim of the orbit.

Orbit

⊐ **Summary Bite.** The orbit is comprised of several bones, including portions of the frontal, maxilla, ethmoid, palatine, sphenoid, zygoma, and lacrimal. Its concavity houses the eyeball (orb) muscles, vessels, nerves, and connective tissue in the living.

The orbit is a complex cavity formed by seven bones: the maxilla, frontal, ethmoid, palatine, zygomatic, sphenoid, and lacrimal bones (Figs. 6-1 and 6-2). It houses the eyeball (orb) and its associated muscles, vessels, nerves, and connective tissues. The medial walls of the orbits are parallel to each other (and to the sagittal suture), whereas their lateral walls are positioned approximately 45 degrees from their medial walls. Consequently, each orbit is widest anteriorly and narrowest posteriorly and may be envisioned to have the shape of a truncated pyramid (see Fig. 6-14 and Chapter 10).

The anterior-most aspect of the orbit (or its base), known as the **rim**, is formed by three bones: the frontal, zygoma, and maxilla. The entire superior aspect of the rim is formed by the frontal bone, which is interrupted by the **supraorbital foramen** (or, frequently, the "notch") located medially. This foramen transmits the supraorbital vessels and nerves. Most of the medial and about half of the inferior rim are formed by the maxilla, specifically its frontal and part of its orbital processes. The remaining inferior portion and most of the lateral portion of the rim are formed by the zygoma. The remainder of the orbit will be described in relation to its roof, floor, lateral and medial walls, and apex.

The **roof** of the orbit is formed by a shelf of the frontal bone known as the **orbital plate**. Two depressions are located anteriorly on the roof; the smaller medial one, known as the **trochlear fovea**, houses a small cartilage associated with the superior oblique muscle of the eye, and the larger depression, the laterally positioned **lacrimal fossa**, accommodates the lacrimal gland. The roof is completed posteriorly by a small portion of the lesser wing of the sphenoid bone.

The **lateral wall** is composed of the greater wing of the sphenoid bone posteriorly and the zygomatic bone anteriorly. The line of fusion between the roof and the lateral wall is incomplete posteriorly, creating the **superior orbital fissure**, which is bounded also by the lesser wing of the sphenoid bone and the orbital plate of the frontal bone. The superior orbital fissure is traversed by cranial nerves III, IV, VI, and the ophthalmic

division of V, as well as small arterial branches and the superior ophthalmic vein. Similarly, a gap between the lateral wall and the floor of the orbit, the **inferior orbital fissure**, is formed by the greater wing of the sphenoid bone, the maxilla, the palatine bone, and the zygoma. The inferior orbital fissure transmits the maxillary division of cranial nerve V, the zygomatic nerve, infraorbital vessels, and the vein to the pterygoid plexus.

The **floor** of the orbit is composed of the maxilla, palatine bone, and zygoma. In the middle of the floor, mostly on the orbital plate of the maxilla, is a depression, the **infraorbital groove**, which communicates with the **infraorbital foramen** via the **infraorbital canal**. The infraorbital vessels and nerve leave the orbit through the infraorbital canal.

The **medial wall** of the orbit is formed by four bones: the maxilla, lacrimal, ethmoid, and sphenoid bones. Bordering the rim of the orbit medially, the frontal process of the maxilla and the lacrimal bone both participate in the formation of a depression, the **fossa** for the **lacrimal sac**. This fossa is continuous inferiorly with the **nasolacrimal canal**. Two small foramina, evident on the medial wall of the orbit at the ethmoidal–frontal suture, are the **anterior** and **posterior ethmoidal foramina**. The anterior ethmoidal foramen transmits the anterior ethmoidal nerve and vessel, whereas the posterior ethmoidal nerve and vessel pass through the posterior ethmoidal foramen.

The **apex** of the orbit consists of a single round opening, the **optic foramen**, through which cranial nerve II, the ophthalmic artery, a branch of the internal carotid artery, as well as the carotid plexus (a sheath of autonomic nerve fibers wrapped around the artery) enter the orbit from the cranial vault.

Nasal Cavity

⊐ **Summary Bite.** The nasal cavity lies in the midline below and between the orbits, covered by the paired nasal bones. Its medial wall is formed by the ethmoid bone, whereas its lateral wall is formed by the zygoma. The frontal bone forms the superior wall, whereas the maxilla forms the floor.

The nasal cavity is below and between the two orbits. Anterosuperiorly, it is covered by the paired **nasal bones**, which articulate with one another in the midline, with the perpendicular plate of the ethmoid internally, as well as with the frontal process of the maxilla and the frontal bone. The nasal bones and the nasal cartilages form the bony and cartilaginous bridge of the nose.

The cavity opens at its anterior extent via the **anterior nasal aperture** (piriform aperture), whose boundary is formed by the two nasal bones superiorly and the maxillae laterally and inferiorly. Inferiorly, at the midline of the anterior nasal aperture, the right and left maxillae fuse, forming a small, bony, nipple-like structure, the **anterior nasal spine**. Posteriorly, the nasal cavity extends to the **posterior nasal aperture**, or **choanae**, where, similarly, the **horizontal plates** of the **palatine bones** fuse in the midline to form the **posterior nasal spines**.

The nasal cavity is divided in the midline into right and left halves by the **nasal septum**, composed of the **perpendicular plate** of the **ethmoid** anteriorly and superiorly and the **vomer bone** inferiorly and posteriorly. The sphenoid, maxillae, and palatine bones also make minor contributions to the bony nasal septum. The floor of each nasal cavity is formed by the horizontal plate of the palatine bone posteriorly and by the palatine process of the maxilla anteriorly.

The **incisive canals** are located at the junction of the vomer with the anterior-most portion of the palatine process of each maxilla. These canals transmit the descending septal arteries and the nasopalatine nerves, which course along on both sides of the nasal septum. The two incisive canals open on the oral palatal surface of the maxillae in the midline just posterior to the interproximal aspect of the central incisors, at the **incisive foramina** housed in the incisive fossa.

The lateral wall of the nasal cavity is rather complex because it contains foramina communicating with the sinuses, **meatuses** (which form air passages in an anteroposterior direction), and their overlying turbinate bones, known as **conchae**.

Several bones, listed in an anteroposterior direction, participate in the formation of the lateral wall: the maxilla, lacrimal, ethmoid, and palatine bones; the medial pterygoid plate of the sphenoid; and the **inferior nasal concha**. The ethmoid bone has turbinate bones, the **superior** and **middle conchae**, protruding into the nasal cavity.

Lateral, deep, and inferior to these conchae are air passages, the meatuses. The **superior meatus** extends as far as the middle concha, and it communicates with the **posterior ethmoid air cells**. The space below and deep to the middle nasal concha and superior to the inferior nasal concha is the **middle meatus**. This meatus communicates indirectly with the anterior ethmoidal air cells, directly or indirectly with the frontal sinus, and with the **maxillary sinus** via the opening (ostium) of the maxillary sinus. The space lateral and inferior to the inferior nasal concha is the **inferior meatus**, which extends as far inferiorly as the floor of the nasal cavity. The **nasolacrimal canal** opens into the anterior portion of the inferior meatus.

Face

Summary Bite. The face is formed by 14 bones: the paired nasal bones, zygoma, lacrimal bones, maxillae, palatine bones, inferior nasal conchae, and the singular vomer and mandible.

The portion of the face between the inferior rim of the orbit and the upper teeth is formed primarily by the maxillae. Just inferior to the rim is the **infraorbital foramen**. Lateral to this is the suture between the **zygomatic process of the maxilla** and the **maxillary process of the zygoma**, with the two processes contributing to the bony cheek prominence (Figs 6-1, 6-2, and 6-6).

The inferior-most aspects of the two maxillae house the 16 maxillary teeth, forming the upper **dental arch** (Figs. 6-1, 6-2, and 6-10). Each maxilla contains a central and a lateral incisor and a canine, whose single root forms a prominent tuberosity on the maxilla, known as the **canine eminence**. Medial to the canine eminence is a fossa superior to the two incisors, the **incisive fossa**, and a similar fossa located lateral to the canine eminence, known as the **canine fossa** (see Fig. 4-3). The maxillary dental arch also houses two premolars and three molars. Teeth of this arch articulate with those of the mandible, the only bone of the skull that possesses the capacity to move.

The right and left halves of the mandible each contain a central and lateral incisor and a canine, whose single root is demarcated on the mandible as the canine eminence. Similarly to the maxillae, medial to this eminence, is the **incisive fossa**. Two premolars and three molars complete the mandibular dental arch. At the level of the second premolar of the mandible is the **mental foramen**, through which the mental nerve and vessels exit the **mandibular canal**.

Occasionally, a line indicating the **mental symphysis** may be observed in the midline inferior to the interdental septum between the two central incisors, extending through the **mental protuberance** or point of the chin. This represents the line of fusion of the right and left halves of the mandible during embryogenesis. The **oblique line**, the **angle**, and the anterior border of the mandible are also evident from this view.

Lateral View

Summary Bite. The lateral view displays the cranial vault with some of the sutures between the various bones making up the cranium, some of the bones of the face, and the bones forming the zygomatic arch.

From the lateral aspect, the skull is viewed in profile. The large cranial vault is evident, as are the bones of the face (Figs. 6-2 and 6-5). Various suture lines may be observed, namely, the **coronal suture**, between the frontal and parietal bones, which ends in the **sphenoparietal suture** at the greater wing of the sphenoid. Another suture, separating the squama of the temporal bone from the parietal bone, is the **squamosal suture**, which arches posteriorly, ending in the **lambdoidal suture** separating the occipital and parietal bones. Continuous with the lambdoidal suture inferiorly is the **occipitomastoid suture**, separating the mastoid portion of the temporal bone from the occipital bone. The anterior border of the temporal squama participates in the formation of the **sphenosquamosal suture**, delineating its fusion with the greater wing of the sphenoid.

Two lines, the **superior** and **inferior temporal lines**, arch across the frontal and parietal bones, indicating sites of attachment of the temporal fascia and temporalis muscle, respectively. This region of the skull lies deep to the zygomatic arch and constitutes the medial wall of a large region known as the **temporal fossa**.

Temporal Fossa

Summary Bite. The temporal fossa is viewed from the lateral aspect and is the depression between the zygomatic arch and the superior temporal lines on the temporal bone indicating the space filled by the temporalis muscle.

The temporal fossa is a space bounded by the zygoma and the zygomatic process of the frontal bone anteriorly and the superior temporal lines superiorly and posteriorly (Figs. 6-5 and 6-6). Inferiorly, its boundary is delineated by the supramastoid crest, the posterior root of the zygomatic arch, a line connecting the posterior and anterior roots of the zygomatic arch, the infratemporal crest of the greater wing of the sphenoid, and its posterior continuation on the temporal bone to the anterior root of the zygomatic arch.

The zygomatic arch marks the boundary of the lateral aspect of this fossa, whereas the bony structures of the skull form its medial wall. The anteromedial aspect of the temporal fossa presents the inferior orbital fissure. The temporal fossa, occupied by muscles, vessels, and nerves, is superior to and continuous with another deep space, the **infratemporal fossa**.

Infratemporal Fossa

Summary Bite. The space deep and inferior to the zygomatic arch, when viewed from the lateral aspect, represents the infratemporal fossa. Medially, it is bounded by part of the maxilla, lateral pterygoid plate of the sphenoid bone, and the pterygomaxillary fissure. This space houses the medial and lateral pterygoid muscles and the insertion of the temporalis muscle.

This space is located inferior and deep to the zygomatic arch. Its contents include the muscles of mastication, their vascular and nerve supply, as well as other structures of the deep face. The anterior boundary of the infratemporal fossa is the infratemporal surface of the maxilla and the deep surface of the zygomatic bone. Medially, it is bounded by the lateral surface of the lateral pterygoid plate of the sphenoid, the maxillary alveolar border, and a gap, the pterygomaxillary fissure. Superiorly, its boundary is the infratemporal crest of the sphenoid (the

boundary between the temporal and infratemporal fossae), the inferior aspect of the temporal squama, and the infratemporal surface of the greater wing of the sphenoid, housing the **foramen ovale** and the **foramen spinosum**.

Posteriorly the infratemporal fossa is poorly defined by the anterior limits of the mandibular fossa, whereas inferiorly it is completely open.

Pterygopalatine Fossa

Summary Bite. The pterygopalatine fossa is viewed from the lateral view and from the lateroinferior view. It lies inside the pterygomaxillary fissure located on the medial wall of the infratemporal fossa between the pterygoid process of the sphenoid and the posterior aspect of the maxilla. The pterygopalatine fossa transmits the maxillary vessels.

Entrance into the pterygopalatine fossa is gained via a gap, the **pterygomaxillary fissure**, which transmits the maxillary vessels. This fissure is located on the medial wall of the infratemporal fossa and is formed by the interval between the pterygoid process of the sphenoid and the convex posterior aspect of the maxilla.

The fossa is pyramidal in shape and is enclosed by three bones, the maxilla and palatine bones, and the pterygoid process of the sphenoid (Fig. 6-6). It communicates with the interior of the skull through the **foramen rotundum**, transmitting the maxillary branch of the trigeminal nerve; with the orbit via the inferior orbital fissure; and with the nasal cavity by the **sphenopalatine foramen**.

Extending posteriorly from this fossa is the **pterygoid canal**, which transmits the nerve of the pterygoid canal. Inferiorly, the fossa becomes constricted and ends in the **pterygopalatine canal** (greater palatine canal) conducting the greater palatine vessels and nerves. The fossa contains an autonomic ganglion and its associations and blood vessels.

Zygomatic Arch

Summary Bite. The zygomatic arch is formed by a suture between part of the zygoma and part of the temporal bone. It may be viewed from the lateral, lateroinferior, frontal, inferior, and lateral oblique aspects. In addition to giving the face form, the contribution of the temporal bone to the zygomatic arch also forms the articular surface for the temporomandibular joint.

The zygomatic arch assists in the formation of the bony prominence of the cheek and provides attachments for the temporalis fascia and the masseter muscle. The zygomatic arch is formed by the **temporal process of the zygomatic bone** and the **zygomatic process of the temporal bone**, which are joined to each other by a suture positioned more or less 45 degrees to the vertical (Figs. 6-2, 6-5, 6-6, and 6-7). Just medial to this suture, in the temporal fossa, the temporalis muscle passes to insert on the mandible.

The zygomatic process of the temporal bone arises from two or (according to some) three roots. The anterior root ends in front of the **mandibular (glenoid) fossa** in a round prominence, the articular eminence, which is the region of articulation of the mandibular condyle with the temporal bone. The posterior root continues further posteriorly, passing above the external auditory meatus and lateral to the mandibular fossa. The **postglenoid tubercle**, a bony structure posterior to the mandibular fossa that assists in preventing backward excursion of the condyle out of the fossa, is considered by some to be the third root of the zygomatic process of the temporal bone.

The zygomatic arch is continuous medially with the **zygoma**, a quadrilateral bone constituting a part of the inferior and lateral borders of the orbit. The superior border is formed by the frontal process of the zygoma and the inferior border by its maxillary process.

The **zygomaticofacial foramen** (frequently two foramina) pierces the body of the zygoma and transmits the zygomaticofacial nerve and vessels. On its orbital aspect, the zygomatic bone presents the two **zygomatico-orbital foramina**, which transmit nerves and vessels to the zygomaticofacial and **zygomaticotemporal** foramina. The latter foramen opens on the medial (temporal) surface of the zygomatic bone, and through it the zygomaticotemporal nerve and vessels enter the temporal fossa.

The zygomatic bone articulates with the zygomatic process of the maxilla, which describes an arched line, the **zygomaticoalveolar crest**, as it curves inferiorly to meet the alveolar portion of the maxilla.

Mastoid and Styloid Processes

Summary Bite. The region just posterior and inferior to the external ear canal is the mastoid process serving as an attachment site for several muscles. Anterior to the mastoid process is a long pointed bone directed inferiorly and anteriorly into the space of the neck. This is the styloid process, which serves as an attachment site for several muscles and ligaments related to movements of the mandible, hyoid bone, tongue, and pharynx.

The **external acoustic meatus** and the surrounding lateral aspect of the tympanic portion of the temporal bone are wedged between the mastoid process and the posterior root of the zygomatic process of the temporal bone just posterior to the mandibular fossa (Figs. 6-5, 6-6, and 6-7). This oval-shaped opening transmits the cartilaginous external ear canal leading to the tympanic membrane.

Behind and inferior to the external acoustic meatus is the **mastoid process**, which serves as a region

of attachment of several muscles. On its posterior aspect the **mastoid foramen** is frequently present, transmitting **emissary veins**. The **styloid process**, located anterior to the mastoid process, is a long, sharp, pointed, icicle-shaped bone directed inferiorly and anteriorly. It gives attachment to several muscles and ligaments that assist in regulation of the excursion and movements of the mandible, hyoid bone, tongue, and pharynx. Between the mastoid and **styloid processes** is a constant foramen, the **stylomastoid foramen**, transmitting the facial nerve.

Posterior View

Summary Bite. The occipital bone and the sagittal and lambdoidal sutures are observed from the posterior view. However, the foramen magnum is not. It may be observed from the lateroinferior view and viewing the base. Many of the muscles of the posterior neck attach to the occipital bone as indicated by the nuchal lines.

When the skull is observed from a posterior view, the **foramen magnum** is not visible. However, it may be observed in a lateroinferior view (Fig. 6-6) and from viewing the base of the skull (Fig. 6-7). The most obvious features present are the posterior aspects of the **sagittal suture** and the **lambdoidal suture**, the former separating the paired parietal bones from each other and the latter acting as the dividing line between the occipital and parietal bones. Occasionally, one or more small islands of bone, known as sutural bones (Wormian bones), are present in the apex of the lambdoidal suture, where it is met by the inferior extent of the sagittal suture. Enclosed by the diverging lines of the lambdoidal suture is the flat, shell-shaped portion of the occipital bone, the squama.

A thick ridge, known as the **superior nuchal line**, extends to bisect the occipital squama into superior and inferior halves. At the midpoint, the right and left superior nuchal lines meet in a bony point, the **external occipital protuberance**.

A thin ridge of bone on the occipital squama, known as the **external occipital crest** or **median nuchal line**, runs directly inferiorly, to terminate at the posteromedial ridge of the foramen magnum. At the midpoint of the external occipital crest, **the inferior nuchal line** extends laterally, representing the superior border of attachment for three muscles of the back of the neck. Occasionally, the **highest nuchal lines**, positioned just above the superior nuchal lines, are also evident. These serve as lines of attachment for the galea aponeurotica.

Superior View

Summary Bite. A superior view of the skull displays an oval shape that is broader posteriorly, being broadest at the parietal eminence. The bones identified from this view are the paired parietal bones and portions of the frontal and occipital bones.

The skull, observed from a superior view, is oval. It is narrower anteriorly and broader posteriorly, where the broadest region is the **parietal eminence**. This view reveals the portions of those bones that form the skullcap, consisting of the frontal squama, two parietal bones, and a small portion of the occipital squama. The frontal eminences and, if present, the metopic frontal sutures are evident. The coronal suture, indicating the border between the frontal and paired parietal bones, is met at its midline by the anterior extent of the sagittal suture at the **bregma**. The sagittal suture separates the right and left parietal bones from each other, terminating posteriorly at the **lambda**, the apex of the lambdoidal suture.

Anterior to the lambda, just lateral to the sagittal suture, are the paired **parietal foramina**, through which **emissary veins** pass. The bones comprising the calvaria (skullcap) are somewhat unusual in that they present two tables of compact bone, the outer and inner plates, which sandwich between them a layer of spongy (cancellous) bone, known as the **diploë**.

Inferior View

Summary Bite. The base of the skull provides a view of the maxillae containing the teeth of the maxillary arch anteriorly, the zygomatic arches laterally, and the superior nuchal line of the occipital bone posteriorly.

The inferior aspect of the skull (the base of the skull) is usually observed with the mandible detached to permit an unobstructed view of the various structures (Fig. 6-7). The anterior-most border includes the maxillary central incisors, whereas the posterior border is said to be the superior nuchal line.

The lateral extent includes the two zygomatic arches and the two mastoid processes. The base of the skull will be examined in three sections: the anterior portion, which extends as far back as the hard palate; the middle portion, which stops at a tangent drawn along the anterior-most point of the foramen magnum; and the posterior portion, which entails the remainder of the base of the skull.

Anterior Portion

Summary Bite. The anterior portion is represented by the 16 maxillary teeth embedded in the maxillary arch, which fuses behind the third molars forming the alveolar tubercle. Superior to this is the maxillary tuberosity. The hard palate forms the roof between the right and left halves of the maxillary arch.

The anterior portion is a flat-topped, dome-shaped region that houses the 16 maxillary teeth arranged peripherally in a horseshoe-shaped configuration (Figs. 6-7 and 6-8). It is the inferior-most portion of the skull, with the exception of the mandible.

The teeth are embedded in the **alveolar arch**, and intruding into the space between any two teeth, known as the interproximal region, is a bony extension, the **interdental septum**. Posterior to the third molars, the buccal and lingual alveolar arches fuse, and the area of fusion is known as the **alveolar tubercle**. Superior to the alveolar tubercle, the broad, posterior extent of the maxilla is the **maxillary tuberosity**.

In the anterior portion (and at this point it should be appreciated that although this view observes the skull upside-down, the descriptive terms refer to the normal anatomic position), the roof is arched and is separated into four segments by two intersecting sutures, the **cruciform suture**. The longer limb of this suture is the combination of the intermaxillary/interpalatine sutures, which separate the **hard palate** into right and left halves. The shorter limb of this suture is made up of the palatomaxillary sutures, which separate the horizontal plates of the palatine bones from the palatine processes of the maxillae.

The anterior-most part of the intermaxillary suture lies in a depression, the **incisive fossa** (not to be confused with the same-named depression on the external aspect of the maxilla), into which the **incisive foramina** opens (Fig. 6-8). The incisive foramen receives the right and left **incisive canals**, each of which transmits the nasopalatine branch of the sphenopalatine artery as well as the nasopalatine nerve.

Posteriorly, on the lateral aspect of the hard palate, normally within the palatomaxillary suture, is the **greater palatine foramen**, through which the greater palatine vessels and nerves pass. Just posterior to this foramen two, or occasionally three, smaller foramina, the **lesser palatine foramina**, are present (Fig. 6-8). They permit passage of the lesser palatine vessels and nerves. These foramina are contained in the **pyramidal process** of the palatine bone, which juts out posteriorly and laterally and is interposed between the **lateral and medial pterygoid plates** of the sphenoid bone.

The posterior aspect of the hard palate ends in a midline, bony projection known as the **posterior nasal spine**, the origin of the muscle of the uvula.

Middle Portion

Summary Bite. The middle portion represents parts of the sphenoid, palatine, temporal, vomer, and occipital bones and their foramina representing passageways for vessels and nerves to move into and out of the skull.

This is the most complex portion of the base of the skull and is composed of parts of the sphenoid, palatine, temporal, vomer, and occipital bones, housing several foramina, which present passageways to and from the exterior of the skull (Fig. 6-7 and 6-8). The pyramidal portion of the palatine bone has already been discussed. It covers a portion of the maxillary tuberosity and is interposed between the alveolar tubercle and the medial and lateral pterygoid plates of the sphenoid bone.

The medial pterygoid plate presents a short, wedge-shaped structure at its inferior free edge, the **pterygoid hamulus**, around which the tendon of the tensor veli palatini muscle passes. This muscle originates in the **scaphoid fossa**, a small depression at the base of the pterygoid processes. Above this fossa, at the root of the medial pterygoid plate, is the opening of the **pterygoid canal (vidian canal)**, through which the like-named nerve passes. Below this fossa is a larger depression, between the lateral and medial pterygoid plates, known as the **pterygoid fossa**. It contains the origins of the medial pterygoid and tensor veli palatini muscles.

Between the right and left medial pterygoid plates is the choana, the posterior entrance into the nasal cavity, which is separated into right and left compartments by the nasal septum. The posterior aspect of this midline septum is the vomer, whose superior, broadened portion, evident in the inferior view, is met by a horizontal projection from the base of the medial pterygoid plate known as the **vaginal process**. This process forms the floor of the **pharyngeal canal**, which transmits the like-named nerve.

Posterior to the vomer is a thick, bridgelike bone, the **basilar portion of the occipital bone**, which flares out laterally as it extends back to the foramen magnum and the **occipital condyles**. A bony protuberance in the middle of the basilar portion of the occipital bone is known as the **pharyngeal tubercle**. It acts as a point of suspension for the entire pharynx, via the pharyngeal raphe. Shallow depressions and slight ridges on either side of the pharyngeal tubercle represent attachments for some of the muscles of the posterior neck.

The occipital bone approximates the jagged **petrous portion** of the temporal bone, which houses the **carotid canal**, through which the **internal carotid artery** gains entrance into the cranial cavity. This canal terminates anteromedially at the apex of the petrous portion of the temporal bone, at the **foramen lacerum**. This foramen, obstructed in the live individual by a cartilaginous plate, is formed by the junction of the temporal, occipital, and sphenoid bones. Small arterial branches to the meninges and emissary veins from the cavernous sinus are said to pass through it.

The petrous portion of the temporal bone articulates anteriorly with the sphenoid, forming a groove that passes backwards and laterally, finally disappearing as a canal in the petrous bone. This groove and

canal house the cartilaginous portion of the auditory tube. A ridge of bone, the **spine of the sphenoid**, forms the lateral border of this groove and is perforated by the **foramen spinosum**, through which the middle meningeal artery and recurrent meningeal branch of the mandibular division of cranial nerve V gains entrance into the cranial cavity.

The **foramen ovale**, located just anterior and medial to the foramen spinosum, pierces the greater wing of the sphenoid and permits the passage of the accessory meningeal artery and the mandibular division of the trigeminal nerve.

Lateral to the foramen ovale is the flat portion of the greater wing of the sphenoid and part of the root of the zygomatic arch of the temporal bone. These form part of the roof of the infratemporal fossa. The lateral border of this table turns upward at nearly a right angle, forming a ridge, the **infratemporal crest**, which marks the boundary between the infratemporal and temporal fossae. The sphenotemporal suture passes diagonally across this ridge. Posterior to this table is a deep depression, housed in the tympanic and squamous portions of the temporal bone, the **mandibular fossa (glenoid fossa)**. This depression accepts the articular disc and, indirectly, the condyle of the mandible, thus participating in the formation of the temporomandibular joint.

The **squamotympanic fissure** passes diagonally across the mandibular fossa. Approximately halfway through its course, a thin wedge of bone, the inferior-most tip of the **tegmen tympani**, protrudes through this fissure, thus creating two new fissures, an anterior (**petrosquamous**) and a posterior (**petrotympanic**) fissure.

The petrotympanic fissure transmits the chorda tympani branch of cranial nerve VII and the anterior tympanic branch of the maxillary artery. The anterior border of the mandibular fossa is represented by the articular eminence of the zygomatic process and the posterior extent by the postglenoid tubercle, which is, according to some, the posterior root of the zygomatic arch. Curving inferiorly and posteriorly from the postglenoid tubercle is the free edge of the tympanic portion of the temporal bone.

Posterior Portion

Summary Bite. The occipital bone and its foramen magnum and occipital condyles, which articulate with the atlas and the mastoid and styloid processes, form most of the posterior portion. Again, many foramina are positioned in the posterior portion.

This portion contains the **foramen magnum**, the **occipital condyles**, the styloid and mastoid processes, and the region of the occipital squama as far superiorly as the superior nuchal line (Figs. 6-5, 6-6, and 6-7). The occipital condyles, which are located on either side of the foramen magnum, articulate with the atlas. Directly in front of and superior to each condyle is the hypoglossal canal, which traverses the bone in a posteromedial direction and transmits cranial nerve XII and a meningeal artery. Just posterior to the condyle is a depression, the **condylar fossa**, which may or may not be perforated by the **condylar foramen**, through which emissary veins pass.

Lateral to the hypoglossal canal is the **jugular foramen**, formed by the **jugular notch of the occipital** and the **jugular notch of the temporal bones**. Several important structures pass through this foramen, namely, cranial nerves IX, X, and XI, the inferior petrosal and transverse sinuses (draining into the jugular bulb, the expanded terminus of the internal jugular vein), and some meningeal arteries.

Just lateral to the large jugular foramen is the small stylomastoid foramen, wedged between the needle-shaped styloid process and the thick, cone-shaped mastoid process, through which cranial nerve VII leaves the skull. The mastoid process also gives rise to several muscles, one of which originates from a deep cleft, the **mastoid notch**, on the medial aspect of the process.

Medial to this cleft is the **groove** for the **occipital artery**. This groove is bordered medially by the **temporo-occipital suture** and laterally by the ridge of bone separating the groove from the mastoid notch. Frequently, above and behind the mastoid process is the **mastoid foramen**, transmitting emissary veins.

The most obvious structure in this part of the base of the skull is the foramen magnum, which transmits the medulla oblongata and associated meninges, the spinal roots of cranial nerve XI, the vertebral arteries, anterior and posterior spinal arteries, and the autonomic fibers traveling on the vertebral arteries. The remaining features of the occipital bone were described in the posterior view.

Internal Aspect of the Skull

The internal aspect of the skull may be divided into two major regions, namely, the superior aspect—that is, the internal surface of the calvaria—and the internal base of the skull.

Internal Surface of the Calvaria

Summary Bite. The calvaria forms the skullcap protecting the superior aspect of the brain. The frontal bone, two parietal bones, and a small portion of the occipital bone comprise the calvaria.

The **calvaria**, or skullcap, is a dome-shaped structure that protects the superior aspect of the brain. It is composed of the frontal bone, the two parietal bones, and

a small portion of the occipital bone. The anteriormost aspect may or may not contain the superior-most extent of the two **frontal sinuses** housed between the external and internal plates of the frontal bone. A thin, wedge-shaped ridge of bone, the **frontal crest**, juts out, its sharp edge pointing posteriorly, to which the **falx cerebri** attaches (Fig. 6-3). The superior aspect of the frontal crest flares out before blending into the surrounding frontal squama. As it flares out, it is grooved, indicating the location of the superior sagittal sinus. This groove, the **sagittal sulcus**, becomes deeper as it continues posteriorly in the midline. The coronal, sagittal, and lambdoidal sutures are also evident.

A few shallow, irregular excavations, the **foveolae granularis**, are present lateral to the sagittal sulcus, indicating the location of the lacunae lateralis, structures associated with arachnoid granulations. The lateral aspects of the cranial vault are grooved by branches of the meningeal vessels (Fig. 6-4).

Internal Base

Summary Bite. The internal base of the skull presents three depressions termed the anterior, middle, and posterior cranial fossae. These depressions house different lobes of the brain.

The internal base of the skull is arranged as three depressions positioned in an anteroposterior direction, each lower than the one preceding it: the **anterior, middle,** and **posterior cranial fossae** (Fig. 6-9).

In the living individual, the internal base and calvaria are lined by a periosteodural membrane, which is reflected onto itself to form venous sinuses (discussed in Chapter 17). These sinuses leave their marks on the bones as grooves, one of which, the sagittal sulcus, was mentioned previously. Additional marks on these bones are caused by the presence of blood vessels (Fig. 6-4), cranial dura, sulci and gyri of the brain, and foramina permitting the passage of structures into and out of the cranial cavity.

Some of the foramina, viewable in the internal base of the skull, were described in the previous section and their contents were noted there. The relative locations of these will be indicated in the present section, but their descriptions will not be repeated because Table 6-2, as well as the previous section, provide that information.

Anterior Cranial Fossa

Summary Bite. The depressions located in the anterior cranial fossa form in the frontal ethmoid and sphenoid bones and house the frontal lobes of the cerebrum.

The anterior cranial fossa is composed of portions of the frontal, ethmoid, and sphenoid bones (Fig. 6-9). The frontal lobes of the cerebrum lie on this floor. The

Table 6-2 Foramine of the Skull and Their Contents

Foramen	Location on Skull	Bone(s)	Location on Bone	Contents
Anterior ethmoidal	Medial wall of orbit	Ethmoidal and frontal	Fronto-ethmoidal suture	Anterior ethmoidal nerve and vessels
Carotid canal	Middle cranial fossa	Temporal	Petrous portion of temporal	Internal carotid artery and associated sympathetic plexus
Cecum	Anterior cranial fossa	Frontal and ethmoidal	Between the base of the frontal crest and crista galli	Emissary veins
Condyloid	Posterior cranial fossa	Occipital	In condylar fossa just behind the condyle	Emissary veins
Greater palatine	Anterior base of the skull	Palatine and maxilla	Between the palato-maxillary suture, lingual to the third molar	Greater palatine vessels and nerve
Hiatus of the facial canal	Middle cranial fossa	Temporal	Petrous portion of temporal, lateral to trigeminal impression	Greater petrosal nerve
Hypoglossal canal	Posterior cranial fossa	Occipital	Directly above the anteror aspect of the occipital condyle	Cranial nerve XII, meningeal branch of the ascending pharyngeal artery
Incisive	Palatal midline	Maxillae	Opens into the incisive fossa just behind the interdental septum between the two central incisors	Nasopalatine nerves and descending septal branches of the sphenopalatine artery
Inferior orbital fissure	Orbit	Sphenoid, maxilla, palatine, and zygoma	Between lateral wall and floor of orbit	Maxillary division of cranial nerve V, zygomatic nerve, infraorbital vessels and veins to the pterygoid plexus, ophthalmic vein
Infraorbital	Inferior to rim of orbit	Maxilla	Inferior to rim of orbit, lateral to nasal aperture, above canine fossa	Infraorbital vessels and nerve
Internal auditory meatus	Posterior cranial fossa	Temporal	Posterior aspect of the petrous portion of temporal	Cranial nerves VII and VIII, nervus intermedius and internal auditory vessels
Jugular	Posterior cranial fossa	Occipital and temporal	Lateral to the foramen magnum, medial to the styloid process	Cranial nerves IX, X, and XI; inferior petrosal and sigmoid sinuses; meningeal arteries; jugular bulb of internal jugular vein
Lacerum	Middle cranial fossa	Temporal, occipital, and sphenoid	Medial to the apex of the petrous part of the temporal; lateral to basilar part of occipital	Covered by cartilaginous plate, which is pierced by meningeal arteries and emissary veins
Lesser palatine	Palate (posterior palatine part)		Pyramidal process of palatine	Lesser palatine vessels and nerves

(continued)

Table 6-2 Foramine of the Skull and Their Contents *(continued)*

Foramen	Location on Skull	Bone(s)	Location on Bone	Contents
Magnum	Posterior cranial fossa	Occipital	Posterior to the clivus	Medulla oblongata and associated meninges, spinal roots of cranial nerve XI, vertebral arteries, anterior and posterior spinal arteries, postganglionic sympathetic fibers
Mandibular	Medial surface of the mandible	Mandible	Medial surface of ramus, inferior to lingula	Inferior alveolar vessels and nerve
Mastoid	Posterior external surface	Temporal	Above and behind the mastoid process near temporo-occipital suture	Emissary veins, mastoid branch of the occipital artery
Mental	Anterior surface of mandible	Mandible	Inferior to interproximal region between first and second premolar	Mental nerve and vessels
Nasolacrimal canal	Anteromedial aspect of orbit	Maxilla and lacrimal	Region of articulation between the frontal process of the maxilla and the lacrimal bone	Nasolacrimal duct
Olfactory	Anterior cranial fossa	Ethmoid	Cribriform plate of ethmoid surrounding the crista galli	Olfactory nerves
Optic	Middle cranial fossa	Sphenoid	Apex of the orbit, between the two roots of the lesser wing of the sphenoid	Optic nerve, ophthalmic artery and associated post ganglionic sympathetic fibers, central artery of retina
Ovale	Middle cranial fossa	Sphenoid	Greater wing of sphenoid, anteromedial to the foramen spinosum	Mandibular division of cranial nerve V, accessory meningeal artery, sometimes the lesser petrosal nerve
Parietal	Anterior to lambda on either side of sagittal suture	Parietal	On superior aspect near the sagittal suture	Emissary vein to superior sagittal sinus, sometimes a branch of the occipital artery
Pharyngeal canal	External base of skull; medial to medial pterygoid plate	Sphenoid and palatine	Between the vaginal process of the sphenoid and the sphenoid process of the palatine	Pharyngeal nerve, pharyngeal artery
Posterior ethmoidal	Medial wall of orbit	Frontal and ethmoidal	Fronto-ethmoidal suture, posterior to the anterior ethmoidal foramen	Posterior ethmoidal nerve and vessels (when present)
Posterosuperior alveolar	Anterior to the pterygomaxillary fissure	Maxilla	Infratemporal surface and maxillary tuberosity	Posterosuperior alveolar nerves and vessels
Pterygoid canal (vidian canal)	Extends from foramen lacerum to pterygopalatine fossa	Sphenoid	Body of sphenoid just above the pterygoid processes	Nerve and vessels of the pterygoid canal (vidian nerve and vessel)

Table 6-2 Foramine of the Skull and Their Contents *(continued)*

Foramen	Location on Skull	Bone(s)	Location on Bone	Contents
Rotundum	Middle cranial fossa	Sphenoid	Greater wing	Maxillary branch of the trigeminal nerve
Sphenopalatine	Medial wall of ptery-gopalatine fossa	Sphenoid and palatine	Between sphenoidal and orbital processes	Sphenopalatine artery and posterior superior nasal brs. (nasopalatine) nerves
Spinosum	Middle cranial fossa	Sphenoid	Spine of the sphenoid	Middle meningeal vessels and recurrent meningeal branch of mandibular division of cranial nerve V
Stylomastoid	Between styloid and mastoid processes	Temporal	Posterior to the base of the styloid process	Facial nerve, stylomastoid vessels
Superior orbital fissure	Postero superior aspect of orbit	Sphenoid and frontal	Between roof and lateral wall, lateral to apex	Cranial nerves III, IV, VI, ophthalmic division of V; sympathetic fibers; branches of middle meningeal artery; recurrent branch of lacrimal artery; superior ophthalmic vein
Supraorbital	Superior rim of orbit	Frontal	Below superciliary arch	Supraorbital nerve and vessels
Zygomaticofacial	Lateral to the infero-lateral angle of the orbital rim	Zygoma	Malar surface, above the origin of zygomaticus major muscle	Zygomaticofacial nerve and vessels
Zygomatico-orbital	Anterior floor of orbit	Zygoma	Orbital surface	Zygomaticofacial and zygomaticotemporal nerves and vessels
Zygomaticotemporal	Temporal fossa	Zygoma	Temporal surface	Zygomaticotemporal nerve and vessels

anterior and lateral extents are formed by the frontal bones, whereas its posterior boundary is formed by the lesser wings and body of the sphenoid.

The frontal bone has a wedge-shaped midline structure, the frontal crest, which ends in a point inferiorly demarcating part of the contribution of the frontal bone to the **foramen cecum**. This foramen, if patent, transmits emissary veins, and it is here that the superior sagittal sinus originates.

The posterior part of the foramen cecum is formed by the ethmoid bone. Just behind this foramen is a triangular wedge of bone, the **crista galli** (cock's comb) of the ethmoid, which provides attachment for the falx cerebri. The base of the crista galli sits in a depression between the two orbital plates of the frontal bone. The floor of this midline depression is known as the **cribriform plate of the ethmoid**. As its name implies, this plate is perforated by numerous **olfactory**

foramina, which transmit the **olfactory nerves** to the **olfactory bulbs** that occupy this depression.

A small, triangular plate of bone extends anteriorly from the body of the sphenoid bone. The apex of this bony triangle, the **ethmoidal spine** of the sphenoid bone, contacts the posterior-most part of the crista galli. Thus, it is interposed between the orbital plates of the frontal bone and the cribriform plate of the ethmoid. The ethmoidal spine blends laterally into the lesser wings of the sphenoid.

Posteriorly, the lesser wings of the sphenoid bone terminate in a curved knife-edge, the inferior aspect of which contains the **sphenoparietal sinus**. The lesser wing of the sphenoid becomes broader medially, ending in the blunt, rounded **anterior clinoid process**, forming a ledge above the middle cranial fossa. This process forms the most anterior attachment of the **tentorium cerebelli**.

Middle Cranial Fossa

Summary Bite. The middle cranial fossa is formed by the lesser wings extending to the greater wings of sphenoid, part of the temporal and parietal bones. The temporal lobes of the brain rest in the floor of the middle cranial fossa. The middle part of the fossa is occupied by the sella turcica, housing the pituitary gland.

The floor of the middle cranial fossa, which supports the temporal lobes of the brain, is at a lower level than and extends anteriorly underneath the anterior cranial fossa. Anteriorly, the middle cranial fossa is limited by the lesser wings of the sphenoid, the anterior border of the **groove** for the **optic chiasma**, and the anterior clinoid processes. Laterally, it extends to the greater wing of the sphenoid, the squamous portion of the temporal, and the inferior part of the parietal bones (Fig. 6-9). Posteriorly, it is limited by the dorsum sellae of the sphenoid and the superior aspect of the petrous portion of the temporal bone.

Most of the center of this fossa is occupied by the **sella turcica** of the sphenoid, spreading anterolaterally and posterolaterally to its wall. The body of the sphenoid is sculpted in the midline to form the sella turcica, whose deepest portion is known as the **hypophyseal fossa**. The anterior wall of the sella turcica, the **tuberculum sellae**, is almost vertical and bears a lateral projection on each side, known as the **middle clinoid process**. The posterior wall of the sella turcica, the **dorsum sellae**, juts up and bears two small, knoblike projections known as the **posterior clinoid processes**. These processes provide attachment for the tentorium cerebelli.

The chiasmatic groove leads laterally into the optic foramen, through which the optic nerve, the central artery of the retina, and the ophthalmic branch of the internal carotid artery, with its associated sympathetic plexus, enter the orbit. Immediately lateral to the optic foramen, the diagonal gap between the lesser and greater wings of the sphenoid is known as the **superior orbital fissure**, which transmits cranial nerves III, IV, VI, and the ophthalmic division of V, along with the ophthalmic veins.

Posterior to the superior orbital fissure is the **foramen rotundum**, through which the maxillary division of the trigeminal nerve exits the cranial fossa. Two additional foramina, the **foramen ovale** and **foramen spinosum**, lie posterolateral to the foramen rotundum in the sphenoid bone.

Medial to the foramen ovale is the **foramen lacerum**, which is, at times, formed into an incomplete canal by a piece of bone, the **lingula**, jutting out posteriorly from the body of the sphenoid. The lingula, at its origin, participates in the formation of a ridge forming the lateral border of a shallow groove for the internal carotid artery. Posteriorly, the lingula

approximates the most medial region of the petrous portion of the temporal bone, the anterior surface of which bears a slight depression known as the **trigeminal impression** (for the trigeminal nerve ganglion).

Lateral to this impression is a small groove on the anterior, deep surface of the petrous portion of the temporal bone. The groove opens posteriorly into a canal, the **hiatus** of the **facial canal**. Above and lateral to the hiatus is a bony prominence, the **arcuate eminence**, overlying the superior semicircular canal. The thin, bony roof of the tympanic cavity partly surrounds (laterally and anteriorly) the arcuate eminence and is known as the **tegmen tympani**.

The superior-most portion of the petrous portion of the temporal bone is a thin ridge, which constitutes part of the posterior border of the middle cranial fossa. This ridge contains the **groove** for the **superior petrosal sinus**.

Posterior Cranial Fossa

Summary Bite. The posterior cranial fossa is both deeper and larger than the other two fossae and houses the brainstem, the cerebellum, and the occipital lobe of the cerebrum. The **foramen magnum** occupies its deepest part. Additionally, the jugular foramina are located in this fossa.

The posterior portion of the internal base of the skull is the posterior cranial fossa. Forming it are parts of the occipital, temporal, and parietal bones plus a small contribution from the sphenoid bone. This fossa houses the brainstem, cerebellum, and the occipital lobe of the cerebrum. The foramen magnum is located at its deepest part.

The remainder of the internal base of the skull is referred to as the **posterior cranial fossa**. It is formed by the occipital, temporal, and parietal bones, along with a small contribution from the sphenoid bone (Fig. 6-9).

Immediately anterior to the foramen magnum, the somewhat concave **clivus** extends upward to articulate with the sphenoid. Along the lateral aspect of this basilar portion of the occipital bone, as it approximates the petrous portion of the temporal bone, is the groove for the **inferior petrosal sinus**. An oval foramen, the **internal auditory (acoustic) meatus**, pierces the posterior face of the petrous temporal bone, leading to the internal ear. Cranial nerves VII and VIII, as well as the internal auditory arteries and veins, pass through it.

Directly inferior to the internal auditory meatus is the large **jugular foramen**, conducting various nerves and vessels. Medial to the jugular foramen is a bony elevation, the jugular tubercle, whose superior surface is grooved for the passage of cranial nerves IX, X, and XI to the jugular foramen.

The **hypoglossal foramen**, leading to the **hypoglossal canal**, pierces the occipital bone just inferior to the jugular tubercle. This canal transmits cranial nerve XII and the meningeal branch of the ascending pharyngeal artery. Occasionally, the condylar canal also pierces the occipital bone, ending at the mouth of the jugular foramen, where it is met by the **groove for the sigmoid sinus**. This groove describes a sigmoid-shaped curve on the occipital and neighboring temporal and parietal bones, where it continues as the **groove for the transverse sinus**. Usually the groove on the left is somewhat shallower than the one on the right. Near the midline of the posterior wall of the posterior cranial fossa, the groove for the transverse sinus makes a 90-degree arc and turns superiorly to end in the **groove for the superior sagittal sinus**.

At the region where the transverse sinus turns superiorly is a large protuberance, the **internal occipital protuberance**, which marks the intersection of two linear bony elevations forming a cross, the **cruciate eminence**. The cruciate eminence divides the region into four concavities. The lower concavities serve as the housing of the two cerebellar hemispheres and are known as the **cerebellar fossae**, whereas the two superior depressions mark the location of the occipital lobes of the cerebrum.

The lower leg of the cruciate eminence, extending from the internal occipital protuberance to the posterior lip of the foramen magnum, is the **internal occipital crest**, which receives the attachment of the falx cerebelli.

MANDIBLE

Summary Bite. The mandible (jaw bone), the only movable bone of the skull, houses the 16 adult mandibular teeth. It is a double-jointed bone articulating with each of the paired temporal bones forming the temporomandibular articulation, thus bringing the lower dental arch into occlusion with the upper dental arch.

The mandible, forming the skeleton of the chin, is one of the largest bones of the skull and the only movable one. The mandible houses the 16 lower teeth and, via its articulation with the temporal bone, brings the lower dentition into intimate contact with the upper dental arch. The mandible consists of a horseshoe-shaped, horizontally placed **body** and two **rami** projecting upward and backward (Figs. 6-1, 6-2, 6-5, and 6-10).

The two rami are suspended from the skull by a series of bilateral ligaments and muscles. These limit the excursion of the bone and simultaneously provide great versatility of motion by permitting a plethora of movements, including opening, closing, protrusion, retraction, lateral excursion, and a limited degree of rotation.

The mandible presents an external and internal surface (Fig 6-10). The **external surface** will be described first. The horseshoe-shaped body presents a fusion line in the anterior midline, between the two central incisors, known as the **symphysis menti** (mandibular symphysis), the inferior extent of which is triangular and is referred to as the **mental protuberance**, or the point of the chin.

The base of the mental protuberance forms the anterior-most portion of the inferior border of the mandible and is somewhat concave in the midline but presents two small, bony projections laterally, the **mental tubercles**. Above the mental tubercles, on either side of the symphysis menti, the body of the mandible presents two slight concavities, the **incisive fossae**.

On the lateral surface, the **mental foramen** is evident, located inferior to the interproximal region between the first and second premolars. It opens in a posterior direction and transmits the mental nerve and vessels.

A line, the **oblique line**, connects the mental tubercle with the anterior border of the ramus. This oblique line is very faint until it reaches the first molar, where it becomes prominent and, at the level of the second molar, begins to arch upward to become continuous with the sharp, anterior edge of the ramus.

Medial to the oblique line, just lateral and distal to the third molar, is a shallow depression, the **retromolar fossa**. Medial to the retromolar fossa is another shallow, triangular depression, the **retromolar triangle**.

The lateral border of the **retromolar triangle** becomes continuous with the **lateral (buccal) alveolar crest**, whereas the medial border is continuous with the **medial alveolar crest** of the third molar. These crests then continue forward to form the buccal and lingual alveolar plates of the mandible. In the interproximal regions, these plates are connected to each other by bony connections, the **interdental septa**.

The **internal surface** in the midline of the body of the mandible bears two, or sometimes four, bony tubercles. The two superior ones are constant and are the mental spines (also referred to as **superior mandibular spines** or **genial tubercles**) from which the genioglossus muscles originate. The two lower tubercles, the **inferior mandibular spines**, serve as the origins of the geniohyoid muscles.

The medial aspect of the body of the mandible bears a bony ridge, the **mylohyoid line**, extending from the symphysis menti to the region of the third molar. The mylohyoid line delineates the origin of the mylohyoid muscle. Superior to the mylohyoid line anteriorly is a shallow fossa, the **sublingual fossa**, whereas the **submandibular fossa** projects posteriorly below this line. Each fossa is named after the major salivary gland that occupies it.

Posterior to the body of the mandible is the ramus. The region where the posterior border of the ramus is continuous with the posterior extent of the base of the mandible is the **angle of the mandible**. The buccal (external) aspect of the ramus is marked with tuberosities and depressions, indicating the site of attachment of the masseter muscle.

Just anterior to the attachment of the masseter is a slight, seldom evident groove on the body of the mandible, the **groove for the facial artery**, indicating the route that artery takes as it curves upward to enter the face. The upward extension of the ramus ends in the **coronoid** and **condylar processes**.

The flattened, triangular coronoid process serves as the insertion for the temporalis muscle. The insertion of this muscle also occupies the anterior border of the ramus on its medial aspect. The condylar process flares out and ends in an articular surface, the **condyle** of the **mandible**, which articulates with the temporal bone.

The region just below the condyle is the **neck of the mandible**, on whose medial aspect the **lateral pterygoid muscle** inserts into a slight depression, the pterygoid fovea. The arciform region between the coronoid and condylar processes is known as the **mandibular notch**, through which the masseteric nerve and vessels pass into the masseter muscle.

Near the middle of the medial surface of the ramus is the **mandibular foramen**, which opens into the **mandibular canal** housing the inferior alveolar nerve and vessels. The opening is guarded anteriorly by a sharp ridge of bone, the **lingula**, whose free apex points posteriorly toward the condyle. The lingula serves as the region of attachment of the sphenomandibular ligament.

Inferior to the lingula is the **mylohyoid groove**, extending from the mandibular foramen in an anteroinferior direction and marking the course of the mylohyoid nerve. The angle of the mandible and the region posterior to the mylohyoid groove presents a roughened, craggy appearance caused by the insertion of the medial pterygoid muscle. (See Figs. 6-11 through 6-13.)

HYOID BONE

Summary Bite. The small, U-shaped hyoid bone is located in the neck above the thyroid cartilage and bridging the centerline of the neck. Several tendons attach to this bone and as many as 10 or 11 muscles attach to each bilateral half.

The hyoid is a small, U-shaped bone that, at first glance, appears insignificant because of its small size (Fig. 6-15). However, each bilateral half gives attachment to three ligaments and as many as 10 and sometimes 11 muscles. This bone is suspended by ligaments and muscles between the temporal bones and the sternum. It consists of five parts: the quadrilateral, median **body (corpus)**, and four **cornua (horns)**, the two **greater** and two **lesser cornua**.

The two greater horns, directed posteriorly, end in a tubercle and are attached by a cartilaginous connection earlier in life. The cartilage ossifies in middle-aged individuals. The lesser cornua, small nipplelike structures pointing cranially and posteriorly, are attached to the articulation of the greater cornua with the body.

Frequently, an anterior midline vertical ridge divides the body of the hyoid bone into right and left halves. The inferior border of the body is flat except for a small, cranially directed midline concavity.

The following muscles attach to the body: genioglossus (via a few tendinous slips), geniohyoid, hyoglossus, levator of the thyroid gland (when present), mylohyoid, omohyoid, sternohyoid, and thyrohyoid. Two ligaments, the hyoepiglottic and thyrohyoid (in part), are also attached to the body of the hyoid bone.

The following muscles are attached to the greater cornu: digastric (via a tendinous loop), hyoglossus, middle pharyngeal constrictor, stylohyoid, and thyrohyoid. The thyrohyoid membrane is attached, in part, to the tubercle of the greater cornu.

The lesser cornu gives attachment to the chondroglossus portion of the hyoglossus muscle as well as to the stylohyoid ligament.

CERVICAL VERTEBRAE

Summary Bite. The seven most superior vertebrae are the cervical vertebrae. The first two, the atlas and axis, are highly modified to permit rotation of the head upon the vertebral column.

There are seven cervical vertebrae, and they constitute the most superior extension of the vertebral column. The superior two, the **atlas** and **axis**, are greatly modified to support the head and permit its rotation at the atlantoaxial joint. The seventh cervical vertebra (C7) is also modified but will not be treated separately here.

Interposed between any two vertebrae is an intervertebral disc, as well as other cartilaginous structures involved in regions of facets to facilitate smooth, frictionless movement and provide cushioning and support for the whole vertebral column.

Typical Cervical Vertebra

Summary Bite. A typical cervical vertebra appears much like thoracic vertebra except that the transverse processes of all cervical vertebrae (except the seventh) are pierced by the large foramen transversarium, housing the vertebral vessels and associated sympathetic plexus.

The typical cervical vertebra, as any other typical vertebra, has a large, anteriorly directed **body** from which the **posterior vertebral arch** is directed dorsally (Fig. 6-16). This arch encloses the **vertebral foramen**. All the vertebral foramina together constitute the **vertebral canal**, which houses the spinal cord, meninges, and associated vessels. The posterior vertebral arch consists of two short, anterior **pedicles** and two broader, posterior **laminae**. Jutting out from the two laminae are two **superior articular processes**, two **inferior articular processes**, two **transverse processes**, and a single posteriorly and inferiorly directed **spinous process**.

The superior and inferior aspects of the pedicles bear **vertebral notches** known as the **superior** and **inferior vertebral notches**. As two vertebrae articulate with each other, the superior notch of the lower vertebra and the inferior notch of the upper vertebra form the **invertebral foramen**, through which the spinal nerves leave the vertebral canal.

The transverse processes of all cervical vertebrae (except the seventh) are pierced by the large **foramen transversarium**, housing the vertebral vessels and associated sympathetic plexus.

The seventh cervical vertebra has a small or doubled foramen transversarium. The superior articular processes project cranially, bearing the posteriorly directed **articular facets**. The inferior articular processes project caudally, with their articular facets directed anteriorly.

The superior surface of the body is somewhat concave and presents an upward-curving lip on either side. The inferior surface of the body is slightly concave in an anteroposterior direction, while being convex in the transverse plane. The bifid spinous process (longest in C7) projects posteriorly and inferiorly.

Atlas

Summary Bite. The first cervical vertebra is greatly modified because it articulates superiorly with the occipital condyles rather than with a superior vertebra. Its body is a modified anterior arch that presents a facet for the

dens of the axis on its dorsal surface, which is retained in the atlas by a ligament. The inferior facets articulate with the superior facets of the axis.

The atlas, or first cervical vertebra, is greatly modified. The body is replaced by an **anterior arch**, whose ventral surface possesses an anterior tubercle, whereas the dorsal surface presents the **facet** for the **dens** of the axis (Fig. 6-17). The anterior arch is connected to the **posterior arch** via the right and left **lateral masses**, which bear the **superior** and **inferior articular facets**. The superior facets articulate with the occipital condyles, and the inferior facets articulate with the superior articular facets of the axis.

The dens is retained in the atlas by the transverse ligament of the atlas, a fibrous sling that is attached to a tubercle on the medial surface of each lateral mass.

The transverse processes of the atlas are very long and bear the foramina transversarium for the passage of the vertebral artery and associated structures. The superior surface of the posterior arch possesses a groove for the passage of the vertebral artery to enter the foramen magnum. The posterior arch ends in the small **posterior tubercle**, representing the remnant of the spinous process.

Axis

Summary Bite. The second cervical vertebra is modified to help form the atlantoaxial joint. The body is modified, forming the toothlike dens which articulates with the anterior arch of the atlas. The spinous process is large and bifid, and it serves for the attachment for the many muscles responsible for head movements.

The axis, or second cervical vertebra, is also modified to participate in the formation of the atlantoaxial joint (Fig. 6-17). The body of the axis is modified superiorly to present a cranial toothlike projection, the **dens**, which is notched posteriorly to accept the transverse ligament of the atlas. Anteriorly, the dens possesses an articular facet that meets the articular facet of the atlas's anterior arch.

The pedicles are modified superiorly because they are overlaid by the superior articular facets, and the vertebral notches of this surface are very shallow. The inferior vertebral notches, however, are very deep. The transverse processes of the axis are short and possess only a single tubercle, but otherwise they are unremarkable. The spinous process is large and bifid, and it serves for the attachment of many muscles responsible for various movements of the head.

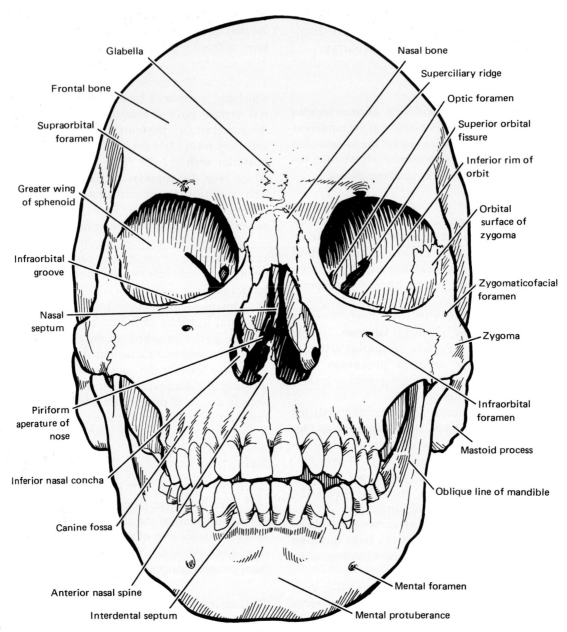

A

Figure 6-1. Frontal view of the skull. *(continued)*

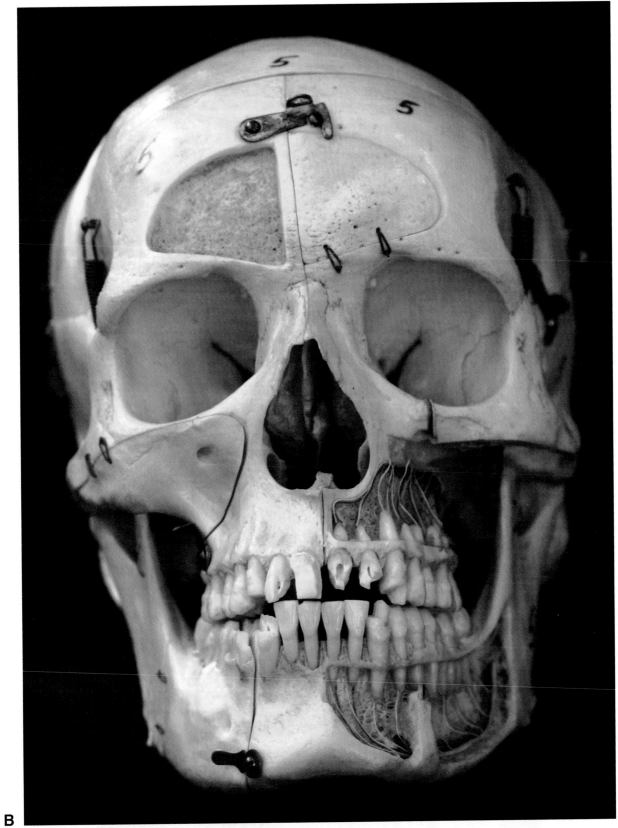

B

Figure 6-1. *(continued)* Frontal view of the skull.

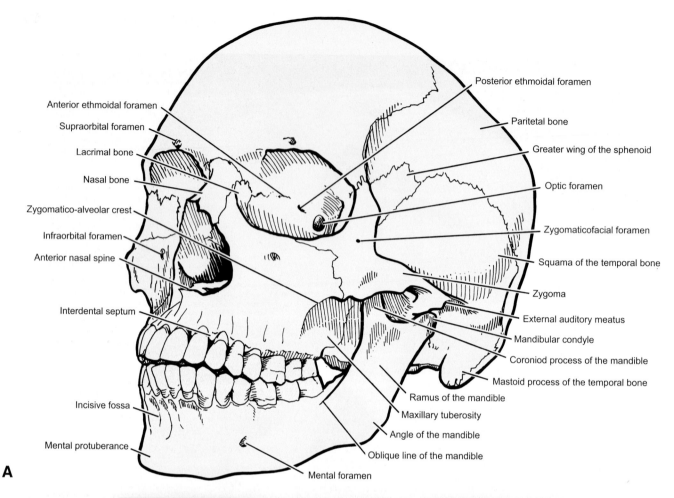

Anterior ethmoidal foramen

Supraorbital foramen

Lacrimal bone

Nasal bone

Zygomatico-alveolar crest

Infraorbital foramen

Anterior nasal spine

Interdental septum

Incisive fossa

Mental protuberance

A

Posterior ethmoidal foramen

Pariteral bone

Greater wing of the sphenoid

Optic foramen

Zygomaticofacial foramen

Squama of the temporal bone

Zygoma

External auditory meatus

Mandibular condyle

Coroniod process of the mandible

Mastoid process of the temporal bone

Ramus of the mandible

Maxillary tuberosity

Angle of the mandible

Oblique line of the mandible

Mental foramen

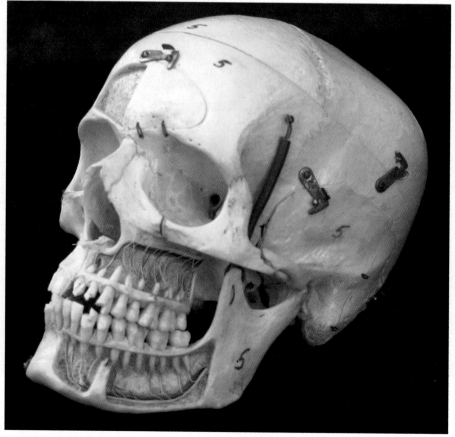

B

Figure 6-2. Anterior oblique view of the skull.

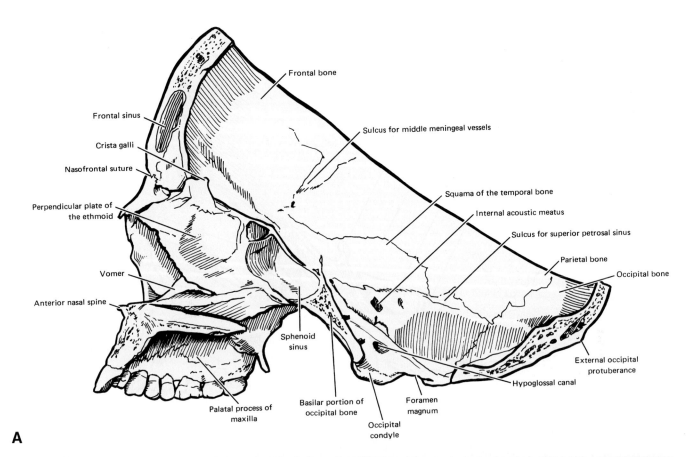

Frontal bone

Frontal sinus

Sulcus for middle meningeal vessels

Crista galli

Nasofrontal suture

Squama of the temporal bone

Perpendicular plate of
the ethmoid

Internal acoustic meatus

Sulcus for superior petrosal sinus

Vomer

Parietal bone

Anterior nasal spine

Occipital bone

Sphenoid
sinus

External occipital
protuberance

Palatal process of
maxilla

Basilar portion of
occipital bone

Hypoglossal canal

Foramen
magnum

Occipital
condyle

A

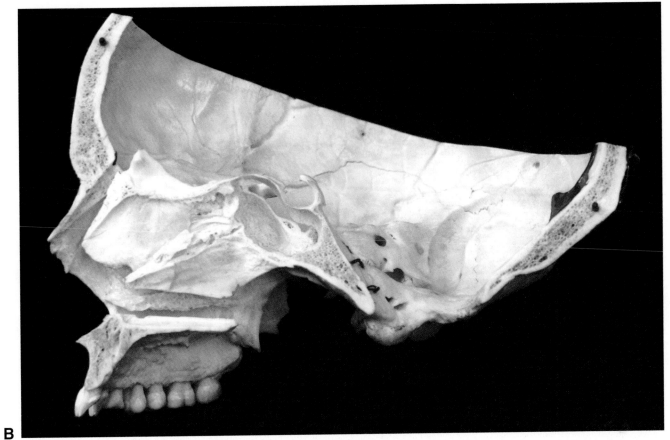

B

Figure 6-3. Median section of the skull with median nasal septum intact.

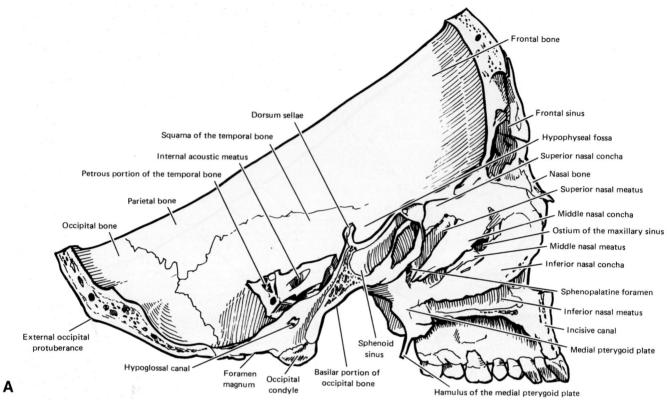

Figure 6-4. Median section of the skull with the median nasal septum removed. *(continued)*

Frontal bone

Dorsum sellae

Squama of the temporal bone

Internal acoustic meatus

Petrous portion of the temporal bone

Parietal bone

Occipital bone

Frontal sinus

Hypophyseal fossa

Superior nasal concha

Nasal bone

Superior nasal meatus

Middle nasal concha

Ostium of the maxillary sinus

Middle nasal meatus

Inferior nasal concha

Sphenopalatine foramen

Inferior nasal meatus

Incisive canal

Medial pterygoid plate

External occipital protuberance

Hypoglossal canal

Foramen magnum

Occipital condyle

Basilar portion of occipital bone

Sphenoid sinus

Hamulus of the medial pterygoid plate

A

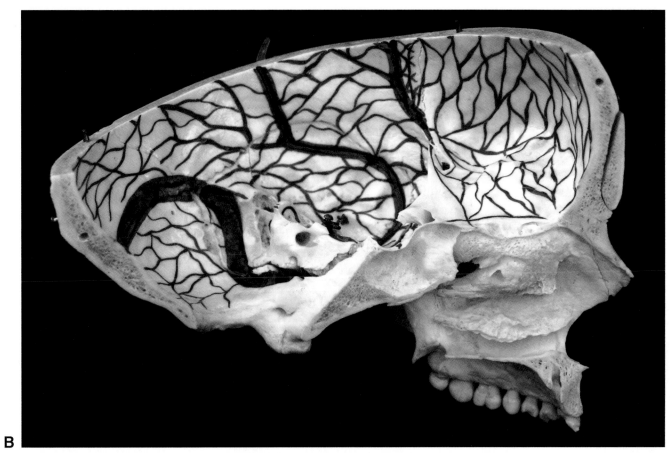

B

Figure 6-4. *(continued)* Median section of the skull with the median nasal septum removed.

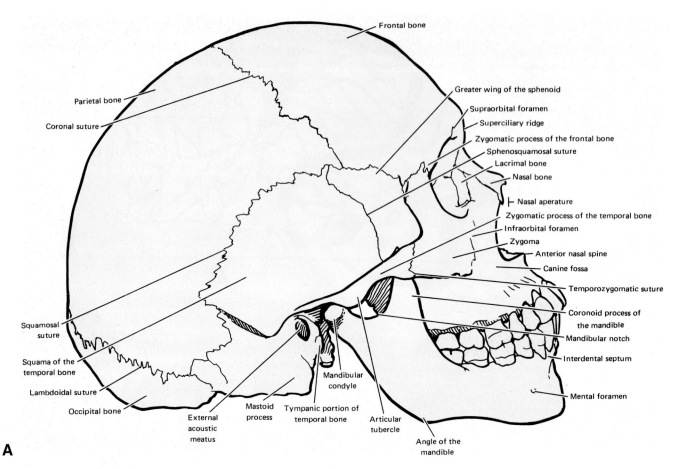

A

Figure 6-5. Lateral view of the skull. *(continued)*

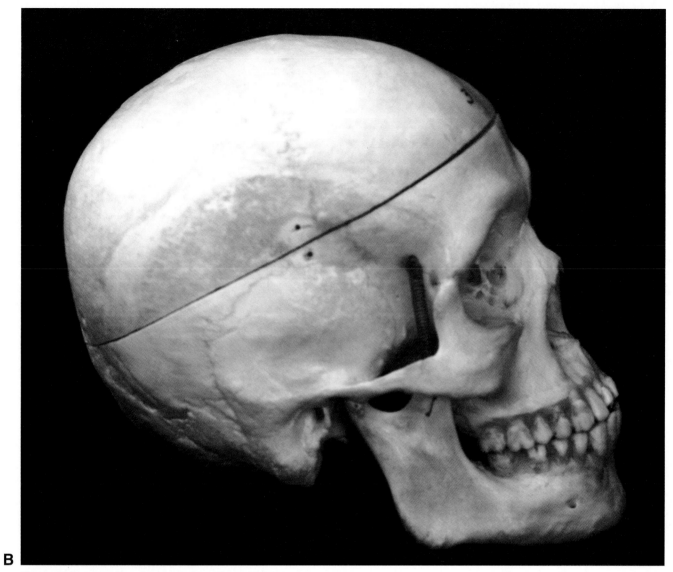

B

Figure 6-5. *(continued)* Lateral view of the skull.

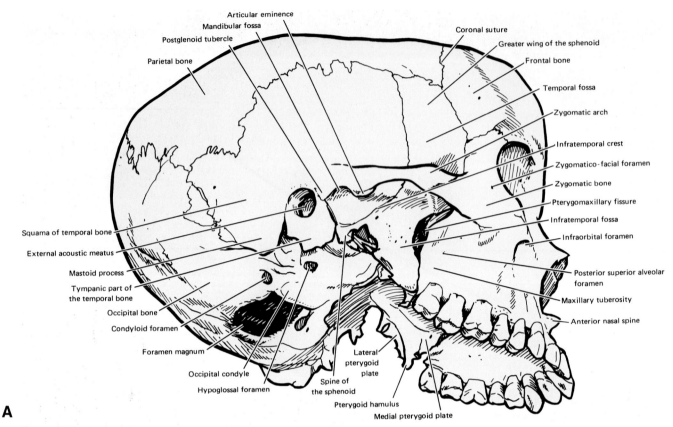

Figure 6-6. Lateroinferior view of the skull. *(continued)*

A

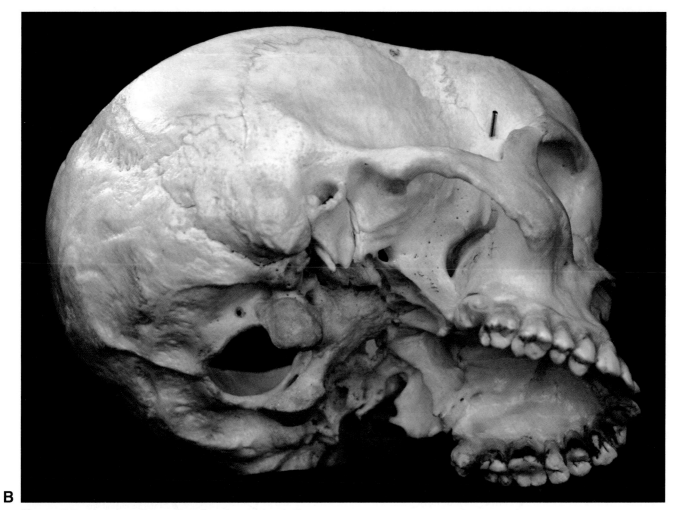

B

Figure 6-6.   *(continued)* Lateroinferior view of the skull.

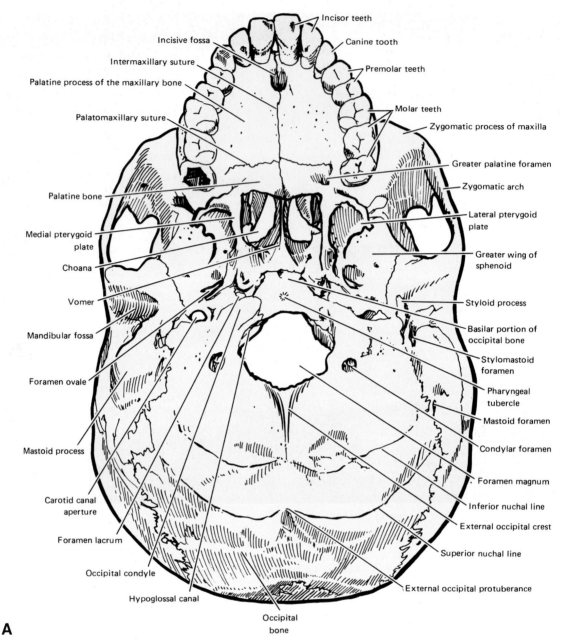

Figure 6-7. Base of the skull. *(continued)*

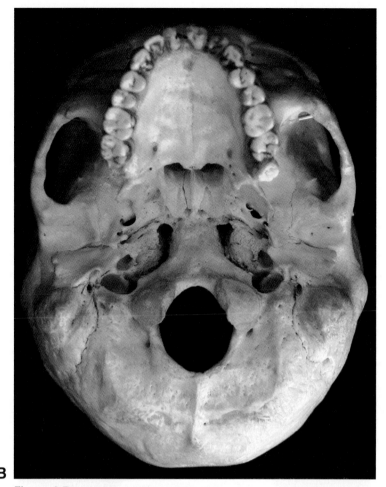

B

Figure 6-7. *(continued)* Base of the skull.

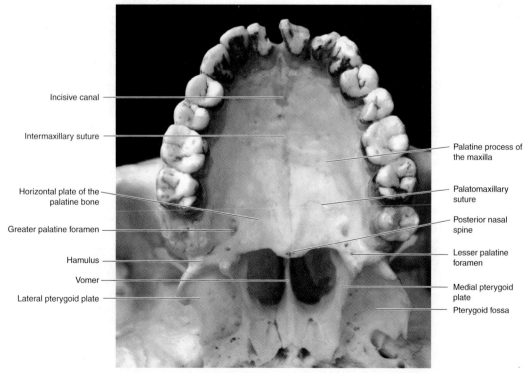

Incisive canal

Intermaxillary suture

Horizontal plate of the palatine bone

Greater palatine foramen

Hamulus

Vomer

Lateral pterygoid plate

Palatine process of the maxilla

Palatomaxillary suture

Posterior nasal spine

Lesser palatine foramen

Medial pterygoid plate

Pterygoid fossa

Figure 6-8. Palate and associated area.

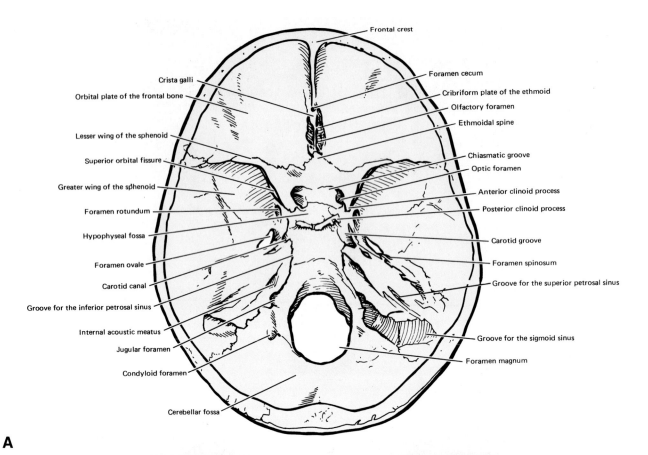

Frontal crest

Crista galli

Orbital plate of the frontal bone

Lesser wing of the sphenoid

Superior orbital fissure

Greater wing of the sphenoid

Foramen rotundum

Hypophyseal fossa

Foramen ovale

Carotid canal

Groove for the inferior petrosal sinus

Internal acoustic meatus

Jugular foramen

Condyloid foramen

Cerebellar fossa

Foramen cecum

Cribriform plate of the ethmoid

Olfactory foramen

Ethmoidal spine

Chiasmatic groove

Optic foramen

Anterior clinoid process

Posterior clinoid process

Carotid groove

Foramen spinosum

Groove for the superior petrosal sinus

Groove for the sigmoid sinus

Foramen magnum

A

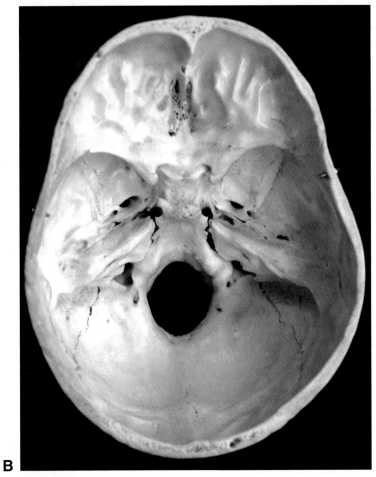

B

Figure 6-9. Internal base of the skull.

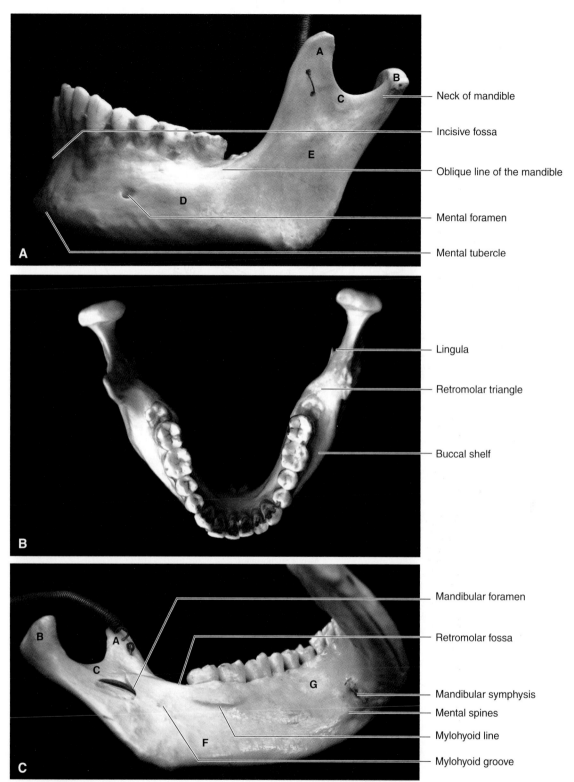

Neck of mandible

Incisive fossa

Oblique line of the mandible

Mental foramen

Mental tubercle

Lingula

Retromolar triangle

Buccal shelf

Mandibular foramen

Retromolar fossa

Mandibular symphysis

Mental spines

Mylohyoid line

Mylohyoid groove

Figure 6-10. Mandible. Lateral aspect (top view). Superior aspect (middle view). Medial aspect (bottom view). **(A)** Coronoid process. **(B)** Mandibular condyle. **(C)** Mandibular notch. **(D)** Body of mandible. **(E)** Ramus of mandible. **(F)** Submandibular fossa. **(G)** Sublingual fossa.

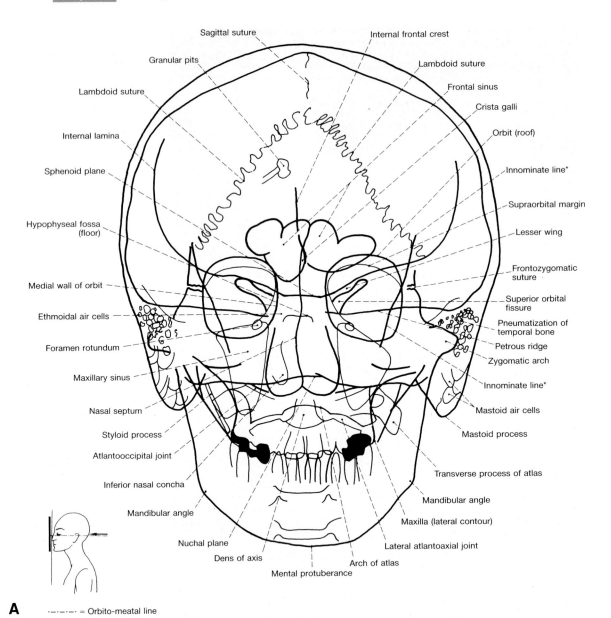

Sagittal suture

Granular pits

Lambdoid suture

Internal lamina

Sphenoid plane

Hypophyseal fossa (floor)

Medial wall of orbit

Ethmoidal air cells

Foramen rotundum

Maxillary sinus

Nasal septum

Styloid process

Atlantooccipital joint

Inferior nasal concha

Mandibular angle

Nuchal plane

Dens of axis

Mental protuberance

Arch of atlas

Lateral atlantoaxial joint

Maxilla (lateral contour)

Mandibular angle

Transverse process of atlas

Mastoid process

Mastoid air cells

Innominate line*

Zygomatic arch

Petrous ridge

Pneumatization of temporal bone

Superior orbital fissure

Frontozygomatic suture

Lesser wing

Supraorbital margin

Innominate line*

Orbit (roof)

Crista galli

Frontal sinus

Lambdoid suture

Internal frontal crest

A   .—.—.—. = Orbito-meatal line

Figure 6-11. Posteroanterior radiograph of the head. *(continued)*

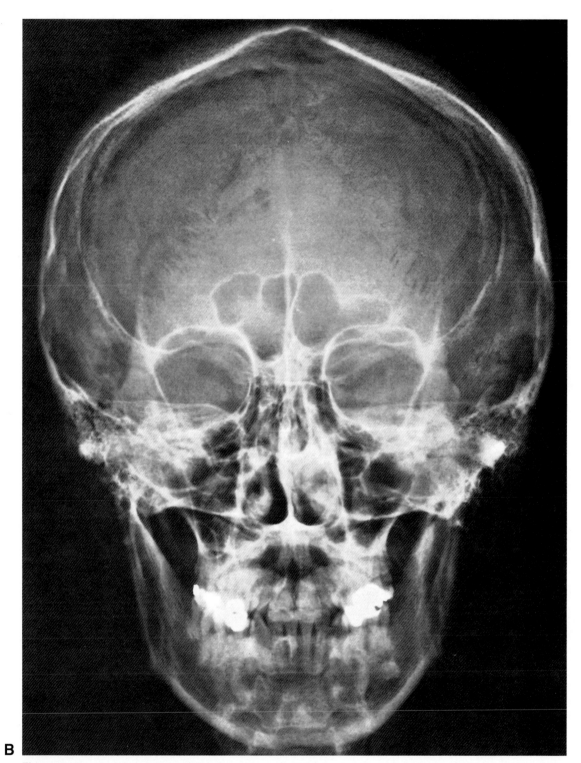

Figure 6-11. *(continued)* Posteroanterior radiograph of the head.

B

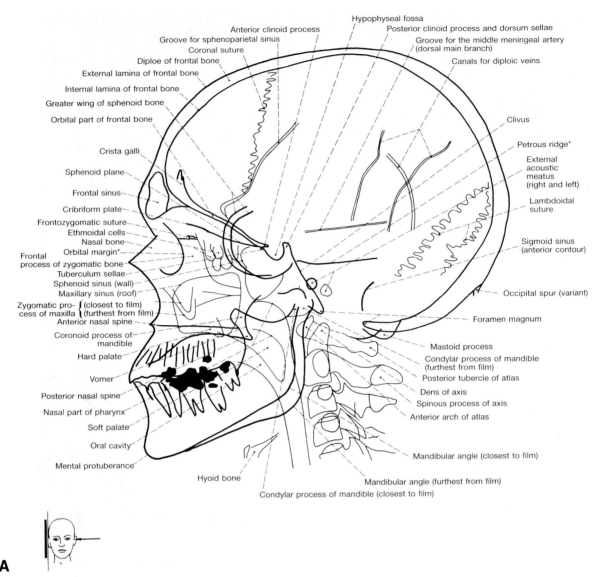

Figure 6-12. Lateral radiograph of the head. *(continued)*

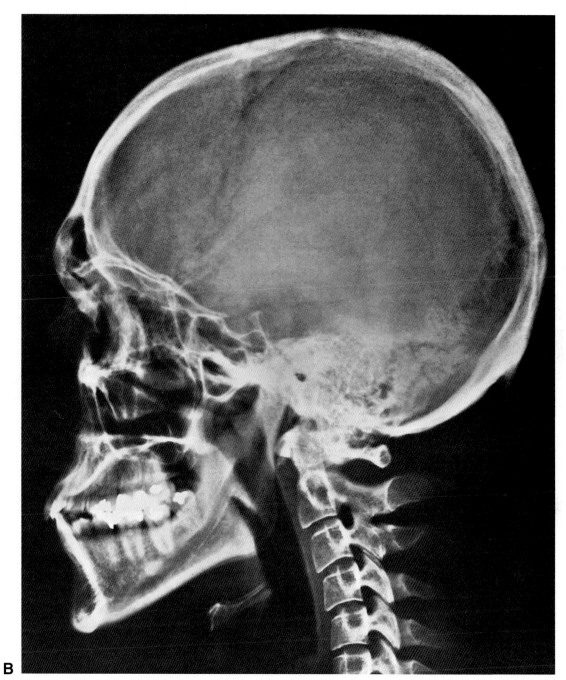

B

Figure 6-12.   *(continued)* Lateral radiograph of the head.

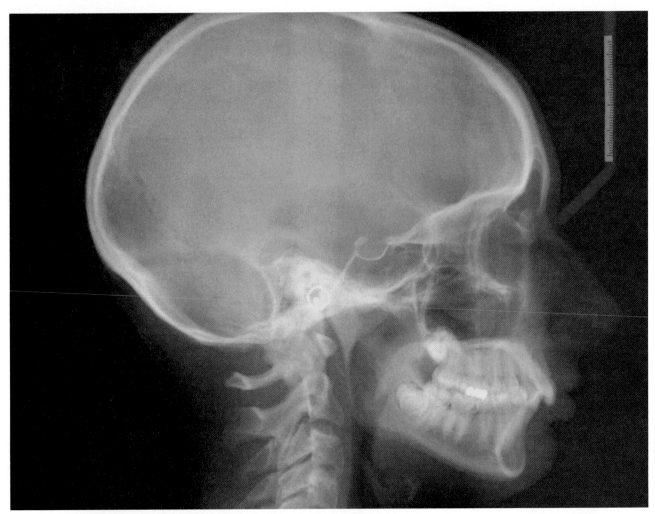

Figure 6-13.   Cephalometric radiograph ready for orthodontic mark-up.

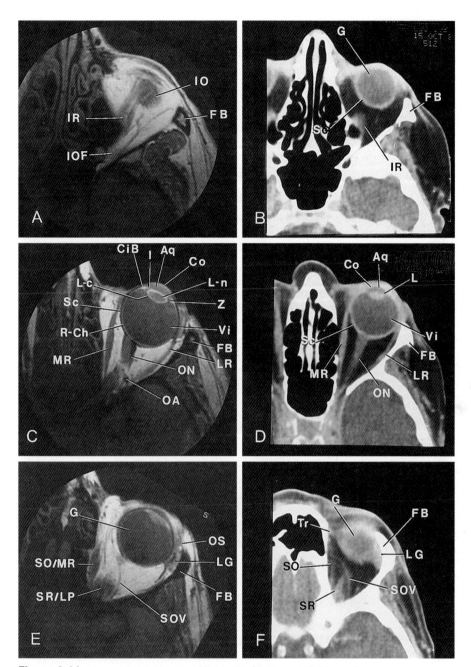

Figure 6-14. Normal axial scans of the orbit. **(A**, **C**, and **E)**. Magnetic resonance scans. **(B**, **D**, and **F)**. Contrast computed tomographic scans. *Aq,* aqueous humor; *Az,* annulus of Zinn; *CiB,* ciliary body; *Co,* cornea; *FB,* frontal bone; *G,* glove; *I,* iris; *IO,* inferior oblique muscle; *IR,* inferior rectus muscle; *L,* lens; *LG,* lacrimal gland; *L-c,* lens cortex; *LEl,* lower eyelid; *L-n,* lens nucleus; *LP,* levator palpebrae muscle; *LR,* lateral rectus muscle; *MR,* medial rectus muscle; *OA,* ophthalmic artery; *OS,* orbital septum; *R-Ch,* retina-choroid; *Sc,* sclera; *SO,* superior oblique muscle; *SO/MR,* superior oblique, medial rectus; *SOV,* superior ophthalmic vein; *SR,* superior rectus muscle; *SR/LP,* superior rectus, levator palpebrae; *Tr,* trochlea; *UEl,* upper eyelid; *Vi,* vitreous; *Z,* zonule.

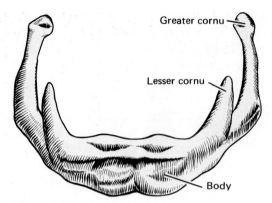

Figure 6-15. Hyoid bone.

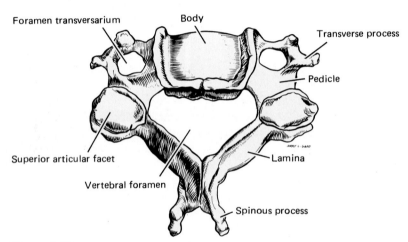

Figure 6-16. Typical cervical vertebra.

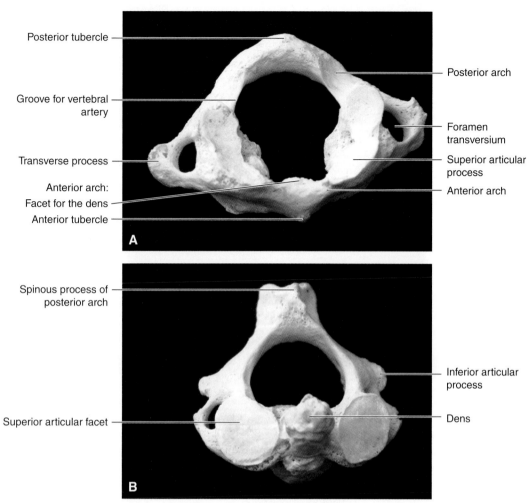

Posterior tubercle

Groove for vertebral artery

Transverse process

Anterior arch:
Facet for the dens
Anterior tubercle

Posterior arch

Foramen transversium

Superior articular process

Anterior arch

A

Spinous process of posterior arch

Superior articular facet

Inferior articular process

Dens

B

Figure 6-17.   Superior views of the atlas (top) and the axis (bottom).

Neck

7

Key Terms

Accessory Nerve possesses two roots, one whose origin is in the brain and another whose origin is in the upper cervical spinal cord. These join together, later to separate. The cranial portion unites with the vagus nerve, whereas the spinal portion of the accessory nerve descends becoming the only cranial nerve to traverse the posterior triangle. It passes through the sternocleidomastoid muscle and then passes deep in the triangle to enter the deep surface of the trapezius muscle, where it forms the subtrapezial plexus. Although motor innervation is provided to both of these muscles by the accessory nerve, proprioception is provided by cervical nerves C2 and C3 for the sternocleiodmastoid and C3 and C4 for the trapezius muscle.

Brachial Plexus is a large complex of cervical spinal nerves that combine, re-form, and divide into anterior and posterior divisions to serve anterior and posterior compartment muscles of the upper limb, with a few contributions to the muscles of the neck. Those of the former are generally the flexors, whereas the latter are the extensors. The spinal nerves making up the plexus arise from C5, C6, C7, C8, and T1. Named peripheral nerves are formed again after the anterior and posterior divisions are completed.

Cervical Sympathetic Trunk Because cervical spinal nerves possess no sympathetic components, the cervical sympathetic trunk represents a continuation of the thoracic sympathetic trunk into the neck. The student will recall that in Chapter 3 the autonomic nervous system was described as a two-neuron chain, and cell bodies of neurons in the cervical sympathetic trunk were said to be located in the intermediolateral cell column of the upper thoracic spinal cord segments. Preganglionic neurons arising from here are seeking postganglionic cell bodies that are located in postganglionic

sympathetic ganglia where synapses will take place. There are three such ganglia located in the cervical sympathetic trunk: superior, middle, and inferior. After synapsing with postganglionic neurons, the axons arising from these ganglia find their way to smooth muscle, cardiac muscle, and glands. Some fibers pass directly, whereas others join a spinal nerve to be distributed to the target.

Deep Fascia of the neck is generally described as surrounding the neck in three distinct layers: investing, prevertebral, and pretracheal. The carotid sheath is made up of contributions of these three layers and it houses the major neurovascular bundle of the neck, namely, the common carotid and internal carotid arteries, the internal jugular vein, and the vagus nerve.

Dorsal and Ventral Primary Rami give rise to the cutaneous branches of the cervical spinal nerves that serve the neck region. Branches of the dorsal primary rami provide cutaneous sensation to the posterior aspects of the neck, whereas branches of anterior primary rami provide cutaneous sensation for the sides and front of the neck. It is interesting to note that the first cervical spinal nerve probably has no cutaneous branches.

Phrenic Nerve is the sole motor nerve to the diaphragm. This nerve arises from the cervical complex, a complex of the first four cervical nerves composed of sensory and motor modalities. Cervical nerves C3, C4, and C5 combine to form the phrenic nerve, which may be observed deep in the posterior triangle lying on top of the anterior scalene muscle. It then passes between the subclavian artery and vein before diving into the thorax on its way to the diaphragm.

Platysma Muscle is the paper-thin sheet of muscle within the superficial fascia of the anterior cervical triangle. It originates

in the superficial pectoral and deltoid fasciae rather than from bone, and proceeds cranially over much of the anterior triangle to insert into the inferior portion of the body of the mandible and into the skin and hypodermis of the face. Although this muscle lies outside the confines of the face, it is still considered a muscle of facial expression because it is innervated by the nerve of the second pharyngeal arch, the facial nerve (VII).

Subclavian Artery is the short, large-diameter artery that ends at the lateral border of the first rib. Its right and left origins differ. The left subclavian arises from the arch of the aorta within the thorax, whereas the right subclavian artery arises deep to the sternoclavicular joint from the terminal of the brachiocephalic trunk. Both arteries ascend into the neck arching between the anterior and middle scalene muscles. The subclavian artery serves as the source of many named arteries serving the structures within the neck. The subclavian artery changes its name at the lateral border of the first rib, where it becomes known as the axillary artery.

Triangles of the Anterior Neck are formed by the sternocleidomastoid muscle as it passes diagonally across the quadrilateral area formed between the anterior border of the trapezius muscle and the anterior midline of the neck, and between the inferior border of the mandible, superiorly, and the superior surface of the middle third of the clavicle, inferiorly. This divides the neck into two principal triangles, the anterior and posterior cervical triangles. Each of these triangles is further subdivided by muscles and bones; thus, each major triangle is made up of several subtriangles. Each triangle possesses its own anatomical component parts, including muscles, veins, nerves, etc. All of the cervical triangles are bilateral (right and left sides) with the exception of the submental triangle, which spans across the midline.

This is the first of several chapters using the regional approach for the examination of the head and neck. The chapter moves from superficial to deeper layers, almost as if the structures were being dissected for the reader. Hence, if a structure passes through the region being discussed, its detailed description will be confined only to that portion that resides in the area being treated. The remainder of that structure will be detailed in the appropriate chapters.

CLINICAL CONSIDERATIONS

Clinical involvement of the cervical region is a complex topic, encompassing, among others, congenital malformations, tumors—both benign and malignant—as well as anatomic considerations during surgical procedures, especially those involving the thyroid gland. The intent of the sections on clinical considerations is not to detail exhaustively the possible clinical significance of each structure located in this area, but merely to illustrate the importance of sound anatomic bases for clinicians dealing with this complicated region.

SURFACE ANATOMY

Summary Bite. The neck is the cylindrical connection between the head and the body. Thus, in addition to its role in supporting the head, it serves as a conduit for vessels and nerves passing between the head and body as well as a passageway for materials entering the digestive system and a passageway for the respiratory system.

The neck is a more or less cylindrical structure connecting the head to the trunk. Anteriorly, it extends from the inferior border of the mandible to the superior surfaces of the manubrium and laterally along the clavicles to the point of the shoulders, or acromion (Fig.7-1).

Posteriorly, it is bounded inferiorly by a somewhat irregular surface, described by an imaginary line drawn between the right and left acromions that passes through the intervertebral disc between the seventh cervical (C7) and first thoracic (T1) vertebra, and superiorly by the superior nuchal line of the occipital bone. The posterior aspect of the neck is composed mostly of muscle masses on either side of the spinous processes of the cervical vertebrae. These muscle masses are more properly considered to be the deep muscles of the back because they function, in addition to supporting the head, in the extension of the atlanto-occipital and other vertebral joints. These muscle masses are covered by the **trapezius muscle**, which contributes to shaping the posterior aspect of the neck.

The anterior midline of the neck presents a bulge whose size reflects sexual dimorphism in that it is considerably larger in males than in females. This prominence is the **larynx** (Adam's apple), specifically the **thyroid cartilage**, whose superior aspect is marked by the easily palpable **thyroid notch**, above which lies the less palpable body and greater cornu of the **hyoid bone**. Inferior to the thyroid notch is the **laryngeal prominence**, which is formed by the fusion of the right and left plates of the thyroid cartilage.

Immediately inferior to the thyroid cartilage is the **cricoid cartilage**, below which the superior two or three cartilaginous rings of the trachea may be palpated. The inferior-most region in the midline of the anterior neck is the **jugular notch** of the manubrium. Tensing the neck reveals the bellies and the tendons of origin of the **sternocleidomastoid muscle** just lateral to this notch. This muscle may be palpated along its entire length as it passes posteriorly and obliquely to insert on the mastoid process of the temporal bone and superior nuchal line of the occipital bones.

Clinical Considerations

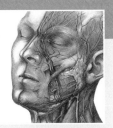

Congenital Malformations

During embryonic development of the head and neck, various congenital malformations may occur. Some of these were detailed in Chapter 5, and the reader is referred to that section.

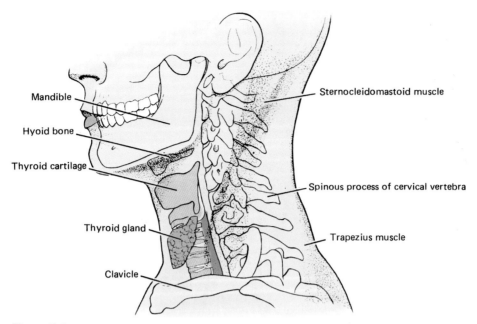

Figure 7-1. Anatomic landmarks of the neck.

SUPERFICIAL STRUCTURES OF THE NECK

Summary Bite. The skin covering the neck overlies the superficial fascia, a connective tissue layer that contains the platysma, a thin sheet of muscle that originates in fascia and inserts upon the mandible and skin of the face. The platysma develops from the second pharyngeal arch; thus, it is innervated by the nerve of the second arch, the facial nerve (cranial nerve VII).

The skin covering the neck is arranged in such a fashion that **Langer lines** run horizontally to encircle it. Deep to the dermis is a very thin fascial layer consisting of an areolar type of connective tissue known as the hypodermis or **superficial fascia**. This superficial fascia envelops the neck, just as the overlying skin does, and contains within it a paper-thin sheet of skeletal muscle, the **platysma** (Fig. 7-2). This muscle originates from the deltoid and pectoralis fasciae and passes cranially, overlying the anterior triangle and the inferior part of the posterior triangle (descriptive divisions of the neck depicted below). The platysma inserts onto the inferior border of the body of the mandible and into the skin and hypodermis of the face. The platysma intermingles with and assists muscles that depress the lower lip and corner of the mouth. The platysma, because it is derived from the second pharyngeal arch, is innervated by the cervical branch of the facial nerve (cranial nerve VII).

Superficial Venous Drainage

Summary Bite. Venous drainage of the superficial neck empties into the external jugular vein coursing deep to the platysma muscle. The course of this vein may be observed in a live individual as it crosses the obliquely oriented sternocleidomastoid muscle. The external jugular vein empties into the subclavian vein at the base of the neck.

The superficial venous drainage consists of the **external jugular vein** and its tributaries, which drain a limited area of tissue—specifically, the region superficial and immediately deep to the investing layer of the deep cervical fascia. It must be kept in mind that venous drainage exhibits great variability in vessel size and routes of distribution. This section details only the classical description.

The external jugular vein is formed by the union of the **posterior auricular** and **retromandibular veins** just posterior to the angle of the mandible, sometimes within the body of the parotid gland. It passes straight down the neck, under the cover of the platysma muscle and associated superficial fascia, superficial to the fleshy belly of the sternocleidomastoid muscle. In its path along this muscle, the external jugular vein crosses the muscle at an oblique angle (Figs. 7-1 and 7-2).

Once the external jugular vein reaches the subclavian triangle, it dives deep to the clavicle to join the **subclavian vein**. Several tributaries join the external jugular vein along its path, from the back of the neck,

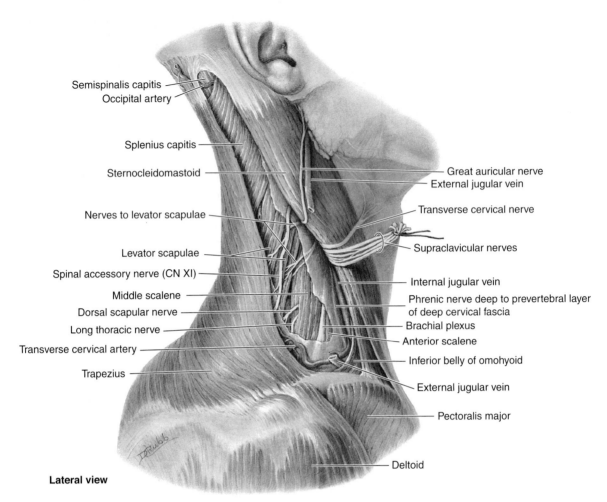

Semispinalis capitis
Occipital artery

Splenius capitis

Sternocleidomastoid

Nerves to levator scapulae

Levator scapulae

Spinal accessory nerve (CN XI)

Middle scalene

Dorsal scapular nerve

Long thoracic nerve

Transverse cervical artery

Trapezius

Great auricular nerve
External jugular vein

Transverse cervical nerve

Supraclavicular nerves

Internal jugular vein
Phrenic nerve deep to prevertebral layer
of deep cervical fascia
Brachial plexus

Anterior scalene

Inferior belly of omohyoid

External jugular vein

Pectoralis major

Deltoid

Lateral view

Figure 7-2. Posterior triangle of the neck (superficial view). The platysma muscle has been reflected to expose veins and cutaneous nerves of the cervical plexus.

and two others, the **transverse cervical** and **supra-scapular veins**. The last two veins drain the region of the shoulder. Another superficial vessel, the **anterior jugular vein**, occasionally empties into the external jugular vein, but usually it joins the subclavian vein directly. Although it lies between the two laminae of the investing fascia, the anterior jugular vein communicates with its corresponding vein on the other side via a venous connection, the **jugular arch**, which occupies the suprasternal space.

Sensory Innervation of the Neck

Summary Bite. Branches of dorsal and ventral primary rami of cervical spinal nerves provide cutaneous innervation to the neck. The cervical plexus is formed by ventral primary rami of C1, C2, C3, and C4. Cutaneous sensation to the front and side of the neck is served by C2, C3, and C4.

Cutaneous innervation of the neck is mediated by branches of the dorsal and ventral primary rami of cervical spinal nerves. It is important to remember the following concepts concerning cutaneous innervation of the neck:

- The first cervical spinal nerve probably has no cutaneous branches.
- The ventral primary rami of C1, C2, C3, and most of C4 form the **cervical plexus**.
- The ventral primary rami of parts of C4, all of C5, C6, C7, and C8, and most of T1 participate in the formation of the **brachial plexus**.
- The cutaneous supply of the side and front of the neck is derived from branches of the cervical plexus (C2, C3, and C4).

Sensation to the back of the neck is mediated by the medial branches of the dorsal primary rami of C2,

C3, C4, and, infrequently, C5. It is not necessary to discuss the posterior neck in this regard.

The front and side of the neck receive their sensory supply from branches of the cervical plexus containing fibers derived from the ventral primary rami of C2, C3, and C4. These branches of the cervical plexus are the lesser occipital, great auricular, transverse cervical, and supraclavicular nerves (Fig. 7-2). These nerves emerge in the posterior triangle, pierce the investing layer of the deep cervical fascia, and distribute to the regions they serve. They all appear very close to each other at the midbelly of the posterior border of the sternocleidomastoid muscle.

The **lesser occipital nerve** (C2) closely follows the posterior border of the sternocleidomastoid as it ascends toward the mastoid process. Near the insertion of this muscle, the lesser occipital nerve perforates the investing layer of the deep cervical fascia, crosses over the sternocleidomastoid muscle, and distributes to the back of the auricle and to the region of the scalp behind and superior to it.

The **great auricular nerve** (C2 and C3) pierces the investing layer of the deep cervical fascia at midbelly of the sternocleidomastoid. It travels obliquely across that muscle, accompanying the external jugular vein in its ascent toward the ear. Shortly before reaching the ear, it bifurcates into an anterior branch supplying sensation to the skin overlying the parotid gland and a posterior branch (or mastoid branch) serving the cutaneous region over the back of the ear and mastoid process.

The **transverse cervical nerve** (C2 and C3) pierces the investing layer of the deep fascia in the vicinity of, but inferior to, the great auricular nerve. It crosses the sternocleidomastoid muscle horizontally under the cover of the platysma, deep to the external jugular vein, where it bifurcates into ascending and descending branches to supply the skin of the anterior triangle of the neck.

The **supraclavicular nerves** (C3 and C4) are the only superficial descending branches of the cervical plexus. These nerves pass deep to the investing layer of the deep cervical fascia as a single trunk, surfacing just inferior to the transverse cervical nerve. The trunk descends deep to the platysma and forms three branches: medial, intermediate, and lateral. These branches perforate the investing layer just cranial to the clavicle and distribute as far inferiorly as the sternal angle and second rib and as far laterally and posteriorly as the skin over the spine of the scapula. Occasionally, one or more of these nerves may be observed to perforate the clavicle.

DEEP FASCIA

Summary Bite. The deep fascia of the neck is organized into three layers: investing, prevertebral, and pretracheal. The carotid sheath, formed by contributions of the three layers, invests the major vessels and cranial nerve X as they are passing between the head and the trunk.

The deep fascia of the neck is usually thought of as being organized into three distinct layers: the **investing**, **prevertebral**, and **pretracheal fasciae**. In addition, the **carotid sheath**, an investment of fascia derived from the component layers of the deep fascia, surrounds the large vessels and nerves that pass between the trunk and the head (Figs. 7-3 and 7-4).

Considerable variation exists in the description of the cervical fascia because there is no precise definition of what constitutes fascia. The descriptions that follow view fascia rather conservatively and presuppose a functional as well as a morphologic basis for this tissue. An important point is that the subdivisions of the cervical fascia form additional compartments and interfascial spaces. One such space, separating the buccopharyngeal and prevertebral fasciae, is the retropharyngeal space, extending from the base of the skull all the way inferiorly into the posterior mediastinum within the thorax (see the "Clinical Considerations" section below).

The **alar fascia**, another minor fascial layer in this area, represents the posterior lamina of the pretracheal fascia and forms a loose, thin connective tissue sheet between the buccopharyngeal fascia and the prevertebral fascia. It terminates laterally in the carotid sheath. An additional minor fascial layer that envelops the infrahyoid muscles is the **fascia of the infrahyoid muscles**.

Investing Fascia

Summary Bite. Investing fascia (superficial layer of the deep fascia) splits into two laminae to "invest" (sandwich) the sternocleidomastoid and trapezius muscles as it surrounds the neck.

The investing fascia, also known as the **superficial layer of the deep fascia**, surrounds the neck and covers the anterior and posterior triangles. It is a thin, though in places rather strong, sheet that is attached along the length of the **ligamentum nuchae** (a strong band of collagenous and elastic fibers along the

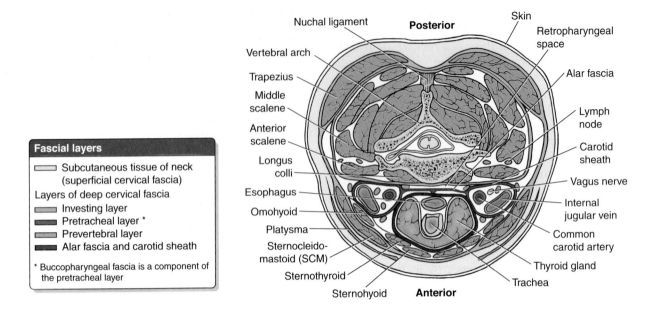

Fascial layers

☐ Subcutaneous tissue of neck (superficial cervical fascia)

Layers of deep cervical fascia

☐ Investing layer
☐ Pretracheal layer *
☐ Prevertebral layer
☐ Alar fascia and carotid sheath

* Buccopharyngeal fascia is a component of the pretracheal layer

Superior view of transverse section (at level C7 vertebra)

Figure 7-3. Cross section of the neck. The view is approximately at the level of the seventh cervical vertebra, illustrating cervical fascia.

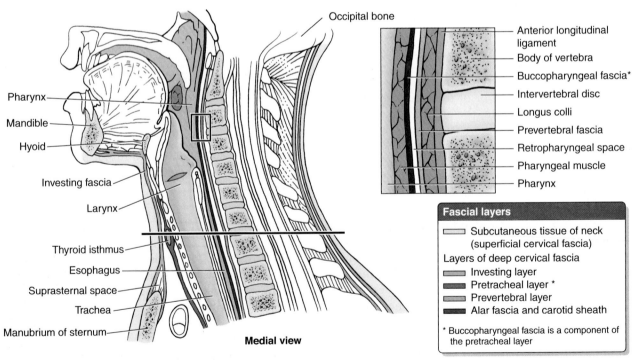

Fascial layers

☐ Subcutaneous tissue of neck (superficial cervical fascia)

Layers of deep cervical fascia

☐ Investing layer
☐ Pretracheal layer *
☐ Prevertebral layer
☐ Alar fascia and carotid sheath

* Buccopharyngeal fascia is a component of the pretracheal layer

Medial view

Figure 7-4. Cervical fascia in midsagittal view.

spines of the cervical vertebrae) and the spine of the seventh cervical vertebra (Figs. 7-3 and 7-4).

As the investing layer proceeds anteriorly, it splits into two laminae around the trapezius muscle, and then fuses into a single layer to split again into two laminae around the sternocleidomastoid muscle. Subsequent to enveloping this muscle, it again fuses into a single layer and continues anteriorly to the front of the neck to join its counterpart from the opposite side. In its passage, it also encompasses the strap muscles of the neck.

The superior attachment of the investing layer includes the external occipital protuberance, the superior nuchal line, and the inferior extent of the mastoid process. Here it splits to enclose the parotid gland, where it continues superiorly as the **parotid fascia**. The superficial lamina of the parotid fascia is attached to the inferior border of the zygomatic arch, whereas the deep lamina extends along the temporal bone to the carotid canal.

A part of this deep lamina is thickened and extends from the styloid process to the mandible and is aptly named the **stylomandibular ligament**. This ligament effectively separates the parotid gland from the submandibular gland.

Inferiorly, the investing layer is attached to the spinous process of the seventh cervical vertebra, the spine of the scapula, the acromion, the clavicle, and the manubrium. In places, it is attached to both the anterior and posterior aspects of the clavicle, and scapula, following the course of the attachment of the sternocleidomastoid and trapezius muscles. The fascia also splits into two laminae to envelop and fix the intermediate tendon of the omohyoid muscle. Immediately above the suprasternal notch, the two laminae of the investing layer remain separated, forming the small **suprasternal space**. This space contains adipose tissue as well as the **jugular arch**, a venous connection between the two anterior jugular veins.

Prevertebral Fascia

Summary Bite. Prevertebral fascia envelops the muscle mass encircling the vertebral column. Where it meets its counterpart from the opposite side as they pass from transverse process of one side to the opposite transverse process along all seven cervical vertebrae, it is weak and contains loose connective tissue forming the "danger space" for spread of infection.

The prevertebral fascia of the cervical fascia envelops the vertebrae and the deep cervical muscle masses surrounding the vertebral column, thus forming the floor of the posterior cervical triangle. Posteriorly, it is attached along the entire length of the ligamentum nuchae, where it merges with the origin of the investing layer (Figs. 7-3 and 7-4).

The prevertebral fascia is attached superiorly to the basilar portion of the occipital bone, as well as to the jugular foramen and to the carotid canal. It passes along the mastoid process of the temporal bone onto the superior nuchal line to the external occipital protuberance, where it meets its counterpart from the opposite side. This cylindrical layer of fascia forms attachments to the anterior surfaces of the transverse processes and bodies of all seven cervical vertebrae. Passing from the transverse process of one side to the other, it forms two laminae, with a loose connective tissue between them. This potential space constitutes the "danger space."

As the prevertebral fascia passes laterally, it covers the deep muscles of the neck as well as all of the cutaneous nerves that eventually pierce it. This fascia attaches to the transverse processes of the cervical vertebrae and continues deep to the trapezius muscle as a thin film of fascia. The accessory nerve is the only cranial nerve lying superficial to the prevertebral fascia. Inferiorly, this fascia continues into the thorax, accompanying the muscles of the neck as these muscles insert onto the bones surrounding the superior thoracic aperture.

Clinical Considerations

Fascial Layers

Fascial layers play an important role in the localization of infection. However, the spaces between fascial layers occasionally communicate with other regions of the body. One such space, between the two laminae of the prevertebral fascia (or, according to some, between the prevertebral and alar fasciae) is the "danger space," serving as a conduit for the spread of infection from the neck into the thorax. Spread of infection via this route can be life-threatening.

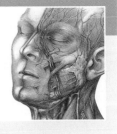

Table 7-1   Muscles of the Back of the Neck

Name	Location	Origin
Trapezius	Most superficial layer covering the back of the neck and upper back	External occipital protuberance, superior nuchal line, ligamentum nuchae, and spinous processes of C7–T12
Splenius capitis	Immediately deep to the trapezius	Ligamentum nuchae; spinous processes of vertebrae C7–T4
Splenius cervicis	Lateral and inferior to splenius capitis	Spines of the vertebrae T3–T6
Iliocostalis cervicis	Back of neck to the angle of upper few ribs	Angles of ribs 3, 4, 5, and 6
Longissimus cervicis	Medial to iliocostalis cervicis	Transverse processes of vertebrae T1–T5
Longissimus capitis	Medial to the longissimus cervicis	Transverse processes of T1–T5 and articular processes of vertebrae C4–C7
Spinalis cervicis	Inconstant	Inferior portion of ligamentum nuchae; spine of vertebrae C7, T1, and T2
Spinalis capitis	Usually fused with the medial part of the semispinalis capitis	Transverse processes of vertebrae T5 and T6
Semispinalis capitis	Deep to the splenius capitis	Transverse processes of vertebrae C7–T6 and articular processes of vertebrae C4–C6
Semispinalis cervicis	Deep to the semispinalis capitis	Transverse processes of T1–T6
Multifidus (cervical portion)	On either side of the spinous process of each cervical vertebra	Articular processes of vertebrae C4–C7
Rotatores longus and brevis spinae (cervical portion)	Dorsal aspect of vertebrae	Transverse processes of C3–C7
Interspinales (cervical portion)	Between the spines of cervical vertebrae	Spine of each cervical vertebra, except C2
Intertransversarii anterior (cervical portion)	Between transverse processes of cervical vertebrae, placed anteriorly	Anterior tubercle of transverse process of vertebrae C2-T1
Intertransversarii posterior (cervical portion)	Behind the intertransversarii anterior	Posterior tubercles of transverse process of vertebrae C2-T1
Obliquus capitis superior	Deep to semispinalis capitis	Transverse process of atlas
Obliquus capitis inferior	Deep to semispinalis capitis and inferior to obliquus capitis superior	Spinous process of axis
Rectus capitis posterior major	Medial to the obliquus capitis superior	Spine of the axis
Rectus capitis posterior minor	Medial to the rectus capitis posterior major	Tubercle of the posterior arch of the atlas

Insertion	Innervation	Action
Lateral ⅓ of the clavicle; acromion, spine, and tubercle of the spine of the scapula	Accessory nerve and ventral primary rami of C3, C4 (proprioception)	Most of its action is on the shoulder in suspending, squaring, shrugging, and pulling it in. It is also a rotator of the scapula. Fixing the shoulder, it assists in pulling the head posteriorly and laterally
Mastoid process of temporal bone and lateral ⅓ of superior nuchal line of occipital bone	Dorsal primary rami of middle cervical nerves	Pulls head back and rotates
Transverse processes of vertebrae C1–C3	Dorsal primary rami of lower cervical nerves	Pulls head back and rotates
Transverse processes of vertebrae C4–C6	Dorsal primary rami of lower cervical nerves	Extends and rotates cervical spine
Transverse processes of vertebrae C2–C6	Dorsal primary rami of cervical nerves	Extends and inclines cervical spine laterally
Posterior aspect of mastoid process of temporal bone	Dorsal primary rami of cervical nerves	Extends and inclines head laterally
Spine of vertebrae C2–C4	Dorsal primary rami of cervical nerves	Extends cervical vertebral column
Lateral to the external occipital crest, between superior and inferior nuchal lines	Dorsal primary rami of cervical nerves	Extends the head
Occipital bone between superior and inferior nuchal lines	Branches of dorsal primary rami of cervical nerves	Extends head and, acting unilaterally, tilts it to one side
Spinous processes of vertebrae C2–C5	Branches of dorsal primary rami of upper thoracic nerves	Extends cervical vertebrae and, acting unilaterally, tilts it to one side
Spine of vertebrae C2–C7	Branches of dorsal primary rami of upper thoracic and cervical nerves	Extends cervical vertebral column, and, acting unilaterally, tilts it to one side
Base of spinous processes of vertebrae above	Branches of dorsal primary rami of cervical nerves	Pulls back spinal column & rotate neck to opposite side
Spine of cervical vertebrae immediately above except C1	Branches of dorsal primary rami of cervical nerves except C1	Extends the cervical spinal column
Anterior tubercles of the transverse processes of vertebrae C1-C7	Ventral primary rami of nerves C2-T1	Tilts the cervical spinal column to one side. Acting in concert with the other side, they fix the cervical spinal column
Posterior tubercles of transverse processes of vertebrae C1-C7	Ventral primary rami of nerves C2-T1	Tilts the cervical spinal column to one side. Acting in concert with the other side, they fix the cervical spinal column
Inferior to the superior nuchal line of the occipital bone	Dorsal primary ramus of suboccipital nerve (C1)	Pulls head back and, acting unilaterally, tilts it to one side
Transverse process of the atlas	Dorsal primary ramus of suboccipital nerve (C1)	Rotates atlanto-axis joint to turn the face laterally
Below and on the inferior nuchal line of the occipital bone	Dorsal primary ramus of suboccipital nerve (C1)	Draws the head back and turns the face laterally
Above superior lip of foramen magnum to inferior nuchal line	Dorsal primary ramus of suboccipital nerve (C1)	Pulls head directly posteriorly

Pretracheal Fascia

Summary Bite. The thin pretracheal fascia, whose posterior lamina is called the buccopharyngeal fascia, surrounds the viscera of the neck as it invests the thyroid gland, larynx, trachea, and the lateral aspect of the esophagus.

The pretracheal fascia forms a small, thin, cylindrical fascial layer surrounding the viscera of the neck. Its posterior lamina is referred to as the **buccopharyngeal fascia**. The pretracheal fascia forms a complete investment for the thyroid gland, and the deep layer of this envelope encircles the larynx and trachea; it also covers the lateral aspects of the esophagus (Figs. 7-3 and 7-4). Posteriorly, the esophagus is separated from the prevertebral fascia by the buccopharyngeal portion of the pretracheal fascia. The superior attachment of the pretracheal fascia is the body and lesser and greater cornua of the hyoid bone, the stylohyoid ligament, medial pterygoid plate of the sphenoid bone, and the pharyngeal tubercle of the occipital bone, where the pretracheal fascia is met by its counterpart from the opposite side. Inferiorly, its boundaries include the oblique line of the thyroid cartilage, and it subsequently merges with the fasciae of the aorta and pericardium. Its fate dorsal to the esophagus is not clear because it merges with the fascial layers of the posterior thoracic wall.

Carotid Sheath

Summary Bite. Contributions from the three layers of the deep cervical fascia form the carotid sheath, which encloses the common carotid artery, the internal carotid artery, the internal jugular vein, and the vagus nerve.

The carotid sheath, a consolidation of connective tissue derived from the three fascial layers of the deep cervical fasciae, encloses the major neurovascular bundle of the neck (Fig. 7-3). Compartments exist within this cylindrical connective tissue sheath that separate constituent parts of the neurovascular bundle. The contents of the carotid sheath are the common carotid artery, the internal carotid artery, the internal jugular vein, and the vagus nerve. The ansa cervicalis, a nerve complex composed of spinal nerves, may be found on the surface of, embedded in, or just within the carotid sheath. Superiorly, the sheath is attached to the area of the jugular foramen and carotid canal, whereas inferiorly it is continuous with the fasciae of the great vessels and heart.

POSTERIOR ASPECTS OF THE NECK

The posterior aspect of the neck is normally presented as a portion of the back in most anatomy texts, thus it will not be presented here since the back is not germane to the thrust of this book.

Two tables are presented to acquaint the reader with the muscles located in the back that are associated with the posterior neck. Table 7-1 presents the muscles located in the back of the neck. The reader can correlate this information with Figs. 7-1, 7-2, and 7-3.

Muscles located in the back of the neck, specifically those forming the suboccipital triangle, are presented in Table 7-2. The reader can correlate the tabular information with the information in Figs. 7-4, 7-5, and 7-6.

TRIANGLES OF THE NECK

Summary Bite. The space between the anterior border of the trapezius muscle and the midline of the neck is divided into two triangles by the sternocleidomastoid as it passes diagonally across this space. The space formed anterior to the sternocleidomastoid muscle is called the anterior cervical triangle, whereas the space located posterior to the sternocleidomastoid muscle is called the posterior cervical triangle. These two major triangles are subdivided into subtriangles by various anatomical landmarks.

The quadrilateral area between the anterior midline of the neck and the anterior border of the trapezius muscle is subdivided into two triangular areas, the anterior and posterior triangles. This division is accomplished by a thick, straplike muscle, the sternocleidomastoid, whose oblique path extends from the manubrium of the sternum to the region behind the ear (Fig. 7-7).

Inferiorly, the **sternocleidomastoid muscle** has two heads of origin, a lateral and a medial, which demarcate a triangular interval between them. Superior to this origin the fibers of the two heads intermingle, forming a thick, muscular belly.

The lateral (clavicular) head springs from musculotendinous fibers attached to the medial one third of the clavicle; it is a flattened, quadrilateral-shaped structure. The medial (sternal) head arises from a conical tendon attached to the anterosuperior border of the manubrium just lateral to the jugular notch.

Table 7-2 Boundaries and Contents of the Suboccipital Triangle

Borders	
Inferior	Obliquus capitis inferior muscles
Medial	Rectus capitis posterior major muscle
Lateral	Obliquus capitis superior muscle
Roof	Dense collangenous and fatty connective tissue deep to the semispinalis capitis muscle
Floor	Atlanto-occipital membrane and the posterior arch of the atlas
Contents	Vertebral artery, suboccipital nerve and its branches, and the greater occipital nerve

The lateral head passes deep to the medial head, and their fibers merge a few centimeters above their origins. The fleshy belly continues to its wide insertion, becoming tendinous just before reaching the mastoid process of the temporal bone and the lateral one half of the superior nuchal line of the occipital bone. This insertion, in conjunction with the medial-most point of insertion of the trapezius muscle, forms the superior apex of the posterior triangle.

The sternocleidomastoid muscle receives motor fibers from the spinal accessory nerve, which pierces the deep surface of its belly. Proprioceptive fibers derived from the second and third cervical spinal nerves also enter the muscle's deep surface.

The sternocleidomastoid acts on the head to approximate the ear of the same side to the shoulder, acting in concert with its counterpart to assist the deep muscles of the back of the neck in flexing the head, thus raising the chin.

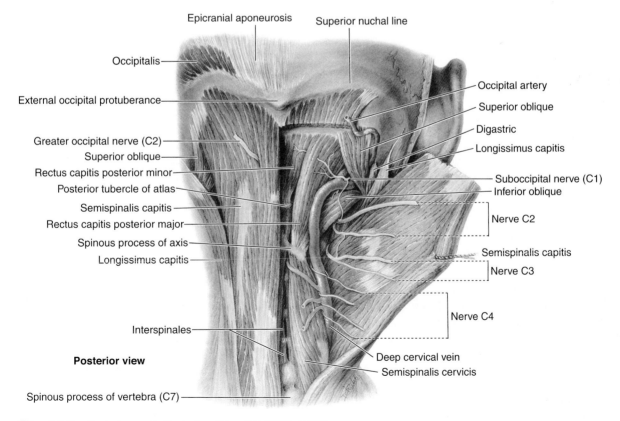

Figure 7-5. Posterior neck displaying the suboccipital region.

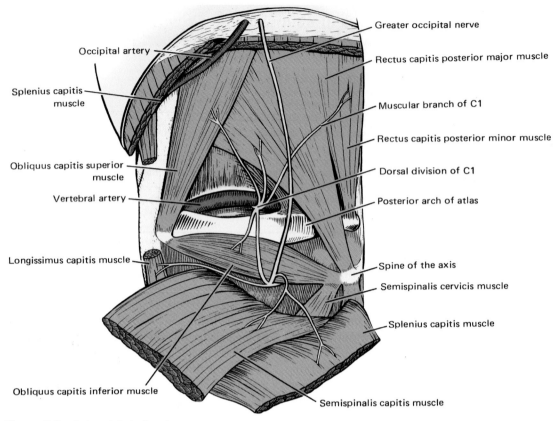

Figure 7-6. Suboccipital triangle.

Labels (clockwise from top):
- Greater occipital nerve
- Rectus capitis posterior major muscle
- Muscular branch of C1
- Rectus capitis posterior minor muscle
- Dorsal division of C1
- Posterior arch of atlas
- Spine of the axis
- Semispinalis cervicis muscle
- Splenius capitis muscle
- Semispinalis capitis muscle
- Obliquus capitis inferior muscle
- Longissimus capitis muscle
- Vertebral artery
- Obliquus capitis superior muscle
- Splenius capitis muscle
- Occipital artery

Clinical Considerations

Torticollis

Torticollis is a condition in which the head is held at an angle, with the ear drawn toward the shoulder of one side. This condition may be either congenital or spasmodic.

It is believed that congenital torticollis is caused by trauma during birth, in which one of the sternocleidomastoids is stretched excessively, causing hemorrhage in the muscle, resulting in fibrous invasion and subsequent shortening of the muscle.

Further complications may arise, such as wedge-shaped cervical vertebrae and muscle atrophy. Spasmodic torticollis usually involves the trapezius, sternocleidomastoid, and perhaps other muscles, all of which undergo spasmodic contractions. The position of the head in this condition mimics congenital torticollis. The defect is not in the muscles but is probably related to neurogenic involvement.

Paralysis of the trapezius may occur if deep wounds in the region of the posterior triangle involve the spinal accessory nerve. Such injury limits the movement of the upper limb to the horizontal position during lifting of the arm. In addition, it causes depression of the shoulder on the affected side.

Referred pain in the region of the shoulder may have its origin in pleurisy that is causing irritation of the phrenic nerve. This situation occurs because the phrenic nerve has the same cervical spinal nerve components as the supraclavicular nerves, and signals transmitted via the phrenic nerve may be interpreted as originating in the area of the shoulder served by the supraclaviculars.

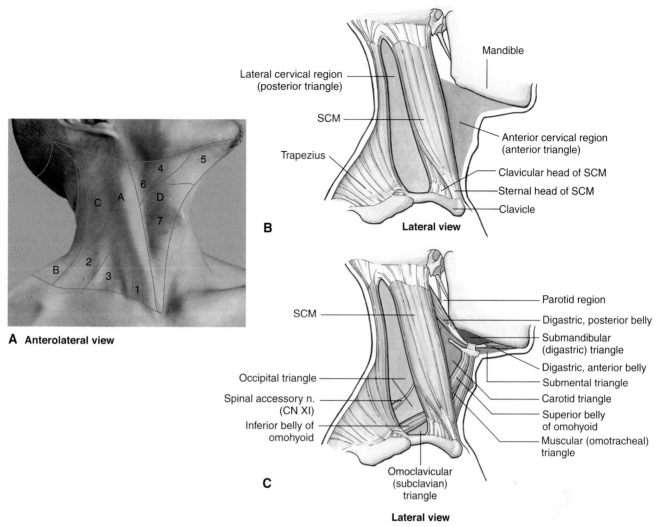

Lateral cervical region
(posterior triangle)

SCM

Trapezius

Mandible

Anterior cervical region
(anterior triangle)

Clavicular head of SCM

Sternal head of SCM

Clavicle

B **Lateral view**

A Anterolateral view

SCM

Occipital triangle

Spinal accessory n.
(CN XI)

Inferior belly of
omohyoid

Omoclavicular
(subclavian)
triangle

Parotid region

Digastric, posterior belly

Submandibular
(digastric) triangle

Digastric, anterior belly

Submental triangle

Carotid triangle

Superior belly
of omohyoid

Muscular (omotracheal)
triangle

C

Lateral view

Figure 7-7. Triangles of the neck.

Muscular and bony structures located in the triangles further subdivide the anterior and posterior triangles into smaller triangular compartments, as is detailed in Table 7-3. The boundaries of the posterior triangle are as follows:

▨ Posteriorly, the anterior border of the trapezius muscle
▨ Anteriorly, the posterior edge of the sternocleidomastoid muscle
▨ Inferiorly, the middle third of the clavicle

A thin, fusiform muscle, the posterior belly of the omohyoid, enters the posterior triangle at its inferoposterior apex. It traverses the lower aspect of this triangle and disappears deep to the sternocleidomastoid, thus subdividing the posterior triangle into an inferior **subclavian** (supraclavicular, omoclavicular) **triangle** and a superior **occipital triangle**.

The limits of the anterior triangle are as follows:

▨ Anteriorly, an imaginary line along the anterior midline of the neck extending from the inferiormost portion of the symphysis menti of the mandible down to the center of the jugular notch of the manubrium
▨ Posteriorly, the anterior edge of the sternocleidomastoid
▨ Superiorly, the inferior border of the mandible

The superior belly of the omohyoid muscle enters the anterior triangle and inserts onto the body of the hyoid bone. The posterior belly of the digastric muscle also enters the anterior triangle, at the interval between the angle of the mandible and the mastoid

Table 7-3 Boundaries of the Cervical Triangles

Name of Triangle	Borders			
	Superior	*Inferior*	*Medial*	*Lateral*
Anterior	Inferior border of the mandible		Anterior midline of the neck from the symphysis menti to the center of jugular notch	Anterior border of the sternocleidomastoid
Submandibular (digastric)	Inferior border of the mandible		Superior border of anterior belly of digastric	Superior border of posterior belly of digastric
Carotid	Inferior border of the posterior belly of the digastric		Superior border of superior belly of omohyoid	Anterior border of sternocleidomastoid
Muscular	Inferior border of superior belly of omohyoid		Anterior midline of the neck from inferior border of body of hyoid to the jugular notch	Anterior border of sternocleidomastoid
Submental		Superior border of body of hyoid bone (between two slings for intermediate tendon of right and left digastrics)		Inferior borders of the anterior bellies of the digastrics
Posterior		Middle one third of the clavicle	Posterior border of sternocleidomastoid	Anterior border of the trapezius
Subclavian (omoclavicular, supraclavicular)	Inferior border of inferior belly of the omohyoid	Middle one third of the clavicle	Posterior border of the sternocleidomastoid	
Occipital		Superior border of the inferior belly of the omohyoid	Posterior border of the sternocleidomastoid	Anterior border of the trapezius

process. It becomes tendinous as it reaches the greater comu of the hyoid bone (near its junction with the body of the hyoid) and is attached to the hyoid bone by a fascial sling.

The muscle, now known as the anterior belly of the digastric muscle, becomes fleshy again and continues to its insertion into the digastric fossa of the mandible. These muscles, in conjunction with the hyoid bone and the inferior border of the mandible, subdivide the anterior triangle into several smaller triangular components:

▨ The anterior and posterior bellies of the digastric muscle enclose a space, the **submandibular triangle** (digastric), just below the body of the mandible.
▨ The posterior belly of the digastric, superior belly of the omohyoid and the anterior border of the

sternocleidomastoid muscles enclose the **carotid triangle**.
▨ The superior belly of the omohyoid, the anterior midline of the neck (and body of the hyoid bone), and the anterior border of the sternocleidomastoid circumscribe the **muscular triangle**.
▨ Finally, the two anterior bellies of the digastric muscle (one on either side) and the intervening body of the hyoid bone delimit the **submental triangle**; this is the only triangle that encompasses both sides of the neck and is, therefore, unpaired.

Posterior Triangle of the Neck

Summary Bite. The posterior triangle is formed by the following structures: anterior border of the trapezius muscle, the lateral border of the sternocleidomastoid muscle, and the middle third of the clavicle. Passage of the inferior belly of the omohyoid muscle across this triangle subdivides it into two subtriangles, the subclavian and occipital triangles.

The boundaries of the posterior triangle are the anterior border of the trapezius, the posterior border of the sternocleidomastoid, and the superior border of the middle one third of the clavicle (Figs. 7-2, 7-7, and 7-8, and Table 7-3).

The inferior belly of the omohyoid muscle crosses the floor of the posterior triangle, subdividing it into the inferiorly located small **subclavian** and the superiorly positioned larger **occipital triangles**.

The posterior triangle is covered by skin, the underlying superficial fascia, and the platysma muscle. It is roofed over by the investing layer of the deep cervical fascia, superficial to which is the external jugular vein and its tributaries, which were described earlier in this chapter.

The cutaneous nerves, derived from the cervical plexus, appear in the posterior triangle and were described previously along with the superficial veins (Fig. 7-2).

Accessory Nerve

The accessory nerve has two component fiber groups: the cranial root derived from the brainstem and the spinal root arising from the spinal cord. The two roots unite and later become separated. The cranial root joins the vagus nerve, whereas the spinal root becomes the distinct peripheral accessory nerve (see Chapter 18).

This nerve then pierces the deep surfaces of the sternocleidomastoid muscle, which it supplies, and emerges in the occipital triangle at the posterior border of that muscle just superior to the appearance of the cutaneous branches of the cervical plexus. The accessory nerve then traverses diagonally across the posterior triangle, passing in the fatty connective tissue between the investing and prevertebral layers of the deep cervical fascia (Figs. 7-2, 7-8, and 7-9). The accessory nerve has no branches in this triangle but dives deep to the trapezius muscle, where it forms the **subtrapezial**

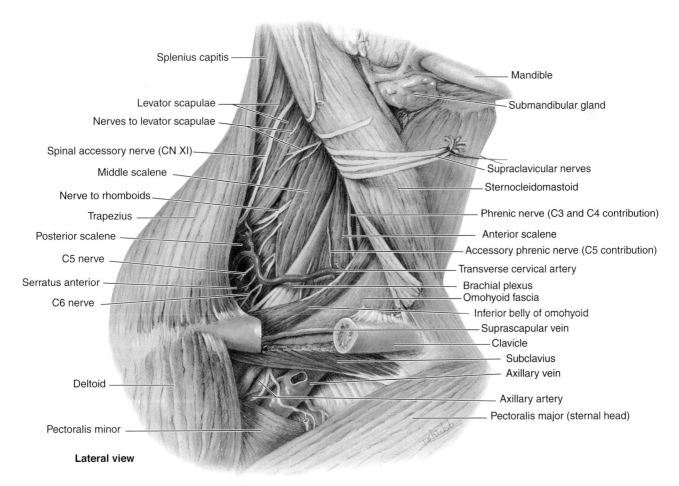

Figure 7-8. Posterior triangle of the neck (deep view).

Table 7-4 Muscles Associated With the Posterior Triangle

Name	Location	Origin
Sternocleidomastoid	Bisects the lateral aspect of the neck	Lateral head: medial one third of clavicle; medial head: manubrium
Platysma	Anterior and posterior triangle of the neck	Epimysium of the deltoid and pectoralis major muscles
Omohyoid	Posterior and anterior triangles of the neck	Superior border of scapula, just medial to the scapular notch
Splenius capitis	Superior apex of posterior triangle	Ligamentum nuchae; spinous processes of vertebrae C7-T4
Levator scapulae	Below floor of posterior triangle	Transverse processes of vertebrae C1–C4
Anterior scalene	Just deep to the clavicular head of the sternocleidomastoid	Transverse processes of vertebrae C3–C6
Middle scalene	Lateral to the anterior scalene	Transverse processes of vertebrae C2–C7
Posterior scalene	Deep and lateral to the middle scalene	Transverse processes of vertebrae C4–C6

plexus in conjunction with spinal nerves C3 and C4 to innervate that muscle. It should be noted that C3 and C4 provide proprioceptive fibers to the trapezius.

Muscles Associated with the Posterior Triangle

Summary Bite. Two groups of muscles are associated with the superficial and deep regions of the posterior triangle. Superficial muscles include the sternocleidomastoid, trapezius, and inferior omohyoid muscles, whereas those forming the floor of the triangle are the prevertebral muscles.

The muscles directly associated with the posterior triangle are the trapezius, the sternocleidomastoid, and the inferior belly of the omohyoid (Table 7-4). In addition, the fascial carpet forming the floor of the posterior triangle lies on a series of muscles that are associated with the triangle although not located in it. These prevertebral muscles are the splenius capitis; the levator scapulae; and the posterior, middle, and anterior scalenes (Fig. 7-8). The trapezius, sternocleidomastoid, and splenius capitis muscles were described earlier.

Omohyoid

The thin omohyoid muscle consists of two bellies, **inferior** and **superior**, that are connected to each other by an intermediate tendon. The inferior belly originates on the superior border of the scapula, just medial to the scapular notch, and passes across the inferior aspect of the posterior cervical triangle, where it is enveloped by the investing layer of the deep cervical fascia (Fig. 7-7). This fascia forms a fascial sling that fixes the intermediate tendon to the clavicle and the first rib. The superior belly of the muscle passes obliquely, deep to the sternocleidomastoid, to emerge in the anterior triangle. It inserts onto the inferior border of the body of the hyoid bone. Branches of the ansa cervicalis (C1, C2, and C3) supply the two bellies of this muscle. The omohyoid acts to depress the hyoid bone, thus countering the actions of the suprahyoid muscles.

Levator Scapulae

The levator scapulae is not properly considered a muscle of the neck. It serves as one of the muscles attaching the superior extremity to the trunk, but its location requires at least a cursory description. It arises from the transverse processes of the first four cervical vertebrae, from where it proceeds as one or more fleshy fascicles along the side of the neck to insert into the medial border of the scapula (Fig. 7-8). It receives its innervation from spinal nerves C3 and C4 directly and from C5 indirectly. The levator scapulae

Insertion	Innervation	Action
Mastoid process of temporal bone and lateral half of superior nuchal line	Accessory nerve and C2, C3 (proprioception)	Unilaterally: approximates ear of the same side to shoulder. In unison with its counterpart: tips head back, raising the chin
Inferior border of body of mandible; skin and hypodermis of face	Cervical branch of the facial nerve	Assists in depressing mandible, corner of the mouth, and lower lip
Inferior border of the body of the hyoid bone	Superior ramus of ansa cervicalis (C1, C2) and the ansa itself (C2, C3)	Depresses the hyoid bone
Mastoid process of temporal; lateral ⅓ of superior nuchal line	Branches of dorsal primary rami of middle cervical spinal nerves	Pulls head back; acting unilaterally, it rotates the head
Medial border of spine of scapula, from superior angle to spine	C3–C5	Elevates scapula; if the scapula is fixed, it tilts head backwards
Ridge and the scalene tubercle of the first rib First rib, between tubercle and groove for subclavian artery Outer surface of second rib	Ventral primary rami of spinal nerves C4–C6 Ventral primary rami of spinal nerves C3–C8 Ventral primary rami of spinal nerves C5–C7	Function in respiration by lifting the thoracic cage. If thoracic cage is fixed, they flex cervical vertebral column to one side or bend it anteriorly when acting in concert

acts to elevate the scapula and, when the scapula is fixed, its contraction tilts the head backward.

Scalenes

The **anterior scalene** is covered, to a great extent, by the clavicular head of the sternocleidomastoid muscle (Fig. 7-8). The anterior scalene originates from the transverse processes of the third through sixth cervical vertebrae. The fibers pass inferolaterally to form a fleshy belly, which inserts as a flat, tendinous sheath on the scalene tubercle of the first rib and on its ridge, just anterior to the groove for the subclavian artery.

Its nerve supply is via branches from ventral primary rami of spinal nerves C4, C5, and C6. The muscle functions in respiration by initially lifting the first rib. If the thoracic cage is fixed, the muscle then flexes the cervical vertebral column to one side. Acting in concert with its counterpart on the other side, the anterior scalene bends the cervical spinal column anteriorly, provided the thoracic cage is immobilized.

Several important anatomic landmarks are associated with the anterior scalene muscle. The subclavian artery is subdivided into three segments as it curves around the deep aspect of this muscle on its

path to the axilla. In addition, the trunks of the brachial plexus traverse the interval between the anterior and middle scalene muscles in passing to the axilla. Moreover, the phrenic nerve lies directly on the anterior scalene muscle, deep to its blanket of prevertebral fascia.

The **middle scalene** muscle is longer than the anterior and originates from the transverse processes of vertebrae C2 through C7 (Fig. 7-8). The fibers become tendinous as the muscle inserts on the first rib between the tubercle and the groove for the subclavian artery.

The middle scalene receives its nerve supply from branches of ventral primary rami of spinal nerves C3 through C8. Its action is the same as that of the anterior scalene (primarily related to respiration).

The **posterior scalene muscle** is the smallest of the three scalene muscles, and it is usually intimately related to the deep and lateral aspect of the middle scalene. The fibers of the two muscles are frequently intermingled so that complete separation cannot be effected.

The posterior scalene originates on the transverse processes of the fourth, fifth, and sixth cervical vertebrae and inserts via a slender, narrow tendon on the external aspect of the second rib. Ventral primary

Table 7-5 Branches of the Cervical Plexus

	Name	Origin	Function
Superficial branches			
Ascending	Lesser occipital	C2	Sensory
	Great auricular	C2,C3	Sensory
	Transverse cervical	C2,C3	Sensory
Descending	Supraclaviculars	C3,C4	Sensory
Deep branches			
Medial	Superior root of ansa cervicalis	C1,C2	Motor
	Branch to geniohyoid and thyrohyoid	C1	Motor
	Branch to rectus capitis lateralis	C1	Motor
	Branch to rectus capitis anterior	C1,C2	Motor
	Branch to longus capitis	C1,C2,C3	Motor
	Branch to longus colli	C1,C2,C3,C4	Motor
	Inferior root of ansa cervicalis	C2,C3	Motor
	Phrenic	C3,C4,C5	Motor and some sensory
Lateral	Branch to trapezius	C3,C4	Proprioception
	Branch to sternocleidomastoid	C2,C3	Proprioception
	Branch to levator scapulae	C3,C4	Motor
	Branch to scalenus medius	C3,C4	Motor

rami of spinal nerves C5 through C7 innervate the muscle, whose action is the same as those of the other two scalenes.

Nerves Associated with the Posterior Triangle

Summary Bite. Cranial nerves C5, C6, C7, C8, and thoracic nerve T1 are, for the most part, trunks forming the brachial plexus (a very large nerve bundle) that serves the entire arm and some of the muscles of the posterior triangle. The cervical plexus is formed by cranial nerves of C1, C2, C3, and C4 and is also present in the posterior cervical triangle.

Brachial Plexus

The ventral primary rami of some spinal nerves appear not to retain their metameric (segmental) identities. Instead, they unite shortly after their origins to form bundles of nerve fibers that become intermixed to form plexuses for redistribution. In this form, the resultant fibers can reach their intended fields, whose original locations became altered.

The **brachial plexus** is one such intermixing of ventral primary rami of spinal nerves C5 through T1 (and occasionally T2). Although the plexus is primarily responsible for innervation of the upper limb and associated structures, it also supplies some muscles of the neck (Fig. 7-8). A thorough discussion of this important plexus is found in any general textbook of anatomy.

Cervical Plexus

Ventral primary rami of the first four cervical spinal nerves participate in the formation of the cervical plexus (Table 7-5 and Fig. 7-9). The ventral primary rami of all but the first cervical spinal nerve bifurcate into ascending and descending branches. These branches then join each other and become united, forming simple loops that lie deep to the prevertebral fascia. Branches arising from the cervical plexus are arranged in a superficial and deep division.

The superficial division is completely sensory and consists of ascending and descending branches. The lesser occipital (C2), great auricular (C2 and C3), and transverse cervical (C2 and C3) comprise the ascending branch, whereas the supraclaviculars (C3 and C4) comprise the descending branches.

The deep division of the cervical plexus is mostly motor, although it does contain sensory components. This division supplies motor innervation to the muscle masses deep to the floor of the posterior triangle, as well as proprioceptive fibers to the sternocleidomastoid and trapezius muscles. Furthermore, the deep division supplies the anterior vertebral muscles. A summary of the specific innervations is in Table 7-5. Two additional important components of this division must be given special consideration: the ansa cervicalis and the phrenic nerve.

Ansa Cervicalis

The **ansa cervicalis** (Figs. 7-9 and 7-13) and its two roots are derived from C1 through C3. The superior

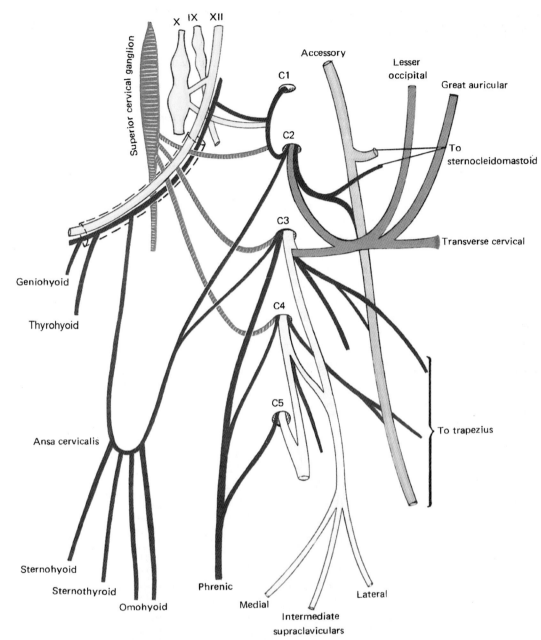

Figure 7-9. Cervical plexus. Note that the cervical sympathetic trunk, vagus nerve, and glossopharyngeal nerve have been cut. The dashed line indicates a segment of the epineurium of the hypoglossal nerve.

root, sometimes incorrectly referred to as the descending hypoglossal, receives fibers from C1 and C2 and the inferior root receives fibers from C2 and C3. Although the superior root of the ansa cervicalis travels for a short distance with the hypoglossal nerve (cranial nerve XII), it does not become a functional part of that nerve.

The superior root joins and travels with the hypoglossal nerve opposite the atlas and descends from that nerve as it passes superficial to the external carotid artery. As the superior root leaves the hy-

poglossal nerve, two filaments (both derived from C1) continue with the hypoglossal nerve for a few millimeters, then branch to supply motor innervation to the thyrohyoid and geniohyoid muscles. The superior root continues to travel superficial to, embedded within, or just inside the carotid sheath.

At the level just below the middle of the neck, the superior root turns posteriorly to form the ansa (loop) in joining with the inferior root, which has descended in the neck alongside the carotid sheath. Four branches arise from the ansa cervicalis to supply motor innervation to the sternohyoid, sternothyroid, and both bellies of the omohyoid muscles.

Phrenic and Accessory Phrenic Nerves

The **phrenic nerve** (C3, C4, and C5), the only motor nerve of the diaphragm, also carries sensory fibers (Figs. 7-8, 7-9, and 7-13). The phrenic nerve passes deep to the prevertebral fascia as it lies on the anterior surface of the anterior scalene muscle.

On its way to distribute to the diaphragm, the phrenic nerve passes between the subclavian artery and vein and then enters the thorax, where it lies anterior to the root of the lung, contacting the fibrous pericardium. The sensory fibers carried by the phrenic nerve serve the mediastinal pleura and the pericardium of the heart.

The **accessory phrenic nerve** (C5) is occasionally present. It descends into the thorax lateral to the phrenic nerve and posterior to the subclavian vein to join the phrenic nerve below the first rib. It also supplies motor fibers to the diaphragm.

Arteries Associated with the Posterior Triangle

 Summary Bite. The subclavian artery, whose right and left origins differ, is the major artery serving the neck. It ascends into the brain and descends into the thorax, serving many structures along its path. It continues into the arm as the axillary artery and, with its branches, is the sole vascular supply to the arm.

Subclavian Arteries

The subclavian artery is a short vessel extending as far laterally as the outer border of the first rib (Fig. 7-10). The origins of the right and left subclavian arteries differ in that the left one arises directly from the arch of the aorta, whereas the right one is one of the terminal branches of the brachiocephalic trunk (see Chapter 21).

The right subclavian artery originates deep to the sternoclavicular joint, and the left subclavian artery originates behind the common carotid artery around the third or fourth thoracic vertebra. Both right and left subclavian arteries travel superiorly to the root of the neck and posterior to the anterior scalene muscle, emerging into the posterior triangle through the interval between the anterior and middle scalene muscles on their way to the lateral border of the first rib, where each artery becomes known as the axillary artery.

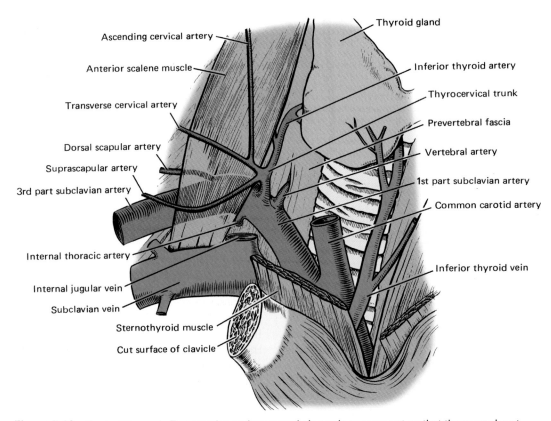

Figure 7-10. Root of the neck. The anterior scalene muscle is made transparent so that the second part of the subclavian artery may be observed deep to it. Note that in this dissection the ascending cervical artery arises from the transverse cervical artery rather than from the more common inferior thyroid artery.

Clinical Considerations

The Subclavian Artery

The **subclavian artery** supplies blood to the entire upper extremity via its continuation, the axillary artery. Uncontrollable bleeding in the upper limb may be stopped by applying pressure with a blunt object on the subclavian artery as it crosses the first rib. The pressure should be directed inferoposteriorly, behind the clavicle, just lateral to the clavicular head of origin of the sternocleidomastoid muscle.

This path, deep to the anterior scalene muscle, permits a convenient division of the subclavian artery into three parts. The first part is from the origin of the vessel to the medial border of the anterior scalene muscle; the second part lies deep to this muscle; and the third part extends from the lateral border of the anterior scalene to the lateral border of the first rib. The branches of the subclavian artery are as follows:

- The vertebral artery, the internal thoracic artery, and the thyrocervical trunk from the first part
- The costocervical trunk from the second part
- The dorsal scapular artery from the third part

Vertebral Artery

The vertebral artery takes its origin from the posterosuperior aspect of the first part of the subclavian artery (Fig. 7-10). It ascends behind the anterior scalene muscle, along the transverse process of the seventh cervical vertebra, and enters the foramen transversarium of the sixth cervical vertebra.

The artery travels through the foramina transversaria of the upper six cervical vertebrae and enters the suboccipital triangle, from where it traverses the foramen magnum to unite with its contralateral vessel to participate in the formation of the basilar artery. Branches arise from the vertebral artery to supply the spinal cord and deep muscles in the vicinity of the suboccipital triangle. The intracranial branches of the vertebral artery are detailed in the description of the brain and spinal cord (see Chapter 17).

Internal Thoracic Artery

The internal thoracic artery originates from the inferior aspect of the first part of the subclavian artery (Fig. 7-10). This artery passes directly inferiorly on the internal anterior thoracic wall just lateral to the margin of the sternum to the sixth or seventh rib, where it bifurcates to form the medially placed superior epigastric and laterally positioned musculophrenic arteries.

Because the internal thoracic artery is a vessel whose distribution is limited to the thorax and abdomen, its branches will not be discussed.

Thyrocervical Trunk

The thyrocervical trunk is a short vessel arising from the superior aspect of the first part of the subclavian artery (Fig. 7-10). Its origin is opposite the point of origin of the internal thoracic artery.

This trunk lies just medial to the anterior scalene muscle, where it trifurcates to form three major branches: the suprascapular, transverse cervical, and inferior thyroid arteries.

The **suprascapular artery** travels obliquely across the anterior surface of the anterior scalene muscle and deep to the sternocleidomastoid, which it supplies. It passes deep to the inferior belly of the omohyoid to reach the scapular notch. Occasionally, the suprascapular artery is a branch of the third part of the subclavian artery.

The **transverse cervical artery** crosses the neck in a fashion similar to, but above, the suprascapular artery. It crosses the floor of the subclavian triangle to travel in company with the spinal accessory nerve and it burrows deep to the anterior border of the trapezius, supplying it and other muscles in the vicinity.

The **inferior thyroid artery** travels superiorly in front of the medial border of the anterior scalene muscle. It then passes deep to the carotid sheath and approaches the inferior aspect of the thyroid gland, which it supplies. The inferior thyroid artery has several small branches, including the terminal ascending and descending branches, both ending in the body of the thyroid gland, as well as muscular branches and the **ascending cervical artery** supplying anterior vertebral muscles of the neck.

Costocervical Trunk

The **costocervical** trunk has different origins on the two sides of the body. On the left, it springs from the posterior aspect of the first part of the subclavian artery, whereas on the right it springs from the posterior aspect of the second part of that artery.

This trunk has two terminal branches: the **superior intercostal artery** and the **deep cervical artery**. The former serves the first and second intercostal spaces, whereas the deep cervical artery is interposed between the first rib and the transverse process of the seventh cervical vertebra. The trunk passes between the semispinalis cervicis and semispinalis capitis, supplying these as well as adjacent muscles, finally anastomosing with the occipital and vertebral arteries.

Dorsal Scapular Artery

The dorsal scapular artery is the only branch arising from the third part of the subclavian artery, although frequently it is a branch of the second part.

The dorsal scapular artery proceeds, anterior to the middle scalene muscle, passing among the trunks of the brachial plexus, to reach the superior angle of the scapula, where it supplies the muscles in the vicinity.

Veins Associated with the Posterior Triangle

Summary Bite. The axillary vein exiting the arm becomes the subclavian vein, which courses for a short distance receiving several venous contributions before joining the internal jugular vein to form the brachiocephalic vein. At this junction the thoracic duct joins on the left side of the neck, whereas the right lymphatic duct joins its counterpart on the right side of the neck.

Subclavian Vein

The subclavian vein is short because it is the continuation of the axillary vein, and it joins the internal jugular vein to form the large brachiocephalic vein (Fig. 7-10).

Thus, the subclavian vein extends from its junction with the internal jugular vein to the external border of the first rib, passing anterior to the anterior scalene muscle, which separates it from the subclavian artery. Here it lies in front of the **subclavius muscle**, which originates on the first rib and inserts on the inferior surface of the clavicle. This muscle, innervated by a branch from the brachial plexus complex, acts as a cushion, protecting the underlying vessels and nerves.

The main tributary of the subclavian vein is the external jugular vein, although frequently the subclavian may receive the dorsal scapular and anterior jugular veins. The left subclavian vein receives lymph from most of the body via the **thoracic duct**, whereas lymph from the remainder of the body is delivered to the right subclavian vein by the **right lymphatic duct**. These lymph vessels pierce the superior aspects of the subclavian veins at the angle of their junctions with the internal jugular veins.

Anterior Triangle

Summary Bite. The anterior triangle is formed by the following: the anterior border of the sternocleidomastoid muscle, the lower border of the mandible, and the midline of the neck. Several muscles coursing through the triangle subdivide it into several subtriangles.

The anterior triangle of the neck is defined by the midline of the neck from the mental symphysis to the jugular notch of the manubrium, the anterior border of the sternocleidomastoid muscle, and the lower border of the mandible. The subdivisions of the anterior triangle are the submandibular, carotid, muscular, and submental triangles, whose borders have been detailed earlier (Fig. 7-7 and Table 7-3).

Clinical Considerations

Fractured Clavicle

The middle third of the clavicle, which forms the base of the posterior triangle, is the most frequently fractured bone in the body. Attached to its deep surface is the subclavius muscle. When the clavicle is fractured it is commonly in the middle third. In this situation, the subclavius muscle affords some protection against a splintered bone from puncturing the neurovascular bundle just deep to the bone. Although the subclavian artery

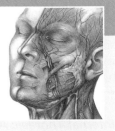

lies behind the anterior scalene muscle just deep to the clavicle, the subclavian vein lying superficial to the anterior scalene muscle makes it especially vulnerable to puncturing by broken bone. The greatest protection against this happening is with the subclavius muscle.

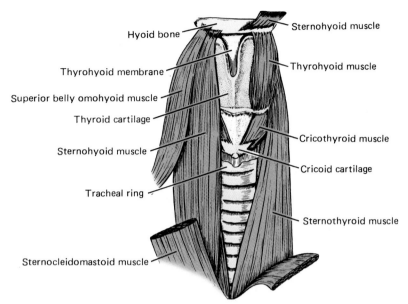

Hyoid bone
Sternohyoid muscle
Thyrohyoid membrane
Thyrohyoid muscle
Superior belly omohyoid muscle
Thyroid cartilage
Cricothyroid muscle
Sternohyoid muscle
Cricoid cartilage
Tracheal ring
Sternothyroid muscle
Sternocleidomastoid muscle

Figure 7-11. Infrahyoid muscles. The thyroid gland has been removed.

Infrahyoid Muscles

Summary Bite. The four pairs of infrahyoid muscles located in the muscular triangle fix and depress the hyoid bone.

Four pairs of straplike muscles represent the infrahyoid muscle group: the sternohyoid, sternothyroid, thyrohyoid, and omohyoid (Fig. 7-11). These muscles act as a group to fix and/or depress the hyoid bone during mastication, deglutition, and speech (Table 7-6).

▨ The **sternohyoid** is a long, thin muscle origina-ting from the posterior aspect of the sternoclav-icular joint region. It ascends to insert onto the inferior border of the body of the hyoid bone just medial to the insertion of the omohyoid muscle.

▨ The **sternothyroid** muscle is wider and shorter than the sternohyoid, under which it lies. It originates on the manubrium of the sternum and inserts on the oblique line of the thyroid cartilage. The sternothyroid muscle also acts to depress the larynx and/or fix it in position.

▨ The **thyrohyoid** muscle lies deep to the sternohyoid. This muscle originates on the oblique line of the lamina of the thyroid cartilage and inserts on the inferior border of the greater cornu and body of the hyoid bone. The thyrohyoid muscle depresses and fixes the hyoid bone, and also raises the thyroid cartilage.

▨ The **omohyoid** muscle was discussed in this chapter's section on the posterior triangle.

Carotid Arteries

The major blood supply of the head and neck is derived from branches originating from the **common carotid artery** (Fig. 7-12; see Chapter 21). This vessel is enclosed by the carotid sheath, which is incompletely subdivided into compartments housing the common and internal carotid arteries, the internal jugular vein, and the vagus nerve.

The common carotid arteries of the two sides have different origins: the right is a branch of the brachiocephalic trunk, whereas the left one branches directly from the arch of the aorta. Consequently, the right common carotid artery is contained wholly within the neck, whereas the left common carotid begins in the upper thorax and enters the neck in the vicinity of the sternoclavicular joint.

The right and left common carotids usually bifurcate approximately at the level of the thyroid cartilage (although this is variable) into an **external** and an **internal carotid artery** (Fig. 7-12). These are considered "terminal branches," hence the common carotid is said to have no branches in the neck.

The common carotid artery is somewhat dilated at its bifurcation, and this expansion is known as the **carotid sinus**. This sinus is a modified region of the vessel, richly innervated by branches of the glossopharyngeal nerve (cranial nerve IX) that serves to monitor blood pressure. An additional structure, the **carotid body**, is also associated with this region of bifurcation. This small, oval, reddish-brown structure lying within the internal carotid artery is innervated by the vagus

Table 7-6 The Infrahyoid Muscles

Name	Location	Origin
Sternohyoid	Anterolateral aspect of neck	Posterior aspect of the sternoclavicular joint area
Sternothyroid	Deep to sternohyoid	Manubrium
Thyrohyoid	Deep to sternohyoid	Oblique line of thyroid cartilage
Omohyoid	Posterior and anterior triangles of the neck	Superior border of scapula just medial to scapular notch

and glossopharyngeal nerves. The carotid body functions as a chemoreceptor monitoring oxygen and carbon dioxide tension, as well as hydrogen ion concentration within the internal carotid artery.

The internal carotid artery has no branches in the neck; instead, it passes through the carotid canal of the temporal bone to enter the cranial cavity. Branches of the internal carotid artery are treated in subsequent chapters.

External Carotid Artery
The external carotid artery has six collateral and two terminal branches.

Branches of the External Carotid Artery

Collateral	Terminal
Superior thyroid	Superficial temporal
Ascending pharyngeal	Maxillary
Lingual	
Facial	
Occipital	
Posterior auricular	

Branches of the external carotid artery that supply regions of the neck are treated in this section. However, branches concerned with the superficial and deep face will be discussed in the appropriate chapters.

Superior Thyroid Artery
The superior thyroid artery is the first branch of the external carotid artery, arising from its ventral aspect just superior to the bifurcation of the common carotid artery (Fig. 7-12).

The superior thyroid artery descends in the neck, accompanied by the same-named vein and the external laryngeal nerve; it reaches the superior pole of the thyroid gland and divides into its terminal branches, some of which anastomose with their counterparts of the other side and with branches of the inferior thyroid artery.

The superior thyroid artery has four named branches—the infrahyoid, sternocleidomastoid, superior laryngeal, and cricothyroid arteries—as well as its terminal anterior, posterior, and occasionally lateral glandular branches at the thyroid gland.

The **infrahyoid artery** is a small vessel that passes deep to the thyrohyoid muscle, caudal to the body of the hyoid bone, and serves that general area.

Clinical Considerations

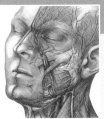

Carotid Sinus Syndrome

Carotid sinus syndrome may result in loss of consciousness due to simple head movements. The syndrome relates to the hypersensitivity of the carotid sinus due to an unknown etiology. Sudden slight pressure changes, such as that occasioned by movement of the head, may result in stimulation of the carotid sinus.

Impulses relayed by the sinus reduce blood pressure and slow the pumping action of the heart, thus decreasing blood supply to the brain, resulting in sudden loss of consciousness.

Insertion	Innervation	Action
Inferior border of hyoid bone	Ansa cervicalis	Depresses and fixes hyoid bone
Oblique line of thyroid cartilage	Ansa cervicalis	Depresses larynx
Greater cornu and body of hyoid bone	C1, via the hypoglossal nerve	Depresses and fixes hyoid bone; elevated the thyroid cartilage when hyoid bone is fixed
Inferior border of body of hyoid bone	Ansa cervicalis	Depresses and fixes hyoid bone

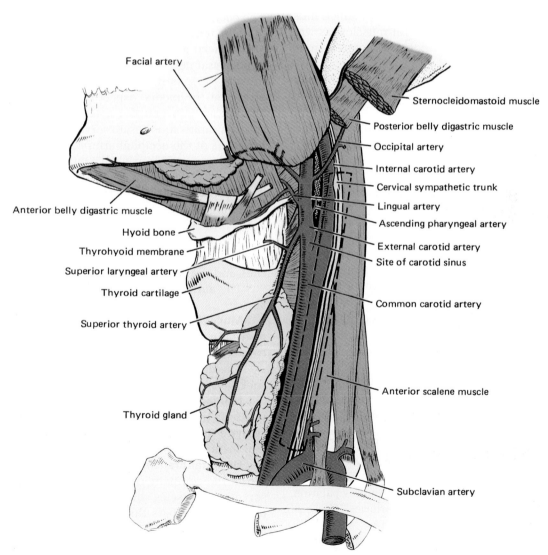

Figure 7-12.   Carotid artery in the neck. The dashed outline indicates the relative position of the internal jugular vein.

The **sternocleidomastoid branch** passes ventral to the carotid sheath and supplies the muscle of the same name on its deep surface.

The **superior laryngeal artery** passes superficial to the inferior constrictor muscle and pierces the thyrohyoid membrane, accompanied by the internal laryngeal nerve, to serve the larynx.

The **cricothyroid branch** is a small vessel that courses along the cricothyroid ligament supplying the same-named muscle and its vicinity. The terminal branches of the superior thyroid artery are discussed later in this chapter in relation to the thyroid gland.

Ascending Pharyngeal Artery

The ascending pharyngeal artery is the smallest branch of the external carotid artery (Fig. 7-12). It arises on the medial aspect of that artery, shortly after the bifurcation of the common carotid, and ascends between the internal carotid and the pharynx. The ascending pharyngeal artery has unnamed muscular branches to the prevertebral muscles, as well as branches supplying additional structures in its vicinity.

This artery has three named branches: the **pharyngeal**, distributing to some muscles of the pharynx and soft palate; the **meningeal**, entering the cranium via several foraminae to vascularize the meninges and bone; and the **inferior tympanic**, supplying the tympanic cavity.

Lingual Artery

The lingual artery often arises in common with the facial artery, then becoming the faciolingual artery (Fig. 7-12). The lingual artery arises near the posterior tip of the greater cornu of the hyoid bone, passes deep to the hypoglossal nerve, then between the middle constrictor and hyoglossus muscles, to supply the muscles of the tongue, tonsil, soft palate, epiglottis, floor of the mouth, and sublingual gland. The branches of this artery are described in Chapter 15.

Facial Artery

The facial artery arises just above (or in common with) the lingual artery and ascends deep to the stylohyoid and posterior belly of the digastric muscles to lie in a groove on the posterior aspect of the submandibular gland (Fig. 7-12). The vessel enters the face by crossing the base of the mandible just anterior to the masseter muscle in the groove for the facial artery. Branches of the facial artery in the neck are the ascending palatine, tonsillar, glandular, and submental arteries. Those of the face will be discussed in Chapter 15.

The **ascending palatine artery** originates near the tip of the styloid process. It ascends between that process and the superior constrictor muscle, then between the styloglossus and stylopharyngeus muscles,

to supply the levator veli palatini, the superior constrictor and neighboring muscles, the soft palate, the tonsils, and the auditory tube.

Glandular branches distribute as three or four vessels to the submandibular gland to supply it and the adjacent area.

The **tonsillar artery** passes between the styloglossus and medial pterygoid muscles and pierces the superior constrictor to supply the palatine tonsil and the posterior tongue.

The **submental artery** arises from the facial artery near the anterior border of the masseter. It follows the base of the mandible anteriorly and turns onto the chin at the anterior border of the depressor anguli oris muscle. The artery supplies muscles it encounters along its passage and anastomoses with several arteries in its vicinity.

Occipital Artery

The occipital artery originates on the posterior aspect of the external carotid artery, just opposite the origin of the facial artery (Fig. 7-12). It passes deep to the hypoglossal nerve and posterior belly of the digastric muscle, lodges in the groove for the occipital artery on the medial aspect of the mastoid process, and passes between the splenius capitis and semispinalis capitis muscles, to serve the back of the head. Branches of the occipital artery are the sternocleidomastoid, mastoid, auricular, muscular, descending, meningeal, and occipital.

The **sternocleidomastoid** branches supply the same-named muscle as two vessels, an upper and a lower branch.

The **mastoid branch** is a small vessel that traverses the mastoid foramen to supply the mastoid air cells and the dura mater in its vicinity.

The **auricular branch** vascularizes the back of the auricle.

Muscular branches of the occipital artery distribute to the digastric, stylohyoid, and splenius capitis muscles.

The **descending branch** serves the muscles of the back of the neck.

Meningeal branches gain entrance to the cranial vault via the condylar and jugular foramina and vascularize the dura and the bones of the posterior cranial fossa.

Occipital branches of the occipital artery distribute in the company of the greater occipital nerve to serve the muscles and tissues of the scalp. Small branches may pass through the parietal foramen to supply the parietal meninges.

Posterior Auricular Artery

The posterior auricular artery is a small branch arising deep to the parotid gland, where it passes between the mastoid process and the cartilaginous external auditory tube.

It vascularizes the parotid gland and the sternocleidomastoid, stylohyoid, and digastric muscles. In addition, the posterior auricular artery has three named branches—the stylomastoid, auricular, and occipital arteries—which are discussed in Chapter 11.

Maxillary and Superficial Temporal Arteries

The maxillary and superficial temporal arteries are the two terminal branches of the external carotid artery. The former and its branches are responsible for the vascularization of the deep face, whereas the latter serves the region of the temple and much of the scalp. These two arteries are discussed in Chapter 8.

Internal Jugular Vein

Summary Bite. The internal jugular vein originates at the jugular foramen and receives blood from the brain, face, and neck on its way to the brachiocephalic vein. It descends in the neck within the carotid sheath.

The internal jugular vein is the main vessel responsible for collecting blood from the brain, the superficial aspects of the face, and the neck. The vessel extends from its dilated origin, the superior bulb housed in the jugular foramen, to its inferior dilation, the inferior bulb terminating in the brachiocephalic vein (Figs. 7-10 and 7-12).

The internal jugular vein is enclosed in the carotid sheath as it travels the length of the neck, and its tributaries pierce this fascia to deliver their blood to the vessel. The internal jugular vein receives blood from the following tributaries: dural venous sinus drainage from within the cranium; the facial vein from the superficial face; the lingual vein from the tongue and floor of the mouth; the pharyngeal, superior, and middle thyroid, and occasionally the occipital veins from the neck.

The pharyngeal and occipital tributaries are treated presently, whereas the remaining vessels are discussed in later chapters. The **pharyngeal veins** arise as small vessels from a plexus of veins, the **pharyngeal venous plexus**, located on the wall of the pharynx. The pharyngeal veins empty into the internal jugular vein in the vicinity of the hyoid bone.

The **occipital vein** arises from the venous network serving the scalp, perforates the fibers of insertion of the trapezius, and enters the suboccipital triangle. Here it empties its contents into a plexus of veins, tributaries of the vertebral and deep cervical veins. Occasionally, the occipital vein, accompanying the same-named artery, travels along the posterior base of the skull to empty into the internal jugular vein or, less frequently, into the posterior auricular vein.

Thyroid Gland

Summary Bite. The thyroid gland is located in the midline of the neck, between the infrahyoid muscles and the thyroid and cricoid cartilages and part of the trachea. It possesses a right and a left lobe connected by an isthmus. The gland is richly vascularized by branches of the external carotid and subclavian, arteries, and occasionally by a branch from the brachiocephalic trunk of the aortic arch. Venous drainage eventually reaches the internal jugular vein.

The **thyroid gland**, an endocrine organ lying deep to the infrahyoid muscles, is situated anteriorly in the neck, partly encircling the superior aspect of the trachea, the cricoid cartilage, and the thyroid cartilage (Figs. 7-10 and 7-12).

Clinical Considerations

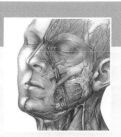

External Jugular Vein

The **external jugular vein** may be used as a venous manometer because in a supine patient the venous blood pressure is not high enough to engorge this vessel much above the clavicle. During failure of the right side of the heart, constriction of the superior venae cavae and increased pressure in the thorax induces a pressure buildup in the venous side of the circulatory system, and this is evidenced by engorgement of the external jugular vein.

Under severe conditions, the vessel may be filled as high as the base of the mandible. This extremely important sign should be recognized by dental professionals using reclining chairs in their practice; the patient should be referred immediately for possible cardiac care.

Clinical Considerations

Thyroid Gland Involvements

Goiter is an abnormal enlargement of the thyroid gland. The incidence of goiter is greater in females than in males.

Occasionally, the enlargement of the thyroid is in an inferior direction, and the condition is referred to as intrathoracic goiter. In this condition, the thyroid physically presses on the trachea and causes breathing difficulties.

Goiter has other serious effects, mainly the overproduction of thyroid hormone. In such a hyperthyroid condition there is a loss of weight, lack of heat tolerance, diarrhea, muscle weakness accompanied by trembling of the upper extremity, insomnia, and exophthalmos. The last condition could be extremely serious, for severe exophthalmos could damage the cornea due to the inability of the eyelids to accommodate the protruded eye, causing drying out of that structure. Exophthalmos may also stretch and damage the optic nerve to the point of blindness.

Hypothyroidism is a condition caused by a greatly reduced production of thyroid hormone. Although no hormone is produced, excessive amounts of thyroglobulin, which is stored as colloid in the thyroid follicles, greatly enlarges the size of the thyroid gland, causing goiter. The symptoms of hypothyroidism are reduced libido, somnolescence, decreased metabolic rate, decreased heart rate and cardiac output, and myxedema, accumulation of body fluids in the interstitial connective tissues.

Cretinism is a disorder caused by excessive hypothyroid state during early childhood. This condition is characterized by mental retardation and greatly reduced physical stature, especially involving skeletal growth.

Thyroidectomy is a serious procedure. Four major considerations must be kept in mind: parathyroid tetani, external laryngeal nerve, recurrent laryngeal nerve, and thyroid crisis. Because the parathyroid glands are located on the deep surface of the thyroid gland, their presence and vascular supply must be established and the glands must not be extirpated along with the thyroid.

Parathyroid removal is not compatible with life, and accidental parathyroidectomy results in parathyroid tetani, whose symptoms are sudden reduction of plasma calcium levels, increased plasma phosphorus levels, and spasmodic muscular contractions, especially in muscles of the larynx, resulting in respiratory obstruction and death.

During thyroidectomy, the external and recurrent laryngeal nerves must be isolated and protected from damage. These two nerves supply the laryngeal musculature and inappropriate handling could damage them, resulting in postoperative hoarseness and even loss of speech.

Bilateral sectioning of the recurrent laryngeal nerve occasionally may result in dyspnea and, unless surgical intervention ensues, even in death.

A treatment for hyperthyroidism is thyroidectomy. One of the postoperative complications that may arise is known as thyroid storm (thyroid crisis), of which the symptoms are high fever, delirium, cardiac arrhythmia, profuse sweating, vomiting, subsequent dehydration, and, if untreated, death.

It is composed of two lobes, laterally positioned, and a centrally placed isthmus connecting the right and left lobes. Frequently, a pyramidal lobe is present that extends from the left lobe near its junction with the isthmus occasionally as far up as the body of the hyoid bone.

Infrequently, a fibromuscular connection exists between the isthmus of the thyroid gland and the body of the hyoid bone. This is known as the **levator thyroideae**. A similar nonmuscular structure, the remnant of the **thyroglossal duct**, may also be present in this location and may bear accessory thyroid tissue.

The thyroid gland has its own connective tissue capsule that subdivides the lobes into numerous lob-

ules. In addition, the gland is loosely ensheathed by laminae of the pretracheal layer of the deep cervical fascia. This connective tissue layer is pierced by blood vessels, which then ramify on the external surface of the connective tissue capsule of the gland. These vessels subsequently enter the substance of the gland within the connective tissue septa, which subdivides the gland into smaller components.

These smaller components are composed of numerous colloid-filled follicles lined by cuboidal cells. The colloid is composed of iodinated thyroglobulins, the storage form of thyroid hormones.

Thyroid hormones stimulate the rate of cellular oxidation. In addition, small clumps of parafollicular cells (C cells) have been noted in the thyroid gland. These cells are responsible for the formation of calcitonin, a hormone that depresses blood calcium levels.

The blood supply of the thyroid gland is exceedingly rich and is derived from the external carotid arteries, the subclavian arteries, and, occasionally, the single thyroidea ima artery, a branch of the brachiocephalic trunk or of the aortic arch.

Superior Thyroid Artery

The superior thyroid artery is usually the first branch of the external carotid artery. It passes inferiorly along the lateral edge of the thyrohyoid muscle, gives off branches as detailed earlier in this chapter, and reaches the superior pole of the lateral lobe of the thyroid gland, where it divides (Fig. 7-12).

The **anterior branch** follows the superior border of the lateral lobe, distributes to its anterior surface, and anastomoses with the anterior branch of the opposite side across the isthmus.

The **posterior branch** follows a similar course on the deep aspect of the lateral lobe, ramifies on that surface, and anastomoses with the inferior thyroid artery, also supplying the parathyroid gland. Occasionally, a lateral branch is present that supplies the lateral aspect of the lateral lobe.

Inferior Thyroid Artery

Branches of the inferior thyroid artery were discussed earlier in the section dealing with the **subclavian artery** (Fig. 7-10). In this section, only its glandular branches are detailed.

As this artery reaches the thyroid gland and forms numerous branches vascularizing the gland, the recurrent laryngeal branch of the vagus nerve passes between these branches. The inferior thyroid artery has two main glandular branches: the **inferior** (supplying the inferoposterior aspect of the gland), which anastomoses with the posterior branch of the superior thyroid artery, and the **ascending branch**, which vascularizes the parathyroid glands. The **thyroidea ima artery**, a small, inconsistent vessel arising either from the brachiocephalic trunk or from the arch of the aorta, supplies the isthmus of the thyroid.

Venous Drainage

The **superior thyroid vein** is a tributary of the internal jugular vein. Its distribution follows that of the superior thyroid artery, hence it drains the area supplied by that vessel.

The **middle** and **inferior thyroid veins** and, to a certain extent, the superior thyroid veins drain the venous plexus formed on the surface of the thyroid gland. The middle thyroid veins deliver their blood to

the internal jugular vein, whereas the inferior thyroid veins drain into the brachiocephalic veins. Occasionally, the right and left inferior thyroid veins form a single vessel just caudal to the isthmus of the thyroid gland. This is the **thyroidea ima vein**, which joins the left brachiocephalic vein.

Parathyroid Glands

Summary Bite. The small endocrine parathyroid glands, usually four in number, are located on the posterior surface of the lateral lobes of the thyroid gland (two superior, two inferior). Their vascular supply is provided by the parathyroid branches of the thyroid arteries. Removal of the parathyroid glands is not compatible with life.

The parathyroid glands are small, oval endocrine glands that lie on the posterior aspect of the lateral lobes of the thyroid gland. Usually, there are two or more on each lobe of the thyroid gland, the **superior** and **inferior parathyroids**.

They are vascularized by branches of the superior and/or inferior thyroid arteries and drained by the middle and inferior thyroid veins. The glands have two major types of cell populations: the principal (chief) cells and the oxyphil cells. The former produce parathyroid hormone (parathormone), a hormone that elevates blood calcium levels. Complete removal of the parathyroids is incompatible with life because all muscles undergo tetany and death results.

Nerves Observed in the Anterior Triangle

Summary Bite. The nerves present in the anterior cervical triangle include the nerves that supply the muscles within the triangle, the vagus nerve and its branches, as well as the cervical sympathetic trunk and its associated ganglia.

Vagus Nerve

Summary Bite. The vagus nerve (cranial nerve X) leaves the internal aspect of the skull via the jugular foramen and, by way of its ganglia, communicates with other nerves in the neck. It serves the pharynx, the larynx, carotid body, soft palate, and the pharyngeal plexus. As it courses through the neck, the trunk of the nerve lies within the carotid sheath.

The vagus or cranial nerve X is the longest cranial nerve in the body, eventually finding its way into the abdominal cavity. It receives detailed treatment in a subsequent chapter; therefore, only its cervical branches are discussed here. The nerve enters the neck as it leaves the jugular foramen (Fig. 7-13; see Chapter 18). Shortly inferior to this foramen, the nerve

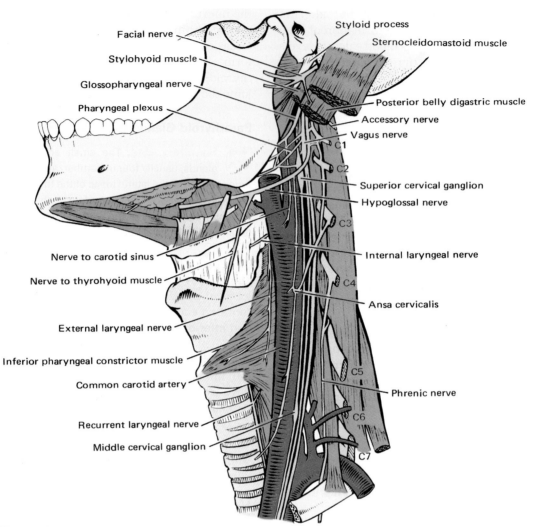

Figure 7-13. Nerve supply to the neck.

Table 7-7	Deep Prevertebral Muscles of the Neck	
Name	**Location**	**Origin**
Longus colli	Anterior surface of vertebral column	Transverse processes of vertebrae C3-T3
Longus capitis	Anterior to longus colli	Transverse processes of vertebrae C3-C6
Rectus capitis anterior	Deep to the longus capitis	Lateral mass and transverse process of the atlas
Rectus capitis lateralis	Just lateral to rectus capitis anterior	Transverse process of atlas

displays a ganglion, the **nodose** or **inferior ganglion**. The vagus communicates with several other nerves through this ganglion.

Branches of the vagus that arise here are:

- **Pharyngeal branches**, which serve the carotid body, pharynx, and some of the soft palate through the pharyngeal plexus.
- **Superior laryngeal nerve**, which bifurcates to form the internal and external laryngeal nerves, which accompany the medial aspect of the internal carotid artery.
- **Internal laryngeal nerve**, which pierces the thyrohyoid membrane in close association with the superior laryngeal branch of the superior thyroid artery to supply the mucous membrane.
- **External laryngeal nerve**, which continues inferiorly, accompanied by the superior thyroid artery. It pierces the inferior pharyngeal constrictor muscle, which it supplies in addition to the cricothyroid muscle, and gives branches to the pharyngeal plexus.
- **Two or three cardiac branches** of the vagus nerve are evident in the neck. These are slender filaments that pass deep to the carotid sheath to ramify in the cardiac plexus.

The **recurrent laryngeal branches** of the vagus differ in their recurring locations on the two sides of the body. On the left side, the nerve originates from the vagus at the aortic arch, makes a hairpin loop around the ligamentum arteriosum, and ascends into the neck in the tracheoesophageal groove. It comes in close contact with the medial aspect of the lateral lobe of the thyroid gland, passes deep to the inferior constrictor, and gains entrance into the larynx, to which it provides sensory and motor innervation.

On the right side of the body, the recurrent laryngeal nerve originates from the vagus at the level of the first part of the subclavian artery, around which it recurs, and ascends in the tracheoesophageal groove. Subsequent to this point, the paths taken by the nerves of the two sides are identical.

Because of the precarious location of the nerve and intimate association with the thyroid gland, surgical procedures involving that gland must include its isolation and strict protection.

Cervical Sympathetic Trunk

Summary Bite. The cervical sympathetic trunk is an extension of the thoracic sympathetic trunk into the neck. The cervical sympathetic trunk possesses three sympathetic ganglia which house postganglionic sympathetic cell bodies. Most postganglionic nerve fibers to the head and neck arise from one of these ganglia.

The cervical sympathetic trunk is the cervical continuation of the thoracic sympathetic trunk (Fig. 7-9; see Chapter 18). It consists of three ganglia connected to each other by short cords. The superior-most of these is the **superior cervical ganglion**, located at the level of the axis and third cervical vertebra. The **middle cervical ganglion**, the smallest of the three, is inconstant and lies at the level of the sixth cervical vertebra. The **inferior cervical ganglion**, located at the level of the seventh cervical vertebra, is often fused with the first (and infrequently with the second and even third) thoracic ganglion, then named the **stellate ganglion**.

The cord intervening between the middle and inferior cervical ganglia splits, forming a loop around the subclavian and occasionally the vertebral arteries. The loop around the subclavian artery is constant and is known as the **ansa subclavia**.

Insertion	Innervation	Action
Transverse processes of vertebrae C5, C6; bodies of vertebrae C2, C3, and C4; and anterior tubercle of atlas	Ventral primary rami of spinal nerves C2-C7	Flexes and rotates neck and bends neck to one side
Basilar part of occipital bone	Ventral primary rami of spinal nerves C1-C3	Flexes the head
Basilar part of occipital bone	Ventral primary rami of spinal nerves C1, C2	Flexes the head
Jugular process of occipital bone	Ventral primary rami of spinal nerves C1-C2	Blends head to one side

Clinical Considerations

Horner Syndrome

During arterial insufficiency of the upper limb, sympathectomy is indicated, whereby the cervical sympathetic trunk is severed. The severance of the sympathetic trunk causes **Horner syndrome**, expressed as the inability to sweat, drooping of the upper eyelid, and constriction of the pupil.

Neurocirculatory compression occurs in an individual when the space between the anterior and middle scalene muscles is reduced in size, thus compressing the subclavian artery and brachial plexus that travel through

this space. Occasionally, the neurocirculatory compression is caused by the presence of a cervical rib or a small slip of muscle, the scalenus minimus, lateral to the anterior scalene. Both of these structures reduce the available space.

The symptoms involved in this syndrome include drooping of the shoulder, pain, paresthesia, or even total lack of sensation and reduced circulation in the upper limb of the affected side.

The cervical sympathetic trunk is embedded in a loose connective tissue layer and positioned between the covering of the prevertebral muscles and the carotid sheath, although often it is located within the deep substance of this structure.

The cervical sympathetic trunk receives no white rami communicantes but does send out gray rami communicantes to each cervical spinal nerve. Preganglionic fibers reach the cervical sympathetic trunk from its thoracic continuation, and these preganglionic fibers synapse in one of these three cervical sympathetic ganglia. Most of the postganglionic fibers of the head and neck originate from these three ganglia.

Superior Cervical Ganglion

The superior cervical ganglion branches into the internal carotid nerve and the pharyngeal branches. The internal carotid nerve arises from the cephalic portion of the ganglion, reaches the internal carotid artery, around which it forms the **carotid plexus**, and travels into the carotid canal to distribute in the cranial cavity.

Communicating branches go to the common and external carotid arteries and distribute to the head. The **pharyngeal branches**, composed of four or more fibers, mingle with branches of cranial nerves IX and X to participate in the formation of the pharyngeal plexus. Other branches also go to some cranial nerves and the cardiac plexus.

Middle Cervical Ganglion

The middle cervical ganglion has three branches, which serve cervical spinal nerves, adjacent viscera, and the cardiac plexus.

Inferior Cervical Ganglion

The inferior cervical ganglion has three branches. **Vertebral branches** are supplied to the vertebral artery, forming the vertebral sympathetic plexus, which serves the head. The other two branches serve lower cervical spinal nerves and supply fibers to the cardiac plexus.

DEEP PREVERTEBRAL MUSCLES OF THE NECK

There are four deep prevertebral muscles of the neck: the longus colli, longus capitis, rectus capitis anterior, and rectus capitis lateralis. These muscles lie deep to the prevertebral fascia, under the floor of the anterior triangle, and function more or less to flex the head and the neck. These muscles are relatively unimportant; hence, their discussion is not warranted. Information concerning their attachments, innervations, and functions is included in Table 7-7.

Superficial Face

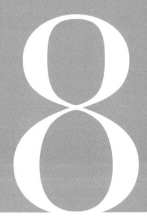

Chapter Outline

Surface Anatomy
Scalp
Muscles
Vascular Supply
Nerve Supply
Clinical Considerations

Face
Muscles
Muscles of the Cheek
Sensory Innervation
Motor Innervation

Blood Supply
Clinical Considerations

Key Terms

Muscles of Facial Expression are unique in that they migrate to their destinations about the scalp, neck, and mostly about the face from second pharyngeal arch mesenchyme and thus receive their motor innervation via the facial nerve (CN VII), the nerve of the second arch. Although most of these muscles originate on bone, most do not insert on bone; rather, they insert into the dermis of the skin and freely intermingle with muscles in their vicinity. Upon contraction, this arrangement and groupings of muscles about the orifices of the face convey movements about these orifices that we interpret as emotions.

Scalp is composed of thick skin normally covered with hair and overlies the eight bones of the cranium. A fibroadipose hy-

podermis overlies the epicranius muscle composed of two bellies with an intervening fibrous connecting sheet, the galea aponeurotica. Deep to this sheet is a facial cleft considered the "danger space" of the scalp. Deep to this is the pericranium—a periostal—covering the bones of the cranial vault. Deep to the skin are the anteriorly positioned frontalis muscle originating from certain muscles of the face and the posteriorly positioned occipitalis muscle originating from the skull bones. Both of these muscles insert into the galea aponeurotica. Because these muscles arise from the second pharyngeal arch they are innervated by the facial nerve (CN VII).

Sensory Innervation of the Superficial Face is provided by all three divisions of

the trigeminal nerve (CN V); thus, the skin of the face is highly sensitive. The ophthalmic division (V_1) serves the forehead and the superior rim of the orbit, upper eyelid, and upper regions and side of the nose. The maxillary division (V_2) serves the inferior rim of the orbit, side of the nose, cheek, and upper lip. The mandibular division (V_3) serves the chin, cheek, the lower lip area about the temporomandibular joint (TMJ), and part of the anterior surface of and about the ear and most of the temple. Additionally, much of the ear and the area about the mandibular ramus are supplied by branches of the cervical plexus. It is to be noted that there is considerable overlap by these branches, thus contributing to the high degree of sensitivity of the face.

Surface Anatomy of the Face includes the 14 bones of the skull making up the face. These bones are overlaid with an assortment of facial muscles, connective tissue, and skin.

The Face Is Highly Vascularized, receiving its vascular supply from several sources. These include branches arising either directly or indirectly from primary branches of the external carotid artery, and from branches arising from the internal carotid artery, namely, the ophthalmic artery. The terminals of these branches form extensive anastomotic networks throughout the face. Because of this fact, facial bleeding is often difficult to control.

Because veins of the face do not possess valves, blood within these vessels may flow in either direction, which provides possible routes for infection about the face, especially the "triangular danger zone of the face." Thus, veins of the face may communicate with the pharyngeal venous plexus of the deep face, which may communicate with the cavernous sinus within the skull. Because of these communications, infections about the face can be very dangerous and life-threatening.

SURFACE ANATOMY

Summary Bite. The eight bones comprising the skeleton of the face are covered by muscles, connective tissue, and skin. The muscles, known as muscles of facial expression, are innervated by the facial nerve because they arise from the second pharyngeal arch.

The bony structures of the skull are overlaid by muscles, connective tissue, and skin that give a characteristic morphology to the face. The facial skeleton, discussed in Chapter 6, may be palpated easily because the overlying soft tissue is very thin over much of its surface.

The mental protuberance can easily be palpated at the chin, as can the body, angle, and ramus of the mandible. The mandibular articulation can be emphasized by repeated opening and closing of the mouth. Proceeding anterosuperiorly from this articulation, the zygomatic arch and zygoma (the prominent portion of the cheek) can be palpated.

The zygomatic bone also forms the lateral and part of the inferior rim of the orbit. The remainder of the inferior rim is formed by the maxilla, whose inferior extent houses the upper dental arch, evident on smiling. Immediately superior to the philtrum of the lip is the fleshy and cartilaginous bulb of the nose. The flexible cartilaginous bridge of the nose becomes immobile near the nasal bones, which lead to the root of the nose, positioned between the two orbits.

Above the superior rim of the orbit, deep to the eyebrows, is the superciliary ridge of the frontal bone, and the forehead is marked by the frontal eminences. The cranium is covered by the scalp and the face is usually considered to be bounded by the anterior hairline of the scalp, the posterior border of the ramus, and the inferior border of the body of the mandible.

SCALP

Summary Bite. The scalp covers the bones of the calvaria and is composed of thick skin and a fibroadipose hypodermis. Deep to this soft tissue is the pericranium, the periosteal covering of the bones which is loosely attached except at the bony sutures.

The scalp is composed of a thick covering of skin and its attending fibroadipose hypodermis overlying the **epicranius** or **occipitofrontalis muscle** with its intervening **galea aponeurotica**, a thick, fibrous aponeurotic connecting sheet. Deep to this sheet is a fascial cleft containing a loose type of connective tissue often considered the "danger space" of the scalp. This tissue separates the aponeurotic sheet from the **pericranium**, the periosteal covering of the bones constituting the vault of the skull. The pericranium is only loosely attached to the underlying hard tissue, except at the sutures, where it is firmly anchored to the intrasutural material.

The vascular and nerve supply of the scalp is tightly bound to the subcutaneous connective tissue, traveling between the muscular aponeurotic layer and the skin.

Muscles

Epicranius Muscle

Summary Bite. The frontalis muscle originates from certain muscles of the face, whereas the occipitalis muscle originates from bones at the base of the calvaria. These two muscles are connected to each other by the intervening tendinous glea aponeurotica.

The **epicranius muscle** is composed of two bellies, the frontalis and the occipitalis, connected to each other by a tendinous aponeurosis, **galea aponeurotica**, whose collagen fibers run in an anteroposterior direction (Fig. 8–1 and Table 8-1).

The **frontalis** is the larger and somewhat fleshier muscle and is not attached to bone. Its fibers originate from the superficial muscles of the orbit and nose (corrugator, procerus, and orbicularis oculi) and insert into the galea aponeurotica somewhat anterior to the coronal suture.

The **occipitalis** originates from bony landmarks—the mastoid process of the temporal bone and the lateral portion of the superior nuchal line of the occipital bone—to insert into the posterior aspect of the galea aponeurotica.

Temporoparietalis

Summary Bite. The temporomarietalis muscle, located on the side of the scalp, is attached to the frontalis and to the auricular muscles of the ear.

The temporoparietalis is a muscle of variable size extending between the frontal belly of the epicranius and the anterior and superior auricular muscles of the ear.

The frontalis and the temporoparietalis muscles are both innervated by the temporal branch of the facial nerve, whereas the occipitalis receives its innervation via the posterior auricular branch of the facial nerve.

These three muscles acting together furrow the forehead, raise the eyebrows, and widen the eyes. The frontal belly acting by itself raises the eyebrow and the temporoparietalis raises the ear.

Vascular Supply

Summary Bite. Blood supply to the scalp arises from two major sources: branches of the external carotid artery and branches from the internal carotid arteries.

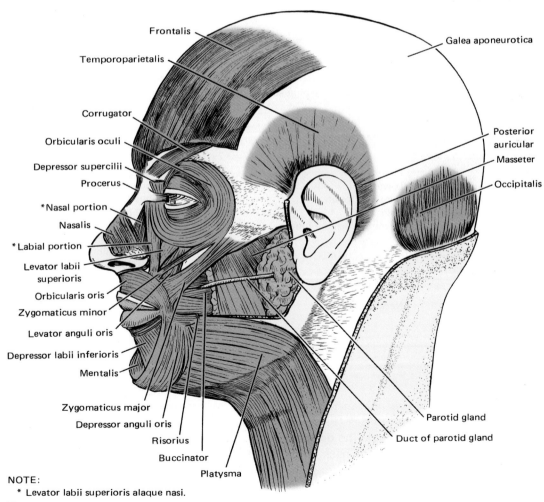

NOTE:
* Levator labii superioris alaque nasi.

Figure 8-1. Muscles of facial expression.

Table 8-1 Muscles of the Face and Scalp

Muscle	Location	Origin
Scalp		
Frontalis	Forehead	Procerus, corrugator, orbicularis oculi
Occipitalis	Back of the head	Mastoid process and superior nuchal line
Temporoparietalis	Temple	Temporal fascia
Ear		
Auricularis anterior	Anterior to ear	Temporal fascia
Auricularis superior	Above ear	Temporal fascia
Auricularis posterior	Behind ear	Mastoid process
Nose		
Procerus	Bony bridge of nose	Fascia of nasal bone
Nasalis	Cartilaginous bridge and wing of nose	Maxilla and alar cartilage
Depressor septi	Lateral to the philtrum	Maxilla
Eye		
Orbicularis oculi	Around the orbit	Nasal process of frontal bone, frontal process of maxilla, medial palpebral ligament, and lacrimal bone
Corrugator	Deep to the orbicularis oculi	Medial aspect of superciliary arch
Mouth		
Levator labii superioris	Upper lip	Zygoma and maxilla just above infraorbital foramen
Levator labii superioris alaque nasi	Upper lip and side of nose	Maxilla, frontal process
Levator anguli oris	Corner of mouth	Canine fossa of maxilla
Zygomaticus major	Cheek and corner of mouth	Temporal process of zygoma
Zygomaticus minor	Cheek and corner of mouth	Maxillary process of zygoma
Risorius	Cheek	Masseteric fascia
Depressor labii inferioris	Lower lip	Oblique line of mandible
Depressor anguli oris	Corner of mouth	Oblique line of mandible
Mentalis	Chin	Incisive fossa of mandible
Orbicularis oris	Circumscribes the mouth	Muscles in the vicinity, maxilla, nasal septum, mandible
Buccinator	Cheek	Pterygomandibular raphe, alveola arches of mandible and maxilla
Neck		
Platysma	Neck and chin	Pectoral and deltoid fascia

Arterial supply to the scalp consists of branches from the external and internal carotid arteries (Fig. 8-2). Branches of the external carotid include the **occipital artery**, supplying the medial aspect of the back of the scalp; the **posterior auricular artery**, supplying the area behind and above the ear; and the **superficial temporal artery**, which vascularizes the lateral aspect of the scalp.

Two branches of the internal carotid artery responsible for vascularization of the anterosuperior aspect of the scalp are the **supraorbital** and **supratrochlear arteries**. Both arteries leave the orbit and ascend over the forehead, supplying it and the top of the scalp.

All of the vessels supplying the scalp freely anastomose with each other. Venous drainage accompanies the arteries, and the vessels are named accordingly.

Insertion	Innervation (Branch of VII)	Action
Galea aponeurotica	Temporal	Wrinkles forehead and raises eyebrow
Galea aponeurotica	Posterior auricular	Tightens the scalp
Galea aponeurotica	Temporal	Elevates the ear
Anterior part of major helix of ear	Temporal	Pulls auricle forward and up
Superior aspect of ear	Temporal	Pulls auricle up
Posteroinferior aspect of ear	Posterior auricular	Pulls auricle back
Dermis above glabella	Buccal	Depresses eyebrows medially
Dermis of nose across bridge and on bulb	Buccal	Dilates nares
Septum and ala of nose	Buccal	Constricts nares
Lateral palpebral raphe, frontalis muscle, corrugator muscle, superior and inferior tarsi	Temporal and zygomatic	Closes the eye
Dermis covering the supraorbital foramen	Temporal and zygomatic	Forms vertical wrinkles between eyebrows
Upper lip	Buccal	Elevates upper lip
Upper lip and alar cartilage	Buccal	Dilates nares and elevates upper lip
Corner of mouth	Buccal	Lifts corner of mouth
Corner of mouth	Buccal	Lifts corner of mouth
Upper lip medial to corner of mouth	Buccal	Elevates upper lip
Corner of mouth	Buccal and mandibular	Draws corner of mouth laterally
Lower lip	Mandibular and buccal	Depresses lower lip
Corner of mouth	Mandibular and buccal	Depresses corner of mouth
Dermis of skin	Mandibular and buccal	Wrinkles chin and protrudes lower lip
Dermis of the lips and surrounding muscles	Buccal	Closes, purses, and protrudes lips
Muscles of the mouth	Buccal	Compresses cheek
Inferior border of body of mandible, skin of face	Cervical	Depresses mandible, corner of mouth, and lower lip

Nerve Supply

Summary Bite. Cutaneous branches of the third cervical and greater occipital nerves serve the posterior scalp, whereas the lateral scalp is served by the auriculotemporal and zyogmaticotemporal nerves. The anterior scalp is served by the supraorbital and supratemporal nerves.

The cutaneous nerves of the scalp follow the main vascular elements (Fig. 8-3). The posterior aspect of the scalp is served by the third occipital and greater occipital nerves. Laterally, the scalp receives its cutaneous innervation via the lesser occipital and auriculotemporal nerves, posterior and anterior to the ear, respectively.

The region in the vicinity of the temple is supplied by the zygomaticotemporal nerve, and the forehead and midline of the scalp are served by the supraorbital and supratrochlear nerves.

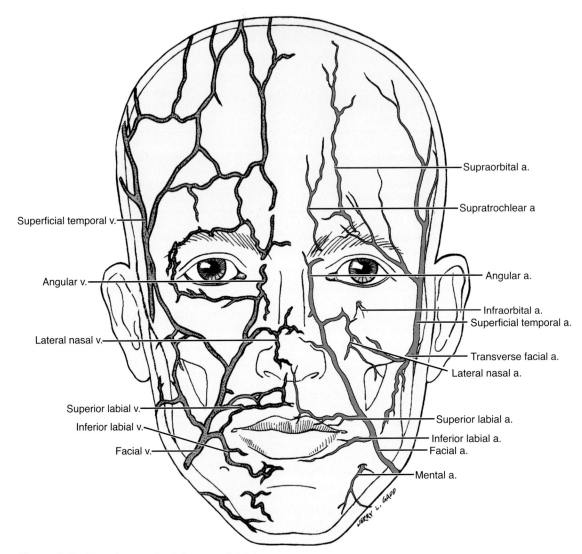

Figure 8-2. Vascular supply of the superficial face.

Clinical Considerations

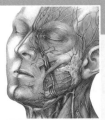

Scalp

Bleeding in the scalp is extremely difficult to stop and is dangerous. The blood supply is extensive and the vessels pass through fibrous septa of the superficial fascia, which mechanically inhibit vessel contraction.

Hemorrhage in this region has a tendency to be contained in the loose connective tissue, the subaponeurotic layer, deep to the galea aponeurotica. Furthermore, infection may result in a localized abscess that, having no outlet to the surface, may enter the valveless emissary veins of this region, also known as the "danger zone of the scalp," and travel to the diplöe and/or the dural venous sinuses. Such infection may result in osteomyelitis, thrombosis, and possibly death.

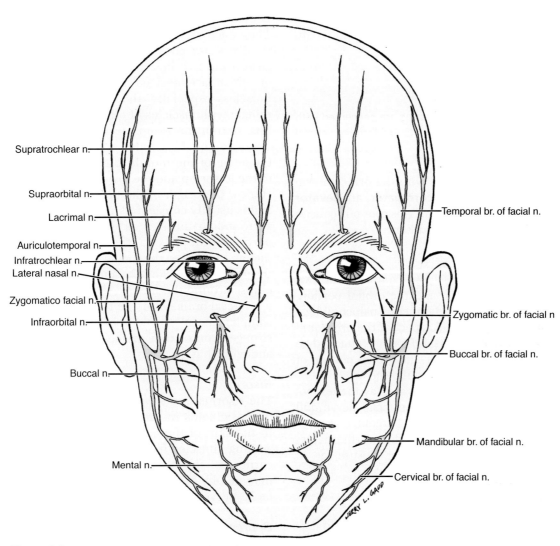

Figure 8-3. Nerve supply of the superficial face.

FACE

Muscles

Summary Bite. Muscles of the face and scalp develop from the second pharyngeal arch and, consequently, receive their motor innervation from the facial nerve (CN VII), the nerve of the second pharyngeal arch.

The muscles of the face (and scalp) are derived from the second pharyngeal arch (hyoid arch) mesenchyme that migrates to its final destination (Fig. 8-1). Considering the origin of these muscles, it is not surprising that they receive motor innervation from branches of the facial nerve (CN VII).

Rather than inserting into bone, these muscles insert into the dermis of the skin, thus their orchestrated

contractions convey various shapes to the face that we interpret as emotions. It is important to understand that fascicles of these muscles intermingle with each other, and they tend to act in groups to control the orifices around which they are grouped, such as the orbit, nose, and mouth. It is according to this grouping that they are described.

Muscles of the Ear and Nose

Summary Bite. Auricular muscles attach to and are capable of moving the external ear but are not often used and thus lose their tone. Three separate muscles of the nose are capable of flaring the nostrils, depressing the eyebrows, and constricting the nares.

The three external muscles of the ear are the **auricularis anterior**, **superior**, and **posterior**. Similarly, the three muscles of the nose are the **procerus**, **nasalis**, and **depressor septi**. These two groups of muscles are fairly inconsequential; pertinent information concerning them is found in Table 8-1.

Muscles Surrounding the Orbit

Summary Bite. Three muscles are concerned with opening and closing the eyelids and forming vertical wrinkles between the eyebrows.

The three muscles concerned with the orifice of the eye are the **orbicularis oculi**, **corrugator**, and **levator palpebrae superioris**. The last of this group is considered in the Chapter 10, Eye and Ear.

Orbicularis Oculi

The orbicularis oculi muscle is composed of two parts, the palpebral portion and the orbital portion. The former originates from the medial palpebral ligament (attached to the medial aspect of the orbit) and inserts into the lateral palpebral raphe (attached to the lateral aspect of the orbit). The orbital portion of the muscle describes an oval around the orbit.

The orbicularis oculi is innervated by the temporal and zygomatic branches of the facial nerve and acts to close the eyelid completely. Forceful closure is mediated by the orbital portion, whereas the palpebral portion is responsible for light closure, as in blinking.

Corrugator

The corrugator (supercilii) muscle is located deep to the superomedial aspect of the orbicularis oculi, at the medial aspect of the eyebrow. It originates at the medial extent of the superciliary arch and inserts into the skin of the eyebrow.

It is innervated by the temporal and zygomatic branches of the facial nerve; the combined actions of the paired muscles approximate the eyebrows, producing frowns.

Muscles Surrounding the Mouth

Summary Bite. Muscles functioning around the mouth include those elevating the upper lip as well as dilating the nares, lifting and depressing the corners of the mouth, depressing the lower lip, drawing corners of the mouth laterally, protruding the lower lip, and closing, pursing, and protruding the lips.

The muscles of the mouth act to alter the shape of the orifice. Their fibers of insertion intermingle with each other; therefore, they share a commonality of action and almost always act in concert.

Orbicularis Oris

The orbicularis oris completely encircles the mouth. Its fibers are positioned at various depths and angles in the two lips. Fascicles of this muscle, some of which are derived from those of neighboring muscles—especially the buccinator—freely intermingle with fascicles of other muscles acting on the lips, permitting extensive movability. Many of the fibers of the buccinator cross over each other at the angle of the mouth so the upper fibers proceed to the lower lip and the lower fibers to the upper lip. Hence, the origin of the orbicularis oris is complex and is usually considered to be from the fibers of the surrounding muscles as well as from the alveolar portion of the maxilla, the septum of the nose, and the area lateral to the incisive fossa of the mandible. Insertion is into the skin and into itself, forming an ellipse around the mouth.

Buccal branches of the facial nerve innervate this complex muscle, which closes the lips and, during stronger contraction, purses them, as in osculation and whistling.

Risorius

The risorius is a small, horizontally placed muscle that originates in the masseteric fascia and inserts in the skin of the corner of the mouth. This is the smiling muscle; it is responsible for drawing the corners of the mouth laterally. The risorius is innervated by buccal and mandibular branches of the facial nerve.

Depressors of the Lip

The **depressor labii inferioris** is quadrangular in shape. It originates on the medial extent of the oblique line of the mandible and inserts into the skin of the lower lip. It acts to depress the lower lip.

The **depressor anguli oris (triangularis)** originates on the oblique line of the mandible and inserts into the skin of the corner of the mouth and depresses it, expressing sadness.

The **mentalis** is a small muscle of the chin. Its origin is in the incisive fossa of the mandible, and it inserts into the skin of the chin to wrinkle it and also to protrude the lower lip, as in drinking.

The **platysma** was previously detailed in Chapter 7. All of the muscles of this group, except the platysma, are innervated by the buccal and mandibular branches of the facial nerve.

Elevators of the Lip

Five muscles elevate the lip and corner of the mouth. The **levator labii superioris alaque nasi** is the most medial of these muscles, originating from the frontal process of the maxilla passing inferiorly along the side of the nose. It then splits into a medial and a lateral portion to insert into the wing of the nose and into the upper lip. This muscle functions in dilating the nostril and raising the upper lip.

The **levator labii superioris** originates from the maxilla and zygoma just inferior to the orbit. Its fibers pass across the infraorbital foramen to insert into the upper lip, lateral to and intermingling with the fibers of the levator labii superioris alaque nasi. The levator labii superioris elevates and protrudes the upper lip.

The **levator anguli oris** lies deep to the levator labii superioris. It originates below the infraorbital foramen, from the canine fossa of the maxilla, to insert into the corner of the mouth. This muscle elevates the angle of the mouth and assists in the formation of the nasolabial furrow.

The **zygomaticus minor**, a slender muscle arising from the maxillary process of the zygomatic bone, inserts just lateral to the insertion of the levator labii superioris muscle. This muscle elevates the upper lip. It also assists in the formation of the nasolabial furrow.

The **zygomaticus major** is the lateral-most muscle of this group. It originates on the temporal process of the zygomatic bone and inserts into the corner of the mouth. This muscle elevates the corner of the mouth and pulls it laterally.

All of the five muscles acting to elevate the lips are innervated by the buccal branches of the facial nerve.

Muscle of the Cheek

The **buccinator**, a quadrangule-shaped muscle occupying the space between the mandible and the maxilla, is the primary muscular component of the cheek. It lies deep to the muscles of facial expression and is separated from them by the buccopharyngeal facia and the buccal fat pad. The parotid duct pierces the substance of this muscle to enter the oral vestibule.

The buccinator originates on the maxilla and mandible, specifically on the buccal surfaces of the alveolar processes in the vicinity of the three molars, and from the **pterygomandibular raphe**, a collagenous tendinous inscription attached to the pterygoid hamulus and the mylohyoid line of the mandible. This raphe is interposed between the buccinator and superior pharyngeal constrictor muscles.

The buccinator inserts into the fleshy corner of the lip in such a fashion that the upper fascicles and the lower fascicles decussate at the corner of the mouth and insert into the lower and upper lips, respectively, becoming fibers of the orbicularis oris. The highest and lowest fascicles, however, continue without decussation into the upper and lower lips, respectively.

The buccinator muscle acts to press the mucosa of the cheek against the teeth, thus aiding in mastication and deglutition. In addition, it assists in distending the oral vestibule and forcefully expelling air, as in blowing dust particles off a surface. The buccal branch of the facial nerve innervates this muscle.

Sensory Innervation

Summary Bite. Sensory innervation to the face is supplied by all three divisions of the trigeminal nerve (CNV). Additionally, areas about the mandibular ramus and the ears are served by sensory branches of the cervical plexus.

Sensory innervation of the greater part of the face is mediated by branches of the ophthalmic, maxillary, and mandibular divisions of the trigeminal nerve (Fig. 8-3; see Chapter 18).

In addition, the region superficial to the angle of the mandible, the posterior aspect of the inferior portion of the ramus, and most of the ear are supplied by the great auricular and, to a lesser extent, the lesser occipital branches of the cervical plexus, as discussed in Chapter 7.

The branches of the trigeminal nerve supplying sensory innervation to the superficial face follow:

Ophthalmic (V$_1$): lacrimal, supraorbital, supratrochlear, infratrochlear, external nasal
Maxillary (V$_2$): infraorbital, zygomaticofacial, zygomaticotemporal
Mandibular (V$_3$): auriculotemporal, buccal, mental

Ophthalmic Division (V$_1$)

Summary Bite. The ophthalmic division (V$_1$) of the trigeminal nerve enters the face through the orbit as several branches to provide sensation for the upper eyelid and the region superior and lateral to the orbit. Another branch exits the lower rim of the orbit to serve the eyelids and the area about the face and side of the nose.

The **lacrimal nerve** leaves the superolateral aspect of the orbit as the palpebral branch and enters the upper eyelid to distribute to the lateral half of that structure and the conjunctiva of the eye. The frontal nerve bifurcates in the orbit to form the **supraorbital** and **supratrochlear nerves** (Fig. 8-13; see Chapter 18).

The supraobital nerve leaves the orbit via the supraornbital foramen (or notch) after supplying a branch to the frontal sinus. The supratrochlear nerve passes superior to the trochlea and leaves the orbit medial to the supraorbital foramen. These two nerves supply sensation to the upper eyelid, the conjunctiva, and the medial half of the forehead and scalp.

The **infratrochlear nerve**, a branch of the nasociliary nerve, leaves the orbit by passing between the middle palpebral ligament of the eye and trochlea to innervate the medial half of the eyelids, the medial angle of the eye, and the side of the nose.

The **external nasal nerve**, a branch of the anterior ethmoidal branch of the nasociliary nerve, leaves the nasal cavity at the distal end of the nasal bone. This nerve provides sensation to the middle of the bridge and part of the ala of the nose.

Maxillary Division (V₂)

> **Summary Bite.** The maxillary division (V₂) of the trigeminal nerve enters the face via the infraorbital foramen, providing sensation to the skin of the lower eyelid, nose, upper lip, and mucosa of the labial vestibule.

The **infraorbital nerve** is a continuation of the maxillary division of the trigeminal nerve. After coursing through the floor of the orbit, the **infraorbital nerve** enters the face via the infraorbital foramen, where it forms a tuft of nerves that may be categorized into three groups: inferior palpebral branches, serving the skin of the lower eyelid and conjunctiva; external nasal branches, providing sensory innervation to the side and mobile septum of the nose; and superior labial branches, supplying the upper lip and mucosa of the superior labial vestibule (Figs. 8-3 and 8-4; see Chapter 18).

The zygomatic branch of the maxillary division of the trigeminal nerve bifurcates to form the **zygomaticotemporal** and **zygomaticofacial nerves**. The former enters the superficial face a little superior to the zygomatic arch and supplies sensation to the region of the temple. The latter emerges in the superficial face by way of the zygomaticofacial foramen to serve the skin over the zygomatic bone.

Mandibular Division (V₃)

> **Summary Bite.** The mandibular division (V₃) of the trigeminal nerve provides sensation via several branches to the temporomandibular articulation, the anterior aspect of and about the ear, skin of the temple, skin over the cheek, buccal vestibule and gingival to the corner of the mouth, chin, lower lip and oral vestibule, and the mandibular teeth and supporting tissues.

The **auriculotemporal nerve** is a branch of the posterior trunk of the mandibular division of the trigeminal nerve (Figs. 8-3 and 8-4; see Chapter 18). It appears in the superficial face just behind the temporomandibular articulation, where it gives rise to the anterior auricular branches serving the anterolateral surface of the ear, and superficial temporal branches to the region of the temple up to the coronal suture.

The **buccal nerve** lies on the surface of the buccinator muscle as it emerges from beneath the masseter muscle. The buccal nerve provides sensation to the cheek and, on piercing the buccinator muscle, supplies sensation to the mucosa of the buccal vestibule and buccal surfaces of the gingivae as far anteriorly as the corner of the mouth.

The **mental nerve** enters the superficial face via the mental foramen of the mandible to serve the chin, the lower lip, and the surrounding mucosa of the oral vestibule.

Motor Innervation

> **Summary Bite.** The muscles of facial expression are derived embryologically from the second pharyngeal arch, and thus receive motor innervation from the facial nerve (CN VII), the nerve of that arch.

Facial Nerve VII

The facial nerve, the nerve of the second pharyngeal arch, leaves the cranial cavity via the internal acoustic meatus and travels in the temporal bone along with the vestibulocochlear nerve. After separating from the vestibulocochlear nerve and giving several branches within the temporal bone, it emerges through the stylomastoid foramen (Figs. 8-3, 8-4, and 11-1; see Chapter 18).

A **posterior auricular branch** arises from the trunk, then passes posterior to the ear on its way to innervate the occipitalis and posterior auricular muscles.

The main stem of the facial nerve then supplies fibers to the stylohyoid muscle and the posterior belly of the digastric muscle before entering the deep aspect of the parotid gland. Here it subdivides into the temporofacial and cervicofacial divisions, which combine to form a loop within the substance of the parotid gland.

It is from this loop that the five terminal branches of the parotid plexus arise to supply motor fibers to the muscles of facial expression (Fig. 8-4 and Table 8-2).

Temporal branches, the superior-most of these, supply the muscles in the region of the temple and part of the forehead.

Zygomatic branches fan out to serve muscles in the area of the prominence of the cheek to the lateral angle of the eye.

Buccal branches, the largest of all the branches and serving the greatest area, course across the masseter and buccinator muscles to innervate muscles of the upper lip and nose.

Mandibular branches pass deep to the depressor anguli oris and platysma. Although there is no

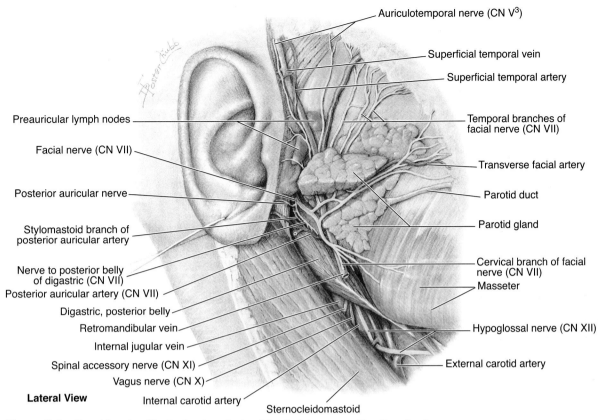

Figure 8-4. Parotid region illustrating terminals of the facial nerve exiting the gland.

universal agreement, most anatomists believe the buccal branches assist the mandibular branches in supplying the muscles of the lower lip.

Cervical branches pass deep to and innervate the platysma muscle.

Blood Supply

The face is a very vascular region because it receives its blood supply from the external carotid artery and its major branches. Additional blood is received from branches of the internal carotid artery.

Table 8-2	Branches of the Facial Nerve in the Superficial Face
Branches*	Muscles Innervated
Temporal	Auricularis anterior; auricularis superior; frontalis; orbicularis oculi; corrugator
Zygomatic	Orbicularis oculi; corrugator
Buccal	Procerus; nasalis; depressor septi; zygomaticus major; zygomaticus minor; levator labii superioris; levator anguli oris; levator labii superioris alaeque nasi; risorius; orbicularis oris; buccinator
Mandibular	Depressor anguli oris; depressor labii inferioris mentalis; risorius
Cervical	Platysma

*Because of individual variation, there is disagreement regarding innervation to the muscles of facial expression, especially those surrounding the mouth. In many instances, buccal branches assist mandibular branches in innervating the muscles surrounding the lower lip.

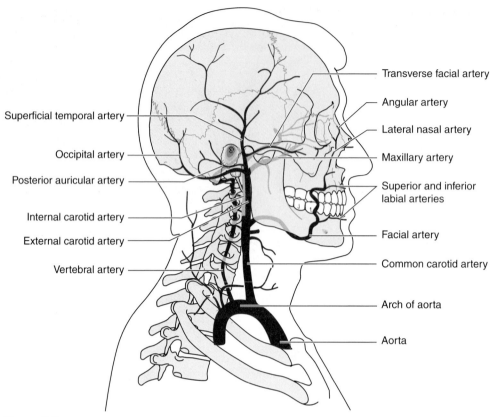

Figure 8-5. Arteries of the head and neck.

The labels in the figure are:
- Transverse facial artery
- Angular artery
- Lateral nasal artery
- Maxillary artery
- Superior and inferior labial arteries
- Facial artery
- Common carotid artery
- Arch of aorta
- Aorta
- Superficial temporal artery
- Occipital artery
- Posterior auricular artery
- Internal carotid artery
- External carotid artery
- Vertebral artery

Arterial Supply

Summary Bite. Arterial blood supply to the face is provided by smaller branches of primary branches of the external and internal carotid arteries (Fig. 8-5). Anastomotic networks form over much of the area, ensuring that the face has a very rich blood supply.

Vascular supply of the superficial face is derived from branches directly or indirectly arising from the external carotid artery as well as from branches of the ophthalmic artery, a branch of the internal carotid artery.

Terminal branches of these vessels form an extensive anastomotic network permeating the superficial aspect of the face. Some of these vessels travel with like-named nerves, and their distribution follows that of their nerve counterparts.

Facial Artery

The facial artery is a branch of the external carotid artery; its cervical branches were described earlier. This artery crosses the mandible to enter the face just anterior to the masseter muscle, lying in the groove for the facial artery on the mandible.

In the face, the artery travels superficially, just under the cover of the platysma muscle. It passes, via

a tortuous path, deep to the zygomaticus major, risorius, and levator anguli oris muscles to the corner of the mouth. Here, it ascends lateral to the nose to terminate as the angular artery at the medial corner of the eye.

Branches of the facial artery in the face are the inferior labial, superior labial, lateral nasal, and angular arteries.

Superior and inferior labial arteries arise near the corner of the mouth. The superior labial artery courses between the orbicularis oris and the mucous membrane of the upper lip to serve the upper lip, whereas the inferior labial artery courses deep to the depressor anguli oris to serve the lower lip. The superior labial artery also provides small branches to the wing (ala) and bulb of the nose.

The **lateral nasal artery** arises near the wing of the nose to supply that structure and the bridge of the nose. The **angular artery** is the terminal continuation of the facial artery, supplying the tissues in the vicinity of the medial corner of the eye.

Superficial Temporal Artery

The superficial temporal artery, one of the terminal branches of the external carotid artery, arises near the level of the earlobe. The vessel branches pro-

Clinical Considerations

Facial Artery Compression

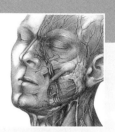

Applying pressure to the facial artery as it passes over the inferior border of the mandible just anterior to the angle will diminish blood flow to that side. However, it must be remembered that because of the many anastomoses on the face, the flow cannot be completely stopped in an area where one of its branches may have been lacerated.

fusely at its cranial-most aspect to supply the region superficial to the zygomatic arch as far medially as the lateral corner of the eye as well as the temple and the lateral aspect of the scalp.

The **transverse facial artery**, a branch of the superficial temporal, accompanies and supplies the parotid duct in its path across the masseter muscle. In addition, it sends branches to the parotid gland and other soft tissues in the vicinity.

The remainder of the arterial supply of the superficial face is derived from either the maxillary artery, a terminal branch of the external carotid artery, or from the ophthalmic artery, a branch of the internal carotid artery.

Branches of the Maxillary Artery

The **maxillary artery**, lying deep to the ramus of the mandible in the infratemporal fossa, provides vascularization of the face through some of its branches. Only those serving the superficial face are described here; the other branches are treated in subsequent chapters.

Branches of the maxillary artery supplying the superficial face are the infraorbital, buccal, and mental arteries.

The **infraorbital artery**, a branch of the third or pterygopalatine portion of the maxillary artery, passes through the infraorbital fissure to lie in the floor of the orbit. It travels in the infraorbital canal and enters the superficial face via the infraorbital foramen to distribute to the lower eyelid, the upper lip, and the area between these two structures.

The **buccal artery**, a branch of the second or pterygoid portion of the maxillary artery, makes its appearance on the face on the superficial surface of the buccinator muscle to supply it, the connective tissue of the cheek, and the mucosa of the buccal vestibule.

The **mental artery** arises from the inferior alveolar branch of the maxillary artery. The mental artery enters the face via the mental foramen of the mandible to supply the soft tissues of the chin.

Branches of the Ophthalmic Artery

Branches of the ophthalmic artery supplying the face are the zygomaticofacial, supraorbital, supratrochlear, and dorsal nasal arteries.

The **zygomaticofacial artery** is derived from the lacrimal branch of the ophthalmic artery. It enters the face via the zygomaticofacial foramen to supply the region of the face superficial to the zygomatic bone.

The **supraorbital and supratrochlear arteries** both arise in the orbit. The former enters the face via the supraorbital foramen (or notch), and the latter makes its appearance medial to the supraorbital notch. These vessels supply the forehead and the scalp.

The **dorsal nasal artery**, a terminal branch of the ophthalmic artery, leaves the orbit at its medial corner to supply the dorsum of the nose.

Venous Drainage

Summary Bite. The superficial face is drained by veins that parallel like-named arteries eventually draining into the facial vein, a tributary of the internal jugular vein. Other veins of the face join the maxillary vein of the deep face to form the retromandibular vein.

Venous drainage of the superficial face is via the supraorbital, posterior auricular, retromandibular, buccal, infraorbital, submental, and superior and inferior labial veins, most of which accompany like-named arteries (Figs. 8-2 and 8-6).

The superficial temporal vein, draining the superficial face, and the maxillary vein, draining the deep face, join to form the retromandibular vein. One additional collecting vein, the facial vein, empties into the internal jugular vein.

Facial Vein

The facial vein serves as the principal venous vessel of the superficial face. It begins in the medial corner of the eye as the angular vein and passes inferiorly, following the course of the facial artery deep to the zygomaticus major and zygomaticus minor muscles,

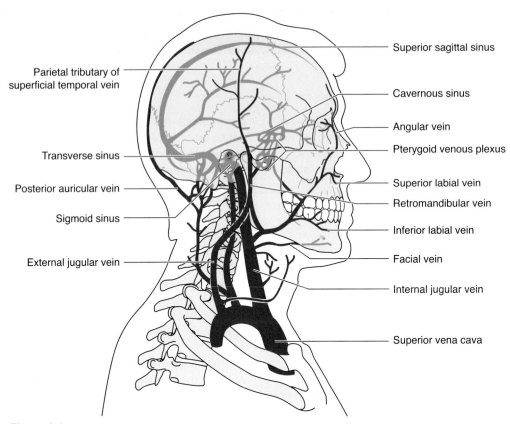

Figure 8-6. Veins of the head and neck.

where it parts company with the artery to empty into the internal jugular vein.

The facial vein communicates with the pterygoid plexus of veins as well as with the ophthalmic veins, both of which present possible passageways to the cavernous sinus due to lack of directional valves.

Superficial Temporal Vein

The superficial temporal vein follows the course of the same-named artery to drain the scalp, temple, and part of the forehead and ear. One of its tributaries is the transverse facial vein, which follows the path of the transverse facial artery.

Clinical Considerations

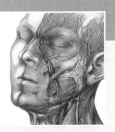

Thrombophlebitis of the Facial Vein

The facial vein does not contain valves; thus, blood flow may pass in either direction and into other venous vessels that may be connected to the cavernous sinus located in the dural venous sinus deep within the cranium. These connections include the superior ophthalmic vein, the pterygoid venous plexus, the inferior ophthalmic vein, and/or the deep facial vein.

Infections in the face, especially in the "triangular danger zone of the face," may cause inflammation of the facial vein and development of thrombophlebitis (clot formation) of the facial vein. Pieces of the infected clot may become free to eventually pass into the cavernous sinus, giving rise to thrombophlebitis of the cavernous sinus, a life-threatening situation if left untreated.

Clinical Considerations

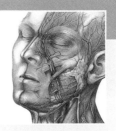

Face

Danger Area of the Face

The area bordered by the upper lip, the lateral aspect of the nose, and the lateral corner of the eye superior to the supraorbital ridge represents the danger area of the face. Squeezing pimples and tampering with boils in this region should be avoided because the area may be drained directly or from communications to the ophthalmic vein, which leads directly into the cavernous sinus of the cranial fossa. Infection may enter the cavernous sinus via this route, resulting in thrombosis, cerebral edema, and possibly death.

Lacerations and Facial Incisions

Because the skin of the face does not possess typical deep fascia, lacerations and facial incisions tend to gape open. Therefore, they must be carefully sutured to minimize scarring.

Bell Palsy

Damage to the facial nerve (or its accidental analgesia during dental procedures) results in paralysis of the muscles of the affected side. Damage may occur during surgical involvement of the parotid gland, infection of the middle ear, knife wounds, or at birth during forceps delivery. Paralysis of the facial muscles results in ptosis of the eye (upper eyelid drooping); depression of the corner of the mouth with accompanying oozing of saliva; speech disorder (especially involving labial sounds); lack of muscle tone; and a sagging, distorted face.

Trigeminal Neuralgia

Trigeminal neuralgia (tic douloureux), an extremely painful, debilitating condition involving pain fibers of the trigeminal nerve, is caused by an unknown etiology but is often associated with dental carious lesions. The pain is often excruciating and is experienced over the face, teeth, gingivae, nasal and paranasal cavities, as well as the external ear canal. These are the areas served by the maxillary and mandibular divisions, although infrequently the area served by the ophthalmic division of the trigeminal nerve may be affected. Treatment varies from alcohol injection into the trigeminal division affected to sectioning of the trigeminal nerve between the pons and the ganglion.

Cranial Fossa

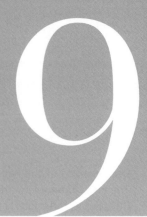

9

Key Terms

Cranial Nerves are 12 in number and originate from the brain and leave the cranial fossa via foramina to seek their targets. Most of the cranial nerves serve structures about the head and neck; however, the vagus nerve, in addition to serving structures in the head and neck, serves structures in the thorax and abdomen. The cranial nerves are named and numbered by convention with Roman numerals [e.g., facial nerve (cranial nerve VII) where the Roman numeral VII indicates the seventh cranial nerve]. Sometimes the cranial nerve is given a CN designation (e.g., CN VII), but this is often left out as one learns that the Roman numerals are used only to number the cranial nerves. The CN designation will normally not be used in this textbook.

Diploic Veins are the veins located between the internal and external compact layers of the bony skull. These diploic veins are in communication with the veins of the scalp, the meningeal veins, the venous sinuses, and with each other.

Dura Mater is the outermost layer of the three meningeal coverings of the brain because it is housed in the cranial fossa. Dura is the thick, collagenous connective tissue layer covering the brain; however, it does not follow the contours of the brain. It consists of two layers: an outer, vascular periosteal layer in contact with the bony skull, and an inner meningeal layer that is in close contact with the arachnoid, the middle meningeal layer covering the brain. The periosteal layer covers the meningeal arteries and

is closely adhered to the skull bones, especially at the bony sutures.

Dural Blood Supply is provided by several meningeal arteries, namely, the anterior, middle, accessory, and posterior meningeal arteries. The anterior meningeal artery branches from a branch of the ophthalmic artery. The middle and accessory meningeal arteries originate from the maxillary artery, whereas the several posterior meningeal arteries arise from the ascending pharyngeal, occipital, and vertebral arteries. These meningeal arteries all arise from arterial vessels outside the cranial fossa and enter it via foramina to vascularize the meninges.

Dural Reflections are formed in the meningeal layer of the dura. These reflections are interposed between certain

152

regions and subdivisions of the brain. For example, the falx cerebri is the dural reflection that is interposed between the right and left halves of the cerebrum; the falx cerebelli is the dural reflection that subdivides the cerebellar fossa into right and left halves; the tentorium cerebelli is the horizontal dural reflection that partially separates the cerebellum from the occipital region of the cerebral hemispheres; and the diaphragma sella is the dural reflection incompletely covering the sella turcica. Additionally, the sensory ganglion of the trigeminal nerve (cranial nerve V) is covered by a dural reflection. These dural reflections assist in protecting the brain. They also form a framework for the arteries, veins, and the dural sinuses.

Dural Venous Sinuses receive venous blood from the meningeal veins, from large veins from the surface of the brain, from most of the named veins of the brain, and from the diploë of the skull. The venous sinuses are not vessels; rather, they are endothelial-lined spaces that collect the venous blood and deliver it to the bulb of the internal jugular vein. From there the blood exits the skull via the internal jugular vein. In addition to receiving venous contributions from several sources, the superior sagittal sinus also receives cerebral spinal fluid from the lacuna lateralis located on either side of the superior sagittal sinus.

Emissary Veins are veins that originate outside of the skull and find their way into cranial fossa to communicate with the dural venous sinuses. Although some of these emissary veins are small and inconstant, the fact that all emissary veins are without valves indicates that the blood flow through them is related to pressure. Thus, they could be passageways of infection from an extracranial to an intracranial direction.

The **cranial fossa**, or the cavity inside the skull, is occupied by the brain and its associated meninges. This chapter discusses the dural lining, its venous sinuses, and cranial nerves that exit the skull. The osteologic characteristics of this region are presented in Chapter 6.

DURA MATER

Summary Bite. The dura mater is the outermost layer of the three meninges covering the brain housed within the cranial fossa. It consists of two layers, a periosteal layer adhering and attaching tightly at bony sutures of the calvaria and a meningeal layer abutting the arachnoid, the middle meningeal layer.

The brain is surrounded by three layers of meninges: a tough, fibrous outer **dura mater** and two delicate layers, the inner-most **pia mater** and the middle, web-like **arachnoid**. The latter two layers are discussed further in Chapter 17, whereas only the dura mater is described here. The dura is a thick, collagenous, coarse investment that does not follow the contours of the brain.

It consists of two layers: the one in intimate contact with the bones of the skull is the **periosteal layer** and the other, in close contact with the arachnoid, is the **meningeal layer**. These two layers adhere closely to one another, except in regions occupied by veins and venous sinuses.

The **periosteal layer** is vascular and is attached to the underlying bone via collagen fibers, known as Sharpey fibers. These attachments are particularly

Clinical Considerations

Cranial Base Fractures

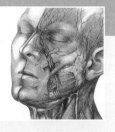

Hard blows to the head may cause hemorrhage in the middle meningeal arteries to collect between the calvaria and the dura forming extradural or epidural hematomas. These events may produce a slight concussion, with recovery followed by drowsiness (perhaps followed by coma) as the mass of blood compresses the brain. The skull must be opened, the blood evacuated, and the ruptured vessels occluded.

Cranial base fractures may rupture the internal carotid artery, producing an arteriovenous fistula, thus permitting blood flow into the cavernous sinus and from there retrograde flow into its tributaries. In this instance, the nerves coursing through the cavernous sinus (cranial nerves III, IV, V₁, V₂, and VI) may become affected. Cranial nerve III is affected first, with pulsating, protruding eyeballs and engorged conjunctiva.

notable at the suture lines, where the dura is firmly bound to the intrasuture materials. The periosteal layer of the dura covers the meningeal arteries, which groove the inner surface of the cranial vault.

Dural Reflections

Summary Bite. The dura does not follow the contours of the brain except at certain areas where its reflections separate subdivisions of the brain, providing additional support and protection. One major dural reflection, the tentorium cerebelli, separates the cerebellum from the cerebrum. The other major dural reflection, the falx cerebri, separates the right and left halves of the cerebrum. Additionally, there are three minor dural reflections.

The meningeal layer of the dura is folded in certain areas, forming incomplete subdivisions of the cranial cavity. These dural reflections are interposed between various parts of the brain, providing it with additional support and protection (Figs. 9-1 and 9-2). The two major folds are the tentorium cerebelli and the falx cerebri, and the three minor folds are the falx cerebelli, the diaphragma sella, and the covering of the trigeminal cave.

Tentorium Cerebelli

The tentorium cerebelli is a horizontally positioned reflection of the meningeal dura that lies between the cerebellum, which it covers, and the occipital region of the cerebral hemispheres, which it supports (Fig. 9-1).

The anterior margin of the tentorium cerebelli is free and concave; it assists in the formation of an oval opening, the tentorial incisure, whose anterior extent is limited by the dorsum sellae of the sphenoid bone. The attachments of the tentorium cerebelli, which fix this structure and make it taut, are as follows:

■ Anteriorly, it is fixed to the anterior and posterior clinoid processes of the sphenoid bone.
■ Laterally, it attaches to the superior edge of the petrous temporal bone.
■ Posteriorly, it is fixed to the periosteal dura attached to the lips of the groove for the transverse sinus of the occipital bone, thus participating in the formation of that sinus.

Falx Cerebri

The falx cerebri is a sickle-shaped fold of the dura. Its inferior edge is free and forms an arc interposed between the two cerebral hemispheres (Fig. 9-1).

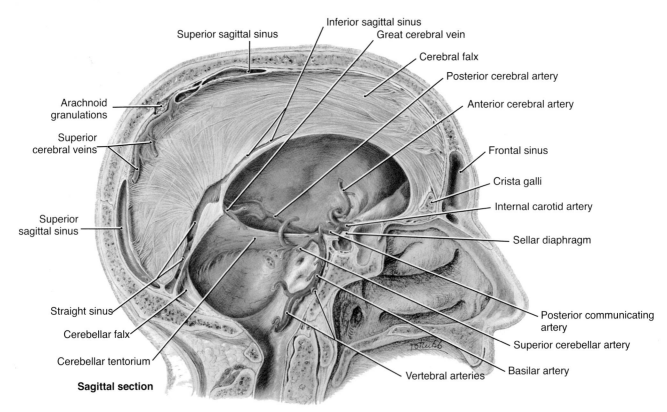

Figure 9-1. Dural reflections (midsagittal view).

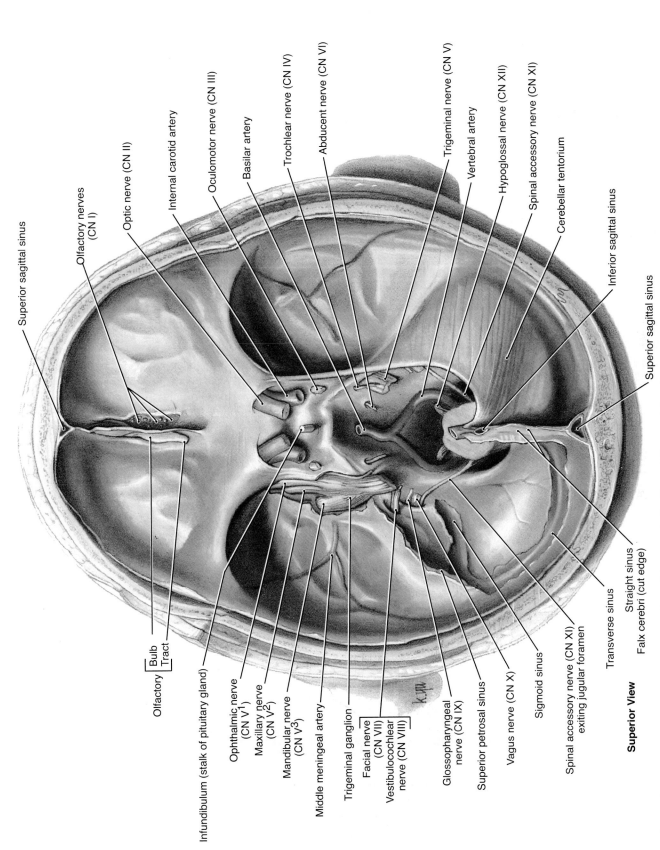

Superior sagittal sinus

Olfactory nerves (CN I)

Optic nerve (CN II)

Internal carotid artery

Oculomotor nerve (CN III)

Basilar artery

Trochlear nerve (CN IV)

Abducent nerve (CN VI)

Trigeminal nerve (CN V)

Vertebral artery

Hypoglossal nerve (CN XII)

Spinal accessory nerve (CN XI)

Cerebellar tentorium

Inferior sagittal sinus

Superior sagittal sinus

Olfactory {Bulb / Tract}

Infundibulum (stalk of pituitary gland)

Ophthalmic nerve (CN V^1)

Maxillary nerve (CN V^2)

Mandibular nerve (CN V^3)

Middle meningeal artery

Trigeminal ganglion

Facial nerve (CN VII)

Vestibulocochlear nerve (CN VIII)

Glossopharyngeal nerve (CN IX)

Superior petrosal sinus

Vagus nerve (CN X)

Sigmoid sinus

Spinal accessory nerve (CN XI) exiting jugular foramen

Transverse sinus

Straight sinus

Falx cerebri (cut edge)

Superior View

Figure 9-2. Major dural venous sinuses and cranial nerves in the floor of the cranial cavity.

▓ Anteriorly, the falx cerebri attaches to the crista galli of the ethmoid bone.

▓ Superiorly, it is fixed to the periosteal dura along the lips of the groove for the superior sagittal sinus, thus participating in the formation of that sinus.

▓ Posteriorly, the falx cerebri is attached to the periosteal dura of the occipital bone, assisting in the formation of the inferior aspect of the superior sagittal sinus.

▓ Inferiorly, it joins to the tentorium cerebelli.

These two meningeal reflections of the dura, the tentorium cerebelli and the falx cerebri, form the straight sinus at their line of intersection. The remainder of the inferior aspect of the falx cerebri is not attached, and this free inferior margin contains the inferior sagittal sinus.

Falx Cerebelli

The falx cerebelli, a small meningeal reflection located deep to the tentorium cerebelli, subdivides the cerebellar fossa into right and left halves. It is attached to the inferior surface of the tentorium cerebelli and is interposed between the two cerebellar hemispheres. The attachments of the falx cerebelli are as follows:

▓ Posteriorly, the periosteal dura of the region of the internal occipital crest, containing the occipital sinus.

▓ Superiorly, the inferior surface of the tentorium cerebelli.

▓ Its anterior edge is free, except at its anterior terminus, where it is attached on either side of the foramen magnum.

Diaphragma Sella

The diaphragma sella is an incomplete covering composed of meningeal dura that acts as a membraneous cover over the sella turcica of the sphenoid bone (Fig. 9-3).

The sella turcica houses the pituitary gland. The diaphragma sella is perforated in the middle, permitting the infundibulum and accompanying vessels of the pituitary gland to pass through it.

Covering of the Trigeminal Cave

The trigeminal ganglion sits on the periosteal (dural) lining in the trigeminal impression on the apex of the petrous portion of the temporal bone. The ganglion is covered by a meningeal reflection, thus transforming the depression into a cave, known as the **Meckel cave**, or the **trigeminal cave**.

Blood Supply of the Dura Mater

▢ **Summary Bite.** Several arteries supply the dura and the calvaria. The middle meningeal artery, a branch of the maxillary artery, is the major artery serving the dura. Smaller areas of the dura are served by branches of the ophthalmic artery anteriorly, whereas branches of the occipital and vertebral arteries serve the dura posteriorly.

The dura mater receives its principal vascularization via the anterior, middle, accessory, and posterior meningeal arteries. It should be noted that these vessels also supply the calvaria.

▓ The **anterior meningeal artery**, derived from the anterior ethmoidal branch of the ophthalmic artery, serves the dura of the anterior cranial fossa.

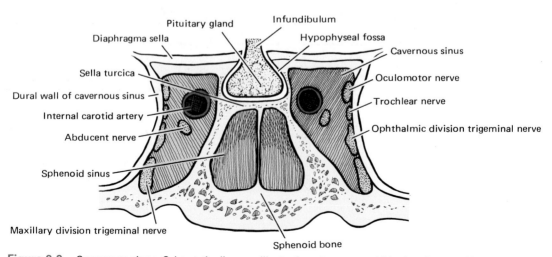

Figure 9-3. Cavernous sinus. Schematic diagram illustrating structures within the sinus and its walls.

The **middle meningeal artery**, the largest of the meningeal vessels supplying the dura, is a branch of the mandibular (or first part) of the maxillary artery and enters the cranial cavity via the foramen spinosum of the sphenoid bone. It grooves the lateral wall of the cranial cavity and divides into branches, forming an arboreal distribution. This vessel and its branches serve the dural lining of the parietal, sphenoid, temporal, and occipital bones. Some of its branches also vascularize the trigeminal ganglion and roots of the trigeminal nerve.

The **accessory meningeal artery**, also a branch of the maxillary artery, gains entry to the cranial fossa through the foramen ovale to vascularize the dura of the trigeminal cave and the trigeminal ganglion.

The **posterior meningeal arteries**, branches of the ascending pharyngeal and occipital arteries, enter the cranial fossa via the jugular foramen, hypoglossal canal, foramen lacerum, and mastoid foramen.

An additional posterior meningeal artery arises from the vertebral artery after that vessel has passed through the foramen magnum. All of these small vessels supply the dura of the infratentorial space of the posterior cranial fossa.

Venous drainage of the dura mater is by the anterior, posterior, and middle meningeal veins, which have distributions similar to their corresponding arteries. The anterior meningeal vein empties into dural sinuses of the anterior cranial fossa; the posterior meningeal veins empty into the posterior dural venous sinuses; and the middle meningeal vein delivers its blood into the sphenoparietal sinus and the pterygoid venous plexus.

Venous Sinuses of the Dura

Summary Bite. Venous sinuses are not vessels but are endothelially lined spaces in the folds of the dura which receive venous blood from emissary veins, the brain, and diploë of the calvaria. They are interconnected and the blood in them eventually reaches the internal jugular vein, which drains blood from the cranial fossa.

The dural venous sinuses are large spaces in comparison to their slender venous tributaries, such as the emissary veins and those that drain the brain and the diploë of the skull. Because the sinuses are endothelially lined spaces between reflections of taut dura mater, their walls are rigid and possess no valves (Figs. 9-1 through 9-3 and Table 9-1).

The sinuses deliver their blood either directly or indirectly via other dural venous sinuses to the **superior bulb of the internal jugular vein** situated in the jugular foramen. The dural sinuses are named superior sagittal, inferior sagittal, straight, occipital, confluence of sinuses, transverse, petrosquamous, sigmoid, cavernous, intercavernous, sphenoparietal, superior petrosal, inferior petrosal, and basilar.

The **superior sagittal sinus**, located in the superior aspect of the falx cerebri, begins as a narrow channel just anterior to the crista galli at the foramen cecum, where it may receive a small emissary vein from the nasal cavity. This sinus receives several of the superior cerebral, dural, diploic, and emissary veins, as well as communications from the **lacunae lateralis**, situated on either side of the superior sagittal sinus, which leaves a depression in the parietal bone. The superior sagittal sinus enlarges in diameter as it passes posteriorly toward its termination to empty into the right transverse sinus.

The **inferior sagittal sinus** occupies the free, inferior margin of the falx cerebri and, draining posteriorly, empties into the straight sinus along with the great cerebral vein.

The **straight sinus** occupies the line of intersection between the falx cerebri and tentorium cerebelli. It receives the great cerebral vein, the superior cerebellar veins, and the inferior sagittal sinus and delivers its blood to the left transverse sinus. Occasionally, the superior sagittal sinus empties into the left transverse sinus and the straight sinus then terminates in the right transverse sinus.

The **occipital sinus** lies in the space between the periosteal and meningeal dura of the falx cerebelli and empties into the confluence of sinuses. The **confluence of sinuses** is a region receiving several of the sinuses into the large dilated space at the internal occipital protuberance. The superior sagittal, straight, and occipital sinuses empty into the confluence, which is then drained by the right and left transverse sinuses.

The **transverse sinus** occupies the dural space at the attached perimeter of the tentorium cerebelli. The sinus of the right side usually receives blood from the superior sagittal sinus, whereas the one on the left usually drains the straight sinus.

The **petrosquamous sinus** is located at the fusion of the temporal squama and its petrous portion. This sinus, the superior petrosal sinus, as well as the diploic, emissary, inferior cerebral, and inferior cerebellar veins also empty into the transverse sinus.

The transverse sinus continues anteriorly as the **sigmoid sinus**, which grooves the temporal, parietal, and occipital bones and empties into the superior jugular bulb of the internal jugular vein.

Table 9-1   Venous Sinuses of the Dura

Sinus	Location	Remarks
Superior sagittal	Superior sagittal sulcus	Receives cerebrospinal fluid from lacunae lateralis
Inferior sagittal	Inferior margin of falx cerebri	Is joined by the great cerebral vein to form the straight sinus
Straight	Intersection of falx cerebri and tentorium cerebelli	Empties into the left (occasionally the right) transverse sinus
Occipital	Occipital bone	Empties into the confluence of sinuses
Confluence of sinuses	At the internal occipital protuberance	Receives blood from the superior sagittal, straight, and occipital sinuses
Transverse	At the attached perimeter of the tentorium cerebelli	Drains the superior sagittal sinus on the right and the straight sinus on the left
Sigmoid	Temporal, parietal, and occipital bones	Continuation of the transverse sinus and empties into the superior jugular bulb
Cavernous	Body of the sphenoid bone lateral to the sella turcica	Internal carotid artery and cranial nerve VI pass through it, whereas cranial nerves III, IV, and V_1 and V_2 are embedded in its lateral wall
Intercavernous (anterior and posterior)	Diaphragma sella	Connect the right and left cavernous sinuses to each other
Sphenoparietal	Inferoposterior ridge of the lesser wing of the sphenoid bone	Empties its blood into the cavernous sinus
Superior petrosal	Superior border of the petrous temporal bone	Drains the cavernous sinus into the transverse sinus
Inferior petrosal	Junction of the occipital clivus and the petrous temporal bone	Drains the cavernous sinus and empties into the superior jugular bulb
Basilar plexus	Basilar portion of occipital bone	Connects the two inferior petrosal sinuses

■ The **cavernous sinus**, a labyrinthine space covered by the meningeal layer of the dura mater, is positioned against the body of the sphenoid bone just lateral to the sella turcica. This sinus receives blood from the orbit via the inferior and superior ophthalmic veins, from the pterygoid plexus of veins via emissary veins, and from the brain via cerebral veins. The sphenoparietal and intercavernous sinuses also empty into the cavernous sinus. This large sinus is drained by the superior and inferior petrosal sinuses, delivering the blood to the superior jugular bulb of the internal jugular vein. Two structures pass through the cavernous sinus, each separately isolated from the bloodstream by endothelially lined fibrous sheaths: the internal carotid artery and the abducent nerve. In addition, several cranial nerves are embedded in the lateral wall of the cavernous sinus: from superior to inferior, the oculomotor and trochlear nerves and the ophthalmic and maxillary divisions of the trigeminal nerve (see Fig. 9-3).

■ The two **intercavernous sinuses** are termed the **anterior** and **posterior intercavernous sinuses**, passing anterior and posterior to the infundibulum, respectively. These connect the right and left cavernous sinuses, thus forming a ring-shaped circular sinus.

■ The **sphenoparietal sinus** is a small sinus passing along the inferoposterior ridge of the lesser wing of the sphenoid bone. It receives small venous contributions from the surrounding dura and empties into the cavernous sinus.

▨ The **superior petrosal sinus** assists in draining the cavernous sinus and empties into the transverse sinus. It passes along the superior border of the petrous portion of the temporal bone. Along its course, it also receives cerebellar, inferior cerebral, and tympanic veins.

▨ The **inferior petrosal sinus** also drains the cavernous sinus and empties directly into the superior jugular bulb. It travels in the inferior petrosal sulcus, a depression created at the juncture of the occipital clivus and petrous temporal bones. The internal auditory veins, cerebellar veins, and smaller veins of the brainstem join the inferior petrosal sinus.

The **basilar plexus** interconnects the two inferior petrosal sinuses. The plexus lies on the basilar portion of the occipital bone and receives blood from the vertebral plexus of veins.

DIPLOIC AND EMISSARY VEINS

Diploic Veins

Summary Bite. The diploë is the cancellous bone containing red bone marrow located between the internal and external tables of compact bone of the calvarium. Veins within the diploë are called diploic veins and they communicate with meningeal veins and veins of the scalp. They drain into the dural sinuses.

The diploic veins are located between the two compact layers of bone that form the vault of the skull. They travel in the diploë and, in adults, communicate with each other, the meningeal veins, veins of the scalp, and the dural sinuses. There are four diploic veins: the frontal diploic vein drains into the superior sagittal sinus; the anterior temporal diploic vein, serves mostly the frontal bone, emptying into the sphenoparietal sinus; the posterior temporal diploic vein is responsible for draining the parietal diploë and emptying into the transverse sinus; and the occipital diploic vein serves the occipital bone delivering blood to the confluence of sinuses directly or to the transverse sinus.

Emissary Veins

Summary Bite. Emissary veins originate outside the skull then enter the skull through foramina, where they communicate with other veins and empty into the dural venous sinuses. Emissary veins do not possess valves; thus, blood flow is directed by pressure, which may serve as a passageway for infections from outside to inside the skull.

The emissary veins, as their collective name implies, serve to connect the veins of the external aspect of the skull with the dural venous sinuses. Although some emissary veins are small and, as such, inconstant, many are significant. It should be noted that because these vessels do not possess valves, blood flow through them responds to pressures within the system. Consequently, they are possible passageways of infection from an extracranial to intracranial direction. The major emissary veins are those described as follows.

The **mastoid emissary** vein links the occipital vein with the transverse sinus via the mastoid foramen. The **parietal emissary vein** interconnects the veins draining the scalp with the superior sagittal sinus by way of the parietal foramen. The deep cervical veins are united with the transverse sinus by the **condyloid emissary vein**, which passes through the condyloid foramen. The venous drainage of the nasal cavity is connected with the superior sagittal sinus via the **emissary vein of the foramen cecum**. The internal jugular vein is interlinked with the cavernous sinus via the **emissary veins of the carotid canal** and the foramen of Vesalius. The pterygoid plexus of veins is united with the cavernous sinus via the **emissary veins of the foramen lacerum and foramen ovale**. The vertebral vein is connected to the transverse sinus by **emissary veins of the hypoglossal canal**.

CRANIAL NERVES

The 12 cranial nerves emanating from the brain leave the cranial cavity via foramina in the cranial fossa (Fig. 9-2; see Chapter 18). During removal of the brain from the cranial cavity, the connections between the brain and the cranial nerves are severed, and these detached nerves may be observed on the floor of the internal base of the skull.

Meningeal Nerves

Summary Bite. Meningeal nerves are the sensory nerves to the dura. They are supplied mostly from all three divisions of the trigeminal nerve (cranial nerve V). Parts of the posterior cranial fossa and roof are supplied with meningeal branches arising from the vagus (cranial nerve X) and hypoglossal nerves (cranial nerve XII) with contributions from upper cervical spinal nerves.

Sensory fibers that supply the dura are called meningeal nerves and are provided mostly by all three divisions of the trigeminal nerve (cranial nerve V). Additionally, dura of the roof and floor of the posterior cranial fossa are supplied with meningeal branches from the vagus (cranial nerve X) and hypoglossal (cranial nerve XII) nerves and, possibly, meningeal fibers of spinal nerves C2 and C3. It is interesting to note that whereas most of the meningeal fibers arise from the cranial nerves while in the cranial fossa, some arise outside the cranial vault and recur back into the cranial fossa via foramina to provide sensation to the dura.

The anterior (rostral)-most nerve structure is the **olfactory tract** and **bulb**, lying just lateral to the crista galli on the cribriform plate of the ethmoid bone. The **olfactory nerve**, the first cranial nerve (I), passes through the perforations of the cribriform plate to enter the bulb as numerous tiny filaments emerging from the olfactory mucosa of the nasal cavity.

The **optic nerve**, the second cranial nerve (II), passes through the optic foramen from the retina of the eye. It continues at the optic chiasma, which rests on the chiasmatic groove of the sphenoid bone just anterior to the infundibulum of the hypophysis.

The **oculomotor nerve**, the third cranial nerve (III), passes through the dura in the vicinity of the cavernous sinus on its way to the orbit via the superior orbital fissure.

The **trochlear nerve**, the fourth cranial nerve (IV), the smallest of the cranial nerves, courses along the free margin of the tentorium cerebelli. It pierces the dura at the posterior clinoid process to pass forward in the lateral wall of the cavernous sinus, eventually to traverse the superior orbital fissure on its way to the orbit.

The **trigeminal nerve**, the fifth cranial nerve (V), the largest of the cranial nerves composed of two roots, is evident just inferior and posterior to the small trochlear nerve. The roots enter the trigeminal cave deep to the dural cover, where the sensory portion displays its sensory ganglion, whereas the motor portion passes deep to that structure. The **trigeminal (semilunar) ganglion** trifurcates into **ophthalmic (cranial nerve V₁), maxillary (cranial nerve V₂),** and **mandibular divisions (cranial nerve V₃),** which leave the cranial cavity via the superior orbital fissure, the foramen rotundum, and the foramen ovale, respectively. The motor root accompanies the mandibular division and, subsequent to passing through the foramen ovale, merges with it.

The **abducent nerve**, the sixth cranial nerve (VI), is noted piercing the dura medial and inferior to the root of the trigeminal nerve. It passes through the cavernous sinus to exit the cranial vault and enter the orbit via the superior orbital fissure.

The two roots of the **facial nerve**, the seventh cranial nerve (VII) and the **vestibulocochlear nerve**, the eighth cranial nerve (VIII), accompany each other into the internal acoustic meatus, under the canopy of the tentorium cerebelli.

The **glossopharyngeal nerve**, the ninth cranial nerve (IX); the **vagus nerve**, the tenth cranial nerve (X); and the **accessory nerve**, the eleventh cranial nerve (XI), all leave the cranial cavity via the jugular foramen. The accessory nerve is composed of a spinal portion ascending through the foramen magnum and a cranial portion with which it unites in the cranial cavity before exiting the cranial vault through the jugular foramen.

The most caudal cranial nerve, the **hypoglossal nerve**, the twelfth cranial nerve (XII), exits the internal base of the skull via the hypoglossal foramen.

The cranial nerves and their distributions are discussed in chapters relevant to their locations. Specific information concerning the individual cranial nerves is detailed in Chapter 18. Also see Figure 17-3 to view the position of the cranial nerves on the ventral surface of the brain.

Eye and Ear

10

Key Terms

Bony Ossicles, located in the middle ear, develop from two sources. The malleus and incus and their associated muscles develop from the first pharyngeal arch, whereas the stapes develops from the second pharyngeal arch. These ossicles are attached to each other in series from the tympanic membrane to the oval window of the cochlea. Vibrations of the tympanic membrane are magnified by the bony ossicles, causing the membrane of the oval window to vibrate and thereby setting the fluid within the spiral cochea in motion. Specialized receptors (neuroepithelial hair cells) within the sensory labyrinth of the organ of Corti are moved by the displacement of the fluid; these mechanical movements are translated into nerve impulses that are transmitted back through the cochlear

division of the vestibulocochlear nerve to the brain for processing.

The Ear serves two functions: balance and hearing. The vestibulocochlear nerve is the cranial nerve serving the ear but, because two separate entities are functioning in the ear, the vestibulocochlear nerve is divided into two divisions: the vestibular division serves the mechanism of balance, whereas the cochlear nerve serves the hearing mechanism. The anatomical structures responsible for the functioning of these two mechanisms develop from the hindbrain and become embedded in the petrous portion of the temporal bone as the inner ear. The middle ear and auditory tube, lined with endoderm, develop from the first pharyngeal pouch, whereas the external

auditory meatus, lined with ectoderm, develops from the first pharyngeal groove. The closing plate between the pouch and the groove forms the tympanic membrane (ear drum) which separates these two developmental regions of the ear.

Intrinsic Muscles of the Eye include those muscles responsible for controlling the aperture of the pupil in the iris and for releasing tension on the lens for accommodation. These intrinsic muscles are innervated by the autonomic nervous system. The sphincter pupillae muscle located in the iris is innervated by parasympathetic nerves, whose postganglionic fibers originate in the ciliary ganglion. The dilatator pupillae muscle located in the iris is innervated by sympathetic fibers whose postganglionic fibers originate in the superior cervical ganglion. The ciliary muscle, whose contractions ease tension on the lens (thus changing its shape) is innervated by parasympathetic postganglionic nerve fibers that originate in the ciliary ganglion.

The Orb is the eyeball. Each orb is set in the bony orbit at an angle such that the optic axis and the ocular axis are not in synchrony with each other. Therefore, two of the extrinsic muscles are located so that this situation can be corrected optically. The superior oblique muscle corrects this by rotating the orb in an inferior–lateral (down and out) position, whereas the inferior oblique muscle rotates the orb in a superior–lateral (up and out) position. These two muscles are innervated by separate cranial nerves. The trochlear nerve (cranial nerve IV) innervates the superior oblique muscle, whereas the oculomotor nerve (cranial nerve III) innervates the inferior oblique muscle. The remaining extrinsic muscles, levator palpebrae superioris and the rectus muscles, are innervated by the oculomotor nerve (cranial nerve III), with the exception of the lateral rectus muscle, which is innervated by the abducent nerve (cranial nerve VI). Secretomotor fibers to the lacrimal gland are supplied by the facial nerve (cranial nerve VII).

Refractive Elements of the Eye include the cornea, aqueous humor, lens, zonula ciliaris, and the vitreous body. These structures, listed from anterior to posterior, refract the light as it passes to the retina. Certain conditions that cause alterations in any of these elements may interfere with visual perception and the vision may become "fuzzy" or less sharp. Scratches on the cornea; high pressure from too much aqueous humor in the anterior chamber; accumulations of pigments or substances in the lens; hardening of the lens; and/or drying and sloughing of cells of the vitreous body as it pulls away from the retina all can have detrimental effects on visual acuity and may even lead to blindness. Some of these conditions include cataracts, glaucoma, and damaged corneas. Fortunately, most of these conditions are reversible by surgical intervention, including transplants.

Vestibular Apparatus is the balancing mechanism that senses the body position in space and during movement. It is housed in the inner ear within the semicircular canals. The saccule and the utricle are located within the membranous labyrinth that lines the bony labyrinth. The membranous labyrinth is filled with endolymph. Located within each of these three separate regions of the vestibular apparatus are specialized receptors (neuroepit hair cells) that detect movement of the contained fluid. This fluid movement is translated into nerve impulses that are transmitted back by way of the vestibular division of the vestibulocochlear nerve to the brain for processing. The semicircular canals are specialized to function in detecting linear, angular, and circular movements, whereas the saccule and utricle function in detecting linear movement of the head.

ORBIT

Summary Bite. The orbit houses the orb (eyeball) and its associated extrinsic muscles, and also contains the lacrimal gland, arteries and veins, cranial nerves II, III, IV, V, VI, and VII, and postganglionic sympathetic nerves. The bony orbit is composed of seven bones: the lacrimal bone and parts of the maxilla, ethmoid, frontal, zygoma, sphenoid, and the palatine bones.

The orbit contains the organ of sight; its associated muscles, nerves, and vessels; and some accessory structures, all of which are embedded in periorbital fat. The bulb of the eye and its associated structures function in unison to receive light rays through the cornea and lens of the eye so the rays may be focused on the posterior wall of the bulb. Here, the retina, with its specialized cells, when stimulated by the light, constructs images and transmits the information to the brain for processing into a complex visual image.

The eye develops from three sources. The retina and optic nerve are outgrowths of the forebrain and are first observable at about 4 weeks of development.

The lens and some of the accessory structures in the anterior portion of the eye are derived from surface ectoderm of the head. Associated structures within the orb, as well as its tunics, are derived from adjacent mesenchyme.

Bony Orbit

Summary Bite. The bony orbit resembles a flattened cone, having a roof, medial and lateral walls, and a floor. The medial walls of the paired orbits are parallel to each other, whereas their lateral walls are directed posteromedially such that, if each were extended, they would converge near the middle of the skull.

The bony orbit, lined by periorbita (periosteum), is conical, with its base located on the superior face and its apex directed posteriorly. The "flattened" cone possesses medial and lateral walls along with a roof and floor (Fig. 10-1 and Tables 10-1 and 10-2).

The medial walls lie nearly parallel to each other on either side of the midline-located ethmoid bone. The lateral walls are directed posteromedially so that, if continued, they would converge near the middle of the skull. For this reason, all structures entering the

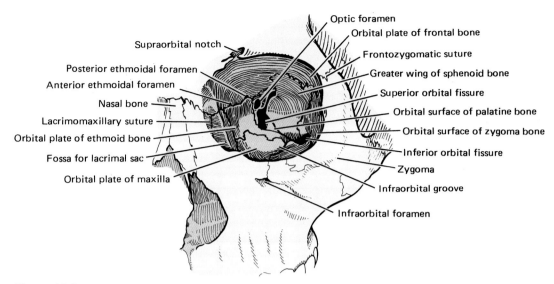

Figure 10-1. Bony orbit.

orbit from its apex are directed laterally from the midline. The attachments of two specific ocular muscles correct for this lateral divergence.

Chapter 6 discusses the bony orbit, so the reader may wish to review that section for details.

Anterior Anatomy

Eyelid

Summary Bite. The eyelids cover and protect the orb from injury. Deep to the skin of the eyelid is the orbicularis oculi muscle. Internally, the eyelids are lined by

conjunctiva, a mucous membrane that reflects onto the sclera (white of the eye). The upper eyelid is larger than the lower due to the presence of the levator palpebrae superioris muscle. Tarsal glands deep to the conjunctiva secrete an oily substance to help seal the eyelids and prevent the overflow of tears. Eye lashes emanate from the free margins of the eyelids.

The eyeball is covered anteriorly by the eyelids, which protect it from injury (Fig. 10-2). The skin of the eyelids covers the circularly oriented **orbicularis oculi** muscle, whereas internally the eyelids are lined by

Table 10-1 Bones of the Orbit

| Region | Bones | | | | | | |
	Maxilla	*Frontal*	*Ethmoid*	*Lacrimal*	*Zygoma*	*Sphenoid*	*Palatine*
Apex						Lesser wing, body	
Floor	Orbital plate				Orbital process		Orbital process
Roof		Orbital plate				Lesser wing	
Medial wall	Frontal process		Orbital lamina	Orbital surface		Body	
Lateral wall					Orbital process	Greater wing (orbital surface)	
Base	Orbital rim	Orbital rim			Orbital rim		

Table 10-2 Communications of the Orbit

Openings Communicating With the Orbit*	Bones of the Orbit						
	Maxilla	Frontal	Ethmoid	Lacrimal	Zygoma	Sphenoid	Palatine
Optic foramen						x	
Superior orbital fissure		x				x	
Inferior orbital fissure	x				x	x	x
Infraorbital canal	x						
Anterior ethmoidal foramen		x	x				
Nasolacrimal sulcus	x			x			
Posterior ethmoidal foramen		x	x				
Supraorbital foramen		x					
Zygomatico-orbital foramen					x		

*When more than one bone is indicated, the opening is at the junction of two or more bones, or in the case of foramina, at a suture.

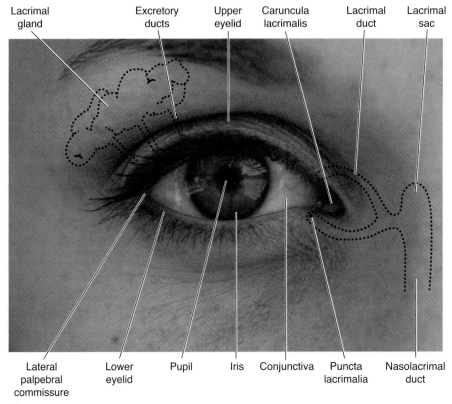

Figure 10-2. External anatomy of the eye.

conjunctiva, a mucous membrane that reflects onto the anterior portion of the sclera. In addition, the upper eyelid possesses the **levator palpebrae superioris** muscle, which makes it larger than the lower eyelid. Everting the eyelid permits observation of the **tarsal glands** deep to the conjunctiva. These glands secrete an oily substance that assists in sealing the margins of the eyelids when they are closed, and this oily substance prevents overflow of tears when the eyelids are open. These glands, along with the **ciliary glands** (modified sudoriferous glands located in the margin), open via small pores onto the margin adjacent to the eyelashes. The eyelashes, arranged in rows of two or three, curve upward and downward on the upper and lower eyelids, respectively.

The opened margins form an elliptical **palpebral fissure** narrowing laterally into an acute lateral palpebral commissure (lateral canthus) and medially into a larger medial palpebral commissure (medial canthus) possessing an enlarged triangular lacus lacrimalis with its caruncula.

Lacrimal Apparatus

Summary Bite. The lacrimal gland is located outside the orb proper, housed in a fossa in the anterosuperolateral aspect of the orbit. It secretes lacrimal fluid (tears) that keeps the cornea moistened as the eyelid moves the fluid to the medial corner of the eye where the fluid is drained by the lacrimal ducts into the lacrimal sac.

The **lacrimal (tear) gland** is located in the lacrimal fossa at the anterosuperolateral aspect of the orbit. The gland secretes fluid that is emptied into the conjunctival sac of the bulb of the eye (Fig. 10-2).

Each time the cornea dries, the eyelids, acting as windshield wipers, move the fluid over the sclera and cornea. The fluid moves medially to the lacrimal ducts, which begin as **puncta** (tiny orifices) at the lateral aspects of the lacus lacrimalis on the medial margins of the eyelids. The fluid passes via these ducts into the **lacrimal sac** located in the groove mostly within the lacrimal bone. The sac represents the upper dilated portion of the **nasolacrimal duct,** which opens into the nasal cavity at the inferior nasal meatus. Secretomotor innervation to the lacrimal gland is supplied by parasympathetic fibers of the facial nerve (cranial nerve VII).

Orb Anatomy

Summary Bite. The orb is spherical structure with a bulge on its anterior surface represented by the transparent cornea. Because of the lateral divergence of the orb in the orbit, the optical axis and the orbital axis do not coincide. Two of the extrinsic muscles of the orb are arranged to compensate for this.

The bulb of the eye is almost spherical, except for its anterior portion, which bulges away from the surface in the region of the eyelids (Fig. 10-3). This anteriorly directed surface projection is the cornea.

The transparent cornea represents a segment of a sphere occupying the anterior one sixth of the bulb, and the remaining opaque bulb represents a more complete segment of a different-sized sphere. The anterior pole of the curvature of the cornea is nearly parallel with the posterior pole of the curvature of the remaining bulb, forming the optical axis. Because of the lateral divergence of the orbit cone, the optical axis and the orbital axis do not coincide. The optic nerve (cranial nerve II) enters the posterior wall of the orb at the orbital axis about 3 mm to the nasal side of the optical axis, represented by the **macula,** the region for greatest visual acuity.

Tunics

Summary Bite. The wall of the orb consists of three separate tunics: the fibrous tunic includes the sclera and cornea; the vascular tunic includes the choroid, ciliary body, and iris; and the retinal tunic, the 10-layered retina.

Clinical Considerations

Conjunctivitis

Conjunctivitis is a mild inflammation of the conjunctiva, which can be either bacterial or an allergic reaction. The sclera and undersides of the eyelids are involved. It is especially prevalent in newborns as they pass through the birth canal. Thus, newborns are immediately given prophylactic antibiotic eye drops to prevent neonatal conjunctivitis. In adults, conjunctivitis is caused mostly by seasonal allergy.

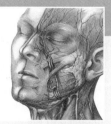

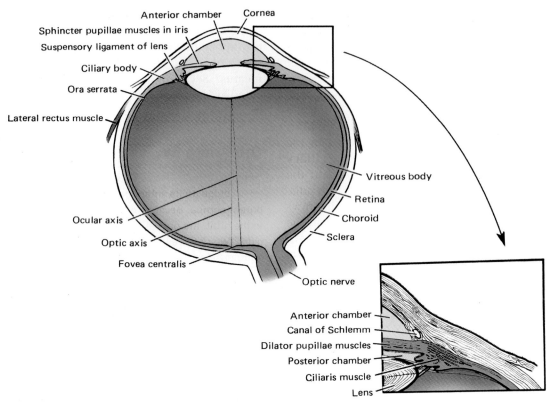

Figure 10-3. Internal anatomy of the globe.

The bulb of the eye is composed of three separate layers fabricated into one wall. The outer covering is the sclera, which is modified anteriorly as the cornea (Figs. 10-3 and 10-4). The middle or intermediate tunic is the pigmented, vascular coat composed of the choroid, ciliary body, and iris. The inner-most tunic is the nervous component, the retina.

Fibrous Tunic

Summary Bite. The tough, fibrous sclera is the white of the eye; it receives attachments of the extrinsic muscles of the eye. The cornea is the anteriorly placed transparent portion of the fibrous tunic.

The **sclera** is a tough, fibrous layer comprising the outer wall of the bulb. It is white and smooth, except where the extrinsic muscles insert into it. Its posterior portion is pierced by the optic nerve, and anteriorly it is covered by the conjunctiva. The anterior portion of the sclera, or the white of the eye, gives way to the transparent, anteriorly bulging **cornea**.

Vascular Tunic

Summary Bite. The vascular tunic is the posteriorly located, highly vascular, darkly pigmented choroid adhering to the sclera and retina. Intermediate between the choroid and iris is the ciliary body and its smooth ciliary

Clinical Considerations

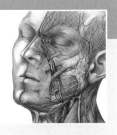

Cornea

The cornea, the transparent, avascular portion of the fibrous tunic of the eye, is highly sensitive and is mostly exposed to the environment. Slight scratches and abrasions of the cornea usually heal without much scarring. However, more severe scarring impedes vision to such a point that a corneal transplant is prescribed. Presently, most transplanted corneas are received from human donors, whereas some transplants are plastic.

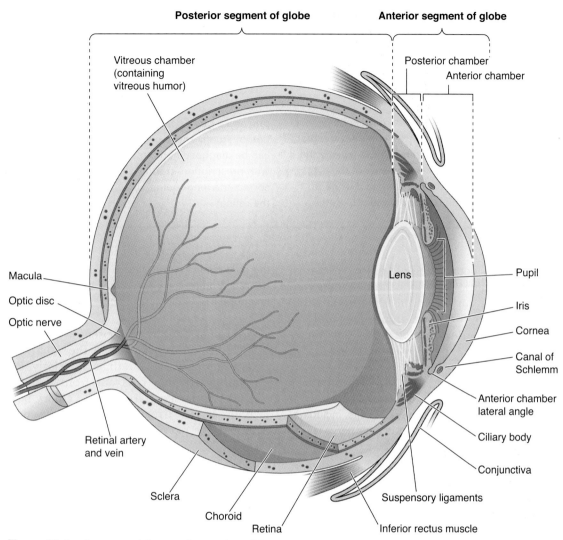

Figure 10-4. Anatomy of the anterior portion of the eye.

muscle attached by suspensory ligaments to the lens. The anteriorly placed, disc-shaped iris contains two separate smooth muscles that regulate the aperture of the pupil in the iris.

The **choroid**, the posteriorly located portion of the intermediate tunic, is a vascular, darkly pigmented layer closely adhering to the sclera and the retina. It is pierced by the optic nerve posteriorly.

The **ciliary body** is a structure located in an intermediate zone between the choroid and the iris portions of the vascular tunic and extends between the most anteriorly located parts of the retina and the iris (Figs. 10-3 and 10-4).

Contained within the ciliary body, as it juts away from the wall, is the ciliary muscle. Radiating out from the ciliary body and attached to the lens are the suspensory ligaments of the lens. The ciliary muscle is smooth muscle and therefore, involuntary. It receives

its innervation via parasympathetic fibers originating in the oculomotor nerve. Contractions of this muscle reduce the tension on the suspensory ligament of the lens, permitting the lens to become more convex, thereby accommodating the eye to focus on objects nearby.

The **iris** is the most anteriorly placed portion of the intermediate tunic. This circular disc, imparted with color from a deep pigmented layer, possesses two separately arranged layers of smooth muscle whose contractions, when stimulated by autonomic nerves, alter the diameter of the hole in the center of the iris, known as the **pupil**.

The iris is continuous with the ciliary body and is connected to the cornea at its periphery. Its location, between the lens and the cornea, separates this space into an anterior chamber in front of it and a posterior chamber behind it (Fig. 10-5). A watery fluid, the **aqueous humor**, is secreted into the posterior chamber of

Clinical Considerations

Myopia and Hyperopia

Changes in the longitudinal dimension of the optical axis will cause images to be focused either anterior (myopia) or posterior (hyperopia) to the retina. This is usually the result of changes in the refractive elements of the eye, notably the cornea, which assumes a slight change in shape or a change in the dimension of the orb. Both processes often occur as a function of aging. These conditions can be diagnosed and treated with prescription-ground glasses that can optically correct the longitudinal dimension of the optical axis to the retina.

the eye by the ciliary body. The fluid passes from this chamber into the anterior chamber through the pupil lying on the anterior surface of the lens. It exits the anterior chamber by draining into the canal of Schlemm, a venous channel located at the junction of the iris and cornea.

Retinal Tunic

Summary Bite. The retina consists of three parts: a nervous portion housing 10 layers of cells, including the photoreceptor rods and cones and the optic nerve layer;

the pars ciliaris is a reduced, thin, non-nervous portion of the retina lining the ciliary body and the non-nervous layer lining the iris as the pars iridica.

The **internal tunic** is composed of the nervous layer of the retina posteriorly and the non-nervous pars ciliaris and pars iridica retinae anteriorly. Posteriorly, the nervous retina fans out from the optic nerve (where it is thickest) to near the ciliary body, where it ends in an irregular margin, the **ora serrata**. Although the nervous portion ends here, a remaining

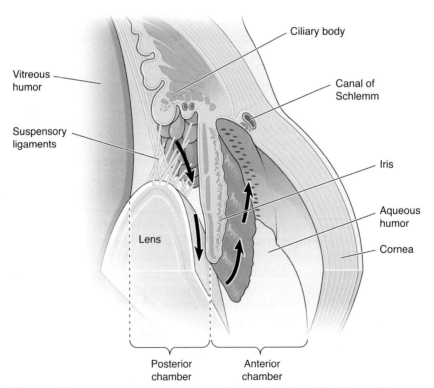

Figure 10-5. Structures within the orbit. Observe that the orbital plate of the frontal bone has been removed, as has the periorbital fascia and fat. The right side represents a superficial dissection and the left side is a deeper view.

Clinical Considerations

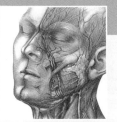

Glaucoma refers to a condition resulting from increased pressure in the anterior chamber of the eye because more aqueous humor is being produced than is being drained off through the venous system. If protracted, the increased pressure can damage the retina, causing blindness. Therapeutic drugs may be used to reduce the production of the aqueous humor.

---

membrane passes over the deep surfaces of the ciliary body and the iris as the pigmented pars ciliaris and pars iridica retinae (Figs. 10-4 and 10-5).

The nervous component of the retina is composed of 10 layers, the outer layer being the pigmented layer next to which lie the specialized receptors of light, the **rods** and **cones**. The rods are more numerous than the cones, except in the area of the **macula** and its centrally depressed **fovea centralis**, where the cones are concentrated, making vision most acute.

No rods or cones are located in the optic disc, which marks the exit of the optic nerve and the entrance of the artery of the retina. This disc represents the only spot on the retina insensitive to light and is thus known as the **blind spot**. The nervous portion of the retina ends at the ora serrata; however, the non-nervous portion continues on as a thin layer known as the pars ciliaris, overlying the deep aspect of the ciliary body and the pars iridica lining the iris.

Space does not permit the discussion of the individual layers of the retina. Further information may be gained from any standard histology textbook.

Refractive Media

Summary Bite. The refractive media permits light rays to pass through them and be refracted to focus on the retina. The refractive media include the cornea, aqueous humor, lens, zonula ciliaris, and the vitreous body.

Refractive media of the eye include (listed in order from anterior to posterior) the cornea, aqueous humor, lens, zonula ciliaris, and vitreous body (Figs. 10-3 and 10-4).

Lens and Vitreous Body

Summary Bite. The lens is a pliable, biconvex body composed of layers of transparent cells. It lies immediately posterior to the iris and is held in place by the suspensory ligaments attached to the ciliary body. The vitreous body is a semigelatinous structure filling the interior of the globe between the lens and the retina to which it is securely adherent.

The cornea and the aqueous humor have been discussed. The lens, a biconvex body that develops from surface ectoderm, is composed of several transparent layers covered by a capsule and retained in position by suspensory ligaments attached to the ciliary body (Fig. 10-5). The transparent zonula ciliaris, ribbonlike fibrils radiating out from the ciliary body to the lens, imparts refractive capability to the lens.

Filling the concavity behind the lens and posterior chamber of the eye is the semigelatinous **vitreous body**, which is the most posteriorly located of the light-refracting structures.

Clinical Considerations

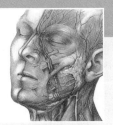

Detached Retina

The 10-layered retina is loosely attached to the choroid layer of the orb and is retained in that position by the vitreous body. Sudden jolts absorbed in the orbit may detach the retina, causing a medical emergency. The detached retina is sightless and will remain so, thus requiring surgical reattachment.

Clinical Considerations

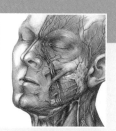

Cataract is an age-related condition where the lens loses its transparency and becomes milky, causing blurred vision. It is the major cause of poor vision and blindness around the world. Modern techniques now permit surgi-

cal placement of plastic lenses resulting in restored vision.

Muscles of the Eye

Extrinsic Muscles

Summary Bite. The extrinsic muscles are seven in number. One muscle operates the upper eyelid, whereas the remaining extrinsic muscles function to rotate the orb in any direction to focus for sight.

There are seven extrinsic muscles of the eye: the levator palpebrae superioris; the superior, inferior, medial, and lateral recti muscles; and the superior and inferior oblique muscles (Figs. 10-5 and 10-6 and Table 10-3).

The **levator palpebrae superioris** originates on the inferior surface of the lesser wing of the sphenoid bone and inserts into the upper eyelid. As previously described, this muscle functions to elevate the upper eyelid. The four **recti muscles—lateral, medial, superior**, and **inferior**—originate from a common tendinous ring surrounding the optic foramen.

Each of these four muscles passes into the orbit and inserts into the sclera of the orb, a few millimeters posterior to the cornea in the position indicated by their names. These muscles function to pull the orb in the direction of the muscle insertion.

It should again be noted that because of the lateral divergence of all structures entering the orbit, the resultant action of the superior and inferior recti muscles are complicated by a slight rotation and medialward deviation.

The **superior oblique muscle** arises from the body of the sphenoid bone immediately above the superior rectus muscle and passes anteriorly to end in a tendinous pully attached to the **trochlear fovea** of the frontal bone. From here, the tendon turns laterally beneath the superior rectus muscle to insert into the sclera between the insertions of the superior and lateral rectus muscles (see Fig. 10-6). Contraction of this muscle directs the eye downward and laterally.

The **inferior oblique muscle** arises from the orbital surface of the maxilla lateral to the lacrimal groove. The muscle passes between the orbital floor and the inferior rectus to be inserted in the sclera

between the insertions of the lateral rectus and superior oblique muscles (see Fig. 10-7). The inferior oblique muscle functions to direct the eye upward and lateralward.

The levator palpebrae superioris, the superior, inferior, and medial recti, and the inferior oblique muscles are all innervated by branches of the oculomotor nerve. The superior oblique muscle is innervated by the trochlear nerve, the sole function of this nerve. Innervation to the lateral rectus muscle is provided by the abducent nerve, another cranial nerve that serves only a single function.

Intrinsic Muscles of the Eye

Summary Bite. The intrinsic muscles of the eye are three in number. These muscles lie within the orb and function to innervate smooth muscles of the ciliary body and the two separate muscles of the iris.

The three intrinsic muscles of the eye are all involuntary. Although the **ciliary muscle** was described with the choroid layer, it will be reviewed here. When the ciliary muscle (attached to the sclera and the ciliary body) contracts, it stretches the ciliary body, thereby releasing tension on the suspensory ligaments and, in so doing, releasing tension on the lens. The effect is that the lens becomes more convex, thus enabling the eye to focus on close objects (this is known as accommodation). Because the ciliary muscle is an involuntary muscle, it is innervated by the autonomic nervous system, specifically by parasympathetic fibers originating in the oculomotor nerve (cranial nerve III). The two remaining intrinsic muscles, both located within the iris, are the sphincter pupillae and dilatator pupillae muscles (Figs. 10-3 through 10-5).

The **sphincter pupillae muscles** are arranged in a circular fashion in the iris around the pupil. Their contraction constricts the pupil. The **dilatator pupillae muscles** are arranged in a radiating band from near the margin of the pupil to the outer walls of the deep surface of the iris. Contractions of this muscle group produce a dilation of the pupil.

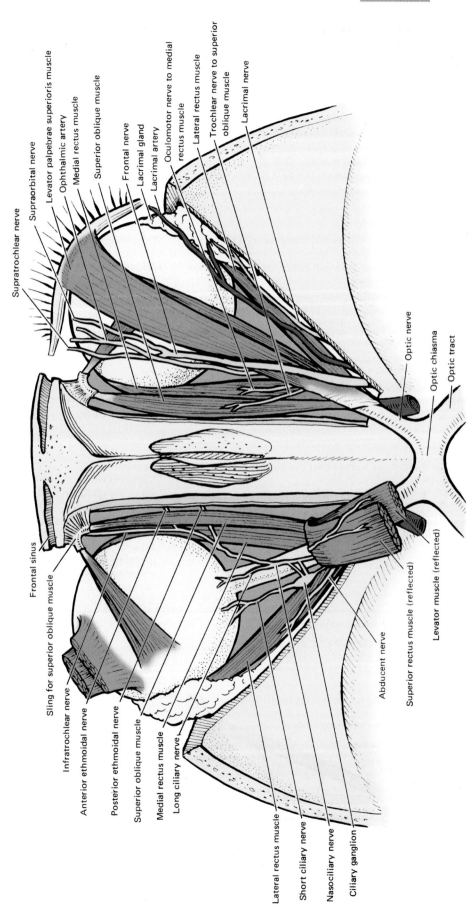

Figure 10-6. External muscles of the eye.

Table 10-3 Muscles of the Eye

Muscle	Origin	Insertion	Innervation	Action*
Levator palpebrae superioris	Orbit roof	Upper eyelid, tarsal plate	Oculomotor	Elevates eyelid.
Extrinsic				
Recti				
Superior	Common tendinous ring surrounding the optic foramen	Superior sclera anterior to equator	Oculomotor	Elevates cornea slightly medialward.
Inferior		Inferior sclera anterior to equator	Oculomotor	Depresses cornea slightly medialward.
Medial		Medial sclera anterior to equator	Oculomotor	Rotates cornea medially.
Lateral		Lateral sclera anterior to equator	Abducent	Rotates cornea laterally.
Obliques				
Superior	Orbit roof	Trochlea to posterosuperior quadrant of sclera	Trochlear	Rotates cornea inferolaterally.
Inferior	Orbit floor	Sclera posteroinferior to superior oblique	Oculomotor	Rotates cornea superolaterally.
Intrinsic				
Ciliary	Located in ciliary body adjacent to iris and attached to suspensory ligament of lens		Oculomotor via ciliary ganglion and short ciliary nerves	Releases pressure on suspensory ligament of lens, permitting it to accommodate.
Pupillae				
Sphincter	Circular band in iris surrounding the pupil		Oculomotor (parasympathetic) via ciliary ganglion and short ciliary nerves	Constricts pupil.
Dilatator	Radiating out in deep layers of iris from pupil		Sympathetic from superior cervical ganglion via long and short ciliary nerves	Dilates pupil.

*Actions described are assuming each muscle is acting alone.

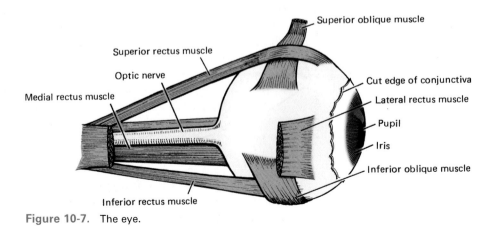

Figure 10-7. The eye.

Both of these muscle groups are innervated by fibers of the autonomic system. The sphincter muscle group is supplied by parasympathetic fibers originating in the oculomotor nerve, whereas the dilatator muscle group is innervated by the sympathetic system, whose postganglionic cell bodies are located in the superior cervical ganglion. It should be mentioned again that the lacrimal gland, which lies within the orbit but outside the orb, is provided with secretomotor fibers from the facial nerve (cranial nerve VII).

Nerves of the Orbit

Summary Bite. Cranial nerves serving the orbit include II, III, IV, V, VI, and VII. Additionally, postganglionic sympathetic fibers serve the orbit.

The orbit possesses nerve components from six cranial nerves: the optic, oculomotor, trochlear, trigeminal, abducent, and secretomotor fibers from the facial. In addition, sympathetic fibers also serve the orbit (Fig. 10-6 and Table 10-3). Each cranial nerve serving the orbit is discussed in detail in Chapter 18 and summarized in Table 18-1.

Optic Nerve
The optic nerve consists of the axons of the ganglionic layer of the retina passing to the brain from the bulb through the optic foramen and to the optic chiasma. Here, certain fibers cross over to the contralateral side to enter the optic tract, whereas other fibers remain on the ipsilateral side to enter the optic tract.

Oculomotor Nerve
The oculomotor nerve enters the orbit through the superior orbital fissure, where it divides into superior and inferior divisions to innervate the intrinsic ciliary and sphincter pupillae muscles and all of the extrinsic muscles except the lateral rectus and the superior oblique.

The superior division sends branches to the levator palpebrae superioris and the superior rectus, whereas the inferior division innervates the medial and inferior recti and the inferior oblique muscles. This division also supplies parasympathetic motor fibers to the **ciliary ganglion**, a parasympathetic terminal ganglion located about 1 cm from the apex of the orbit between the optic nerve and the lateral rectus muscle. Preganglionic parasympathetic fibers synapse on postganglionic cell bodies within the ganglion. The axons of these cell bodies reach the orb via the **short ciliary nerves**, to be distributed to the ciliary and sphincter pupillae muscles (see Tables 10-3 and 18-2).

Trochlear Nerve
The trochlear nerve enters the orbit through the superior orbital fissure on its way to the superior oblique muscle, the only muscle it serves.

Trigeminal Nerve
The **ophthalmic division** of the trigeminal nerve enters the orbit through the superior orbital fissure as three branches: the lacrimal, frontal, and nasociliary nerves, all serving sensory function only (see Tables 18-1 and 18-3).

The smallest branch, the **lacrimal nerve**, runs laterally, superior to the lateral rectus, on its way to supply the lacrimal gland and adjacent conjunctiva with sensory innervation.

This nerve often communicates with a secretomotor postganglionic parasympathetic fiber for the lacrimal gland from the pterygopalatine ganglion.

Preganglionic fibers reach the ganglion from the facial nerve, whereas the postganglionic fibers are distributed to the lacrimal nerve via zygomaticotemporal branches of the maxillary division of the trigeminal nerve.

The **frontal nerve** is the largest nerve of the ophthalmic division. It courses forward above the levator palpebrae superioris muscle. Midway in the orbit, it divides into a medial branch, the supratrochlear nerve, and the laterally oriented supraorbital nerve.

The **supratrochlear nerve** pierces the orbital fascia and supplies the conjunctiva, eyelid, and skin over the medial part of the forehead.

The **supraorbital nerve** exits the orbit through the supraorbital notch or foramen to supply the forehead and scalp. A small twig of this nerve enters the frontal bone to serve the frontal sinus.

The **nasociliary nerve** crosses over the optic nerve on an oblique course to the anterior ethmoidal foramen. It communicates with the ciliary ganglion, where sensory fibers may pass through the ganglion without synapsing on their way to the orb via the short ciliary nerves that carry postganglionic parasympathetic fibers. Other branches, termed **long ciliary nerves** (sensory and postganglionic sympathetic), pass to the orb directly. Branches of the nasociliary nerve enter the anterior and posterior (and occasionally, middle) ethmoidal foramina.

Just before entering the anterior ethmoidal foramen, the **infratrochlear nerve** arises from the nasociliary nerve and passes to the medial angle of the eye, supplying the skin of the eyelids and the side of the nose.

The **anterior** and **posterior ethmoidal nerves** serve the ethmoidal and frontal sinuses. **Internal** and **external nasal branches**, derived from the anterior ethmoidal nerve, supply the mucous membranes of the anterior septum and the skin over the ala of the nose, respectively.

The **maxillary division** of the trigeminal nerve enters the floor of the orbit through the inferior orbital fissure. It is not discussed here because its only contribution to the orbit is a few periosteal branches.

Abducent Nerve

The abducent nerve enters the orbit through the superior orbital fissure, passing laterally to innervate the lateral rectus muscle, the only muscle it serves.

Sympathetic Nerves

Postganglionic sympathetic fibers, whose cell bodies are located in the superior cervical ganglion, find their way into the orbit as communications to several cranial nerves from the **carotid plexus**. They travel to their destination via these routes or via the sympathetic nerve plexus wrapped around the arteries of the orbit.

Nerves destined for the dilatator pupillae muscles reach the orb either by the long ciliary nerves or by passing, with sensory branches from the nasociliary nerve, through the ciliary ganglion and on to the dilatator pupillae muscles located within the iris via the short ciliary nerves.

Vascular Supply

 Summary Bite. The arterial supply to the structures in the orbit, including the extrinsic muscles, retina, ciliary body, and intrinsic muscles, comes from branches of the ophthalmic artery. Superior and inferior ophthalmic veins drain the orbit into the cavernous sinus. The inferior ophthalmic vein communicates with the pterygoid venous plexus.

The **ophthalmic artery** enters the orbit through the optic canal and divides into two groups. The orbital group serves some of the accessory structures to the orb, whereas the ocular group serves the extrinsic muscles and the orb proper, along with the retina, the ciliary body, and the intrinsic muscles (Fig. 10-6).

Superior and **inferior ophthalmic veins** drain the structures of the orbit and empty their contents into the cavernous sinus. The inferior ophthalmic vein also communicates with the pterygoid venous plexus.

EAR

Summary Bite. The ear is a purely sensory organ specialized for the sensations of hearing and balance.

Development

Summary Bite. The internal ear develops from the hindbrain and eventually becomes encased within the petrous portion of the temporal bone. It is composed of two parts: the vestibular apparatus (for balance) and the cochlea (for hearing).

The organ of hearing and balance begins its development shortly after that of the eye. It develops from a thickening of the hindbrain to form the mechanism for balance and the cochlea for hearing, both of which make up the internal ear and eventually become surrounded by the petrous portion of the temporal bone.

The middle ear and auditory tube develop from the first pharyngeal pouch, as described in Chapter 5. Interposed between the endodermal lining of the

Clinical Considerations

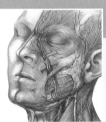

Conductive Hearing Loss

Otitis Media
The auditory tube permits the spread of infection from the nasal cavity into the middle ear cavity. This condition **(otitis media),** resulting from acute infection, may rupture the eardrum and/or may pass into the mastoid air cells. Antibiotics are used to circumvent and treat this condition. Auditory tube obstructions often lead to middle ear infections, especially in children.

Otosclerosis
Occasionally, the stapes becomes immobilized as a result of bony deposits around the oval window. This condition, known as **otosclerosis**, is a major cause of hearing loss, especially in older adults. It is usually correctable by surgical procedures. Both otitis media and otosclerosis, if left untreated, will result in deafness.

auditory tube and the ectodermal lining of the pharyngeal groove is the closing plate, which persists as the **tympanum** (eardrum) (see Fig. 5-4).

It is within this middle ear cavity that the bony ossicles develop. By way of review, the **malleus** (hammer) and its muscle, the **tensor tympani**, develop from first arch mesenchyme, as does the **incus** (anvil). The **stapes** (stirrup) and its muscle, the **stapedius**, develop from second arch mesenchyme. In keeping with the rule that structures developing within an arch are innervated by the nerve of that arch, it then follows that the tensor tympani muscle is innervated by the trigeminal nerve, and the stapedius muscle is innervated by the facial nerve.

External Ear

Summary Bite. The external ear includes the pinna and several extrinsic muscles of the ear, as well as the external audiory meatus to the tympanic membrane.

The external ear comprises the pinna and the external auditory meatus; it develops from the first pharyngeal groove as well as from the tubercles from pharyngeal arches I and II that surround the first pharyngeal groove (Fig. 10-8).

Several muscles develop from the second arch in the vicinity of the ear; thus, all are innervated by the facial nerve. They are the extrinsic muscle group of the pinna, (including the anterior, superior, and posterior auricular muscles) and an intrinsic group (including some six small, insignificant, vestigial muscles that are not described here).

Nerve Supply

Summary Bite. Sensory innervation to the external ear emanates from several sources that overlap the area serviced. These include branches from the cervical plexus and branches from cranial nerves V, VII, and X with contributions from IX.

Sensory innervation to the pinna and the external auditory meatus is broad and overlapping. It includes the great auricular and lesser occipital nerves, originating from the cervical plexus, and branches from several cranial nerves, including the auricular branch of the facial, the auriculotemporal branch of the trigeminal, the auricular branch of the vagus, and perhaps contributions from the glossopharyngeal nerve to the auricular branch of vagus.

Middle Ear

Summary Bite. The middle ear (tympanic cavity), housing the three bony ossicles and their associated muscles, lies within the temporal bone and communicates with the mastoid air cells; it also communicates with the nasopharynx via the auditory tube.

The middle ear or tympanic cavity is a mucous membrane-lined, air-filled space within the temporal bone that communicates with the mastoid air cells through a small opening, and with the nasopharynx via the cartilaginous auditory tube (Fig. 10-8). It is through the latter communication that atmospheric pressure is equalized on either side of the tympanum (see Fig. 4-20).

The rostral end of the tympanic cavity contains the bony ossicles. On the lateral wall, attached to the tympanum by several ligaments, are the malleus and its muscle, the tensor tympani. The stapes and the stapedius muscle are attached by the ligaments to the medial wall, where the footplate of the stapes impinges on the **fenestra vestibuli** (oval window) of the cochlea. Interposed between the malleus and the stapes is the incus, which articulates with both. Vibrations received at the tympanic membrane set the malleus, incus, and stapes in motion because they are articulated together in series. The result is that the vibrations are amplified by about 20 times when the footplate of the stapes articulates with the membrane of the oval window. The tensor tympani muscle attached to the malleus and the stapedius muscle attached to the stapes modulate the vibrations and function as protective measures for the hearing mechanism. The tensor tympani muscle prevents large movement of the malleus during loud sounds that have set the tympanum into heavy vibration. The stapedius muscle prevents large movement of the stapes as it impinges upon the oval window (Table 10-4). Located inferior to the oval window is the **fenestra cochleae** (round window) covered by a membrane; this secondary tympanic membrane is where the hydraulic pressure within the membranous labyrinth is dissipated (Table 10-4).

Vessels and Nerves

Summary Bite. Branches of several arteries provide a rich blood supply to the middle ear. Venous drainage delivers blood to the petrosal sinus and the pterygoid plexus of veins. The tympanic plexus is formed by branches of cranial nerve IX and from sympathetic fibers; it serves the mucous membranes. Cranial nerve V innervates the tensor tympani muscle, whereas cranial nerve VII innervates the stapedius muscle.

Many vessels supply the structures of the middle ear. These vessels arise from several sources, which include tympanic branches from the maxillary, the

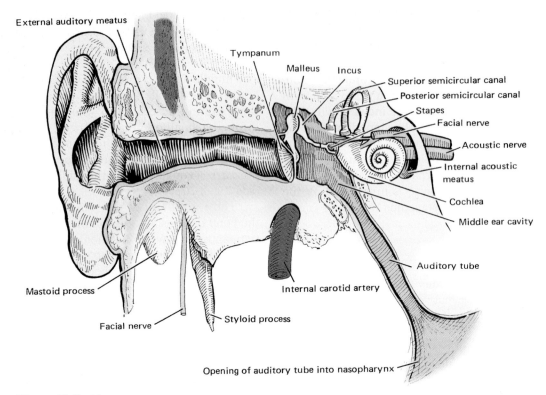

Figure 10-8. The ear.

stylomastoid branch of the posterior auricular, and many small branches from the pharyngeal, middle meningeal, and internal carotid arteries.

Venous drainage generally parallels the arteries to become tributaries of the superior petrosal sinus and the pterygoid plexus of veins.

The **tympanic plexus** of nerves, located in the middle ear, is derived from the glossopharyngeal nerve and sympathetic fibers to serve the mucous membranes. In addition, the cranial portion of the facial nerve enters the bony medial wall of the cavity on its way to the stylomastoid foramen, where it will exit the skull. While there, it gives off a motor branch to the stapedius and to the chorda tympani,

which passes over the tympanic membrane and across the malleus to exit the cavity. The tensor tympani receives its motor innervation from a like-named branch of the mandibular division of the trigeminal nerve.

Inner Ear

Summary Bite. The inner ear, embedded within the petrous portion of the temporal bone, is composed of two separate functional, but interconnected, components. The vestibular system, composed of the vestibule and semicircular canals, functions in balance. The other component, the cochlea, functions in hearing.

Table 10-4 Bony Ossicles and Their Associations

	Attachments				
Ossicle	*Lateral*	*Medial*	*Ligaments*	*Muscle*	*Nerve*
Malleus (Hammer)	Tympanum	Incus	Anterior Superior Lateral	Tensor Tympani	Trigeminal V
Incus (Anvil)	Malleus	Stapes	Posterior Superior		
Stapes (Stirrup)	Incus	Oval window of the cochlea	Annular ligament of base	Stapedius	Facial VII

Clinical Considerations

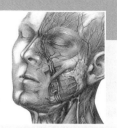

Inner Ear Disorder

Ménière's Disease is an inner ear disorder affecting both the vestibular and cochlear mechanisms. It causes hearing loss, vertigo, dizziness, nausea, tinnitus, and vomiting. It is related to an excess of endolymphatic fluid in the cochlea. It is cyclic and, if left untreated, can result in permanently impaired hearing or complete hearing loss.

The inner ear, entirely embedded in the petrous temporal bone, lies medial to the middle ear. It consists of a bony and a membranous labyrinth. The **bony labyrinth** is composed of the vestibule, semicircular canals, and the cochlea, filled with fluid (perilymph). Suspended within the perilymph is the **membranous labyrinth**, containing its own endolymph (Fig. 10-8).

The **vestibule**, housing the oval window, occupies a central position in the bony labyrinth. Projecting from it, posteriorly and superiorly, are the three **semicircular canals**, arranged so that each canal and its dilated ampulla lies at right angles to the other two. Projecting anteriorly from the vestibule is the **cochlea**, a bony structure turned on itself two and one half times around a central core termed the **modiolus**, giving it the appearance of a snail's shell. Its lateral wall contains the round window.

The membranous labyrinth is composed of the semicircular ducts, the cochlear duct, and two sacs, the utricle and the saccule. The utricle occupies the vestibule and the saccule lies anteroinferior to it. The endolymph from the semicircular ducts is received in the utricle.

Endolymph from the cochlear duct is received into the saccule via the small ductus reuniens. A small endolymphatic duct ending in a blind pouch projects posteriorly and communicates with the saccule and utricle. The cochlear duct separates the cochlea into the scala vestibuli superiorly and the scala tympani inferiorly. These two scalae are in communication near the summit of the cochlea through a tiny pore called the **helicotrema**.

The cochlear duct, composed of a spiral membranous tube, houses the **spiral organ of Corti** in its basilar membrane. The spiral organ receives peripheral nerve endings from that portion of the vestibulocochlear nerve responsible for receiving sensations and transmitting them to the brain for processing into what we perceive as sounds.

Nerves

Summary Bite. The vestibulocochlear nerve (cranial nerve VIII) consists of two divisions: a vestibular division conveying impulses for balance, and a cochlear division conveying impulses for hearing.

Clinical Considerations

Neural Hearing Loss

Nerve deafness is the result of lesions within nerve transmission from the spiral organ of Corti to the brain, as in the case of the formation of a neuroma within the vestibulocochlear nerve. Although this is a benign condition and can be surgically eliminated, hearing may not be recovered. Vestibulocochlear nerve destruction caused by certain drugs and other factors, including intense noise of high frequency for a prolonged period of time, may also lead to loss of hearing.

The **vestibulocochlear nerve**, in company with the facial nerve (cranial nerve VII), enters the internal auditory meatus of the temporal bone. Shortly thereafter, the facial nerve parts company from the vestibulocochlear nerve to enter the facial canal. Recall that it supplies the stapedius with motor fibers and that it gives rise to the chorda tympani. The remainder of the facial nerve will be discussed in later chapters. The vestibulocochlear nerve conveys impulses from the vestibular (balance) and auditory (hearing) mechanisms (Fig. 10-8).

The vestibulocochlear nerve consists of two separate sets of fibers: the **vestibular nerve** for balance, and the **cochlear nerve** for hearing. After entering the meatus as a single nerve, the two separate and enter the membranous labyrinth to terminate as special endings at their receptor sites. For additional information regarding anatomy and the function of the statoacoustic system, refer to anatomy textbooks

Parotid Bed

Key Terms

The Facial Nerve (cranial nerve VII) passes from the stylomastoid foramen to enter the parotid gland. Several arteries and veins pass through the gland on their way to other regions of the head and neck. Also, several cranial nerves that emanate from the brain pass through the gland on the way to their targets. The facial nerve forms a loop inside the substance of the gland. Arising from this loop are the five terminal branches of the facial nerve (temporal, zygomatic, buccal, mandibular, and cervical branches) that leave the gland on the face to provide motor innervation to the muscles of facial expression.

Parotid Duct also known as the Stenson duct, exits the most anterior superficial portion of the gland to travel,

just deep to the skin, over masseter muscle on the lateral aspect of the face. It then dives, at the anterior border of the masseter, into the buccal fat pad. The duct then pierces the buccinator muscle to enter the oral cavity at the parotid papilla located in the buccal vestibule opposite the second maxillary molar. Parotid salivary secretions are delivered into the oral cavity through the parotid papilla.

Parotid Gland is the largest of the three major salivary glands. It is enclosed in its own capsule which is a reflection of the deep fascia. Superficially, the parotid gland is located on the side of the face lying, in part, over the masseter muscle, anterior to the ear and superior to the zygomatic arch. It is irregular in shape

and therefore is wedged in between the ramus of the mandible and the space posterior and medial to it; that space is called the parotid bed. Many fingerlike projections of the parotid gland fill this irregular space with glandular tissue. Thus, there are no definite descriptions as to the extent of the gland within the parotid bed.

Secretomotor Innervation to the Parotid Gland is provided by the parasympathetic component of the autonomic nervous system. The glossopharyngeal nerve (cranial nerve IX) is the nerve of origin for the secretomotor innervation of the parotid gland. Remember that autonomic innervation is a two-neuron chain system with an autonomic ganglion between preganglionic and postganglionic neurons. In this instance, the otic ganglion is that parasympathetic ganglion. Preganglionic nerve fibers originating in the glossopharyngeal nerve reach the otic ganglion where they synapse on postganglionic nerve cell bodies. Postganglionic fibers arising from the ganglion are passed to the auriculotemporal branch of the mandibular division of the trigeminal nerve (V_3) for delivery to the gland, thus effecting secretomotor function.

SUPERFICIAL ANATOMY AND BOUNDARIES

Summary Bite. The parotid bed is an irregular space located between the ramus of the mandible, the external acoustic meatus and the mastoid and styloid processes, the digastric muscles, and sternocleidomastoid muscle.

The space lying between the ramus of the mandible, external acoustic meatus, and mastoid and styloid processes of the temporal bone is known as the **parotid bed** (Fig. 11-1).

The medial extent of this bed is bordered by the posterior belly of the digastric muscle and the muscles attached to the styloid process. Inferiorly, the bed is bounded by the superoanterior border of the sternocleidomastoid muscle. This somewhat irregularly-

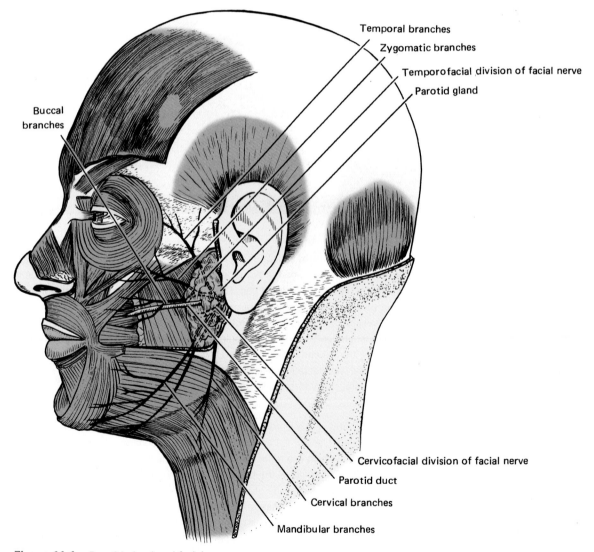

Figure 11-1. Parotid gland and facial nerve.

shaped area houses the parotid gland, which is molded into this space, thus assisting in filling out the contour of the jaw/neck/ear junction.

Representatives of two cranial nerves—the facial nerve and trigeminal nerve—pass through the substance of the parotid gland to reach their destinations in and about the head and neck. Similarly, the external carotid artery and some of its branches course through the gland, as do some of the tributaries forming the external jugular vein.

PAROTID GLAND

Summary Bite. The parotid gland, the largest of the three major salivary glands, is encapsulated by portions of the deep cervical fascia. Part of the gland lies on the lateral surface of the masseter muscle, whereas most of it lies within the parotid bed with fingerlike projections between some muscle masses in the deep face.

The parotid gland is the largest of the three major salivary glands (parotid, submandibular, and sublingual glands) and is enclosed within a capsule that is part of the deep cervical fascia. It is located on the lateral aspect of the face and in the parotid bed (Figs. 11-1 and 11-2).

Because the gland is molded into an irregular space, it is also irregular in shape. The superficial aspect of the gland extends superiorly over the masseter muscle to the zygomatic arch, where an accessory portion of the gland may be detached from the main substance.

Inferiorly, it is mostly confined to the region between the mastoid process, the sternocleidomastoid muscle, and the angle of the mandible, where it extends over the posterior aspect of the masseter muscle.

Medially, the gland extends into the deeper portions of the parotid bed to the styloid process and its attached musculature. Here, a wedge-shaped portion of the gland may intervene between the medial and lateral pterygoid muscles for a short distance. Often, glandular lobes extend into other spaces adjacent to the parotid bed. One such lobe passes between the ramus of the mandible and the medial pterygoid muscle (above that muscle's insertion), whereas other lobes pass between the external auditory meatus and the temporomandibular joint (TMJ) and between the external carotid artery and the superior constrictor muscle of the pharynx.

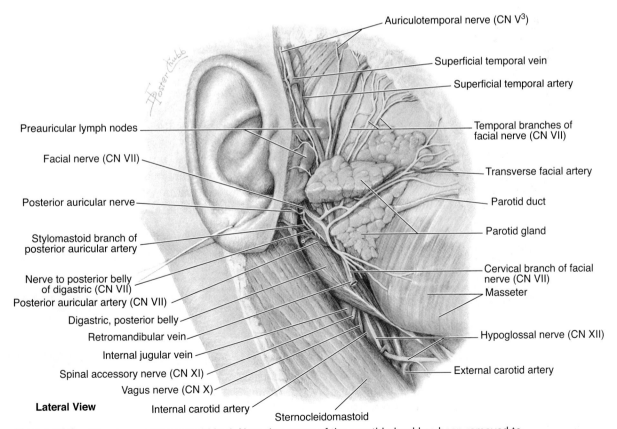

Figure 11-2. Structures of the parotid bed. Note that some of the parotid gland has been removed to expose structures passing through the gland.

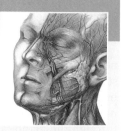

Clinical Considerations

Sialography of the Parotid Duct

Occasionally, calculus accumulations occur in the parotid duct, thereby obstructing salivary flow. Radiologic examination on injecting radiopaque dye into the parotid duct opening (**sialography**) identifies the blocked region, and the obstruction may have to be relieved surgically.

Exiting the anterior aspect of the superficial portion of the gland is the **parotid duct (Stenson duct)**, which passes anteriorly, superficial to the masseter muscle, to dive medially into the buccal fat pad; it pierces the buccinator muscle on its way to the oral vestibule. It delivers the parotid salivary secretions at the opening of the parotid papilla located opposite the second maxillary molar.

Relationships

> **Summary Bite.** Many structures passing between the neck and the head, including arteries and veins as well as several cranial nerves emanating from the brain, pass through the parotid gland.

Because the parotid gland is irregular in shape, possessing many fingerlike projections radiating in several directions from the parotid bed, the gland associates with or engulfs many of the structures passing through this region (Fig. 11-2).

Structures associated with the superficial aspect of the gland include branches of the great auricular nerve originating from the cervical plexus that provide sensory innervation to the region, and small lymph nodes that drain the superficial area.

Structures associated with the deep aspect of the gland, provided it sends projections medial to the styloid process, include the external and internal carotid arteries, the internal jugular vein, and both the vagus and glossopharyngeal nerves.

Several structures pass through the gland. The external carotid artery enters the substance of the gland, and it is there that several of its branches arise, including the posterior auricular, maxillary, and superficial temporal arteries. The retromandibular vein, as well as the veins uniting to form it, also pass through the gland.

The facial nerve (cranial nerve VII), exits the stylomastoid foramen and enters the substance of the gland. While in the gland, the facial nerve forms a plexus before exiting the gland to innervate the muscles of facial expression.

The **auriculotemporal nerve**, a branch of the mandibular division of the trigeminal nerve (cranial nerve V), enters the substance of the gland from its deep aspect along the neck of the mandible and emerges from the gland just inferior to the root of the zygomatic arch. While within the gland, it communicates with the facial nerve and distributes fibers to the gland. The functions of these communications are considered in the next section and in the section in this chapter on the facial nerve.

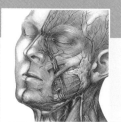

Clinical Considerations

Mumps

Mumps, a viral infection of the parotid gland that causes acute inflammation and profuse swelling of the gland, impinges on the auriculotemporal and great auricular nerves, causing much pain as the gland is pressured during mastication. Occasionally, it causes orchitis, pancreatitis, and encephalitis. Fortunately, this condition has been mostly eradicated as a result of vaccination.

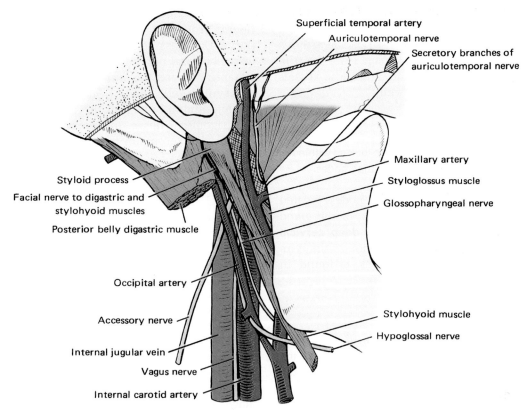

Figure 11-3. Structures deep in the parotid bed. Note that the carotid sheath has been removed to expose the internal carotid artery, the internal jugular vein, and the vagus nerve.

The structures entering the parotid gland exit from its posterior, superior, inferior, and anterior surfaces (Figs. 11-2 and 11-3). The posterior auricular artery exits from the posterior aspect of the gland. The superficial temporal artery and vein, auriculotemporal nerve, and temporal branches of the facial nerve may be observed at the superior margin of the gland. Inferiorly, the retromandibular vein exits the parotid gland just before joining the posterior auricular vein to form the external jugular vein. Emanating from the entire facial margin of the gland are the ter-minal branches of the facial nerve, grouped into five major branches: the **temporal**, **zygomatic**, **buccal**, **mandibular**, and **cervical branches** (see Fig. 11-1).

Vascular supply

 Summary Bite. The posterior auricular artery is the major vascular supply to the parotid gland.

The posterior auricular artery, arising from the exter-nal carotid artery within the substance of the parotid

Clinical Considerations

Parotid Gland

Infections of the parotid gland may be confused with toothache as a result of trigeminal nerve involvement. An inflamed parotid papilla (the orifice of the parotid duct in the oral cavity) may be an indication that the problem may be caused by the parotid gland rather than by a tooth. Diseases of the parotid gland cause pain to be referred to the ear, the TMJ, and the external auditory meatus. This is due to the overlapping of sensory branches of various nerves serving the regions of the parotid bed, ear, and TMJ.

gland, provides branches that vascularize the gland. Additional small glandular branches arising from the superficial temporal and transverse facial arteries also supply the gland. Venous drainage is via the tributaries passing through the gland, and these vessels empty into the external jugular vein.

Lymphatics

Summary Bite. Lymph nodes are located within the gland and drain into the cervical lymph nodes.

Lymph percolating through lymph nodes located superficially and within the substance of the gland is delivered into the **superficial** and **deep cervical lymph nodes**. A more detailed discussion of the lymphatic system of the head and neck is found in Chapter 20.

Innervation

Summary Bite. General sensation to the parotid gland is provided by the great auricular nerve of the cervical plexus. Sympathetic innervation is supplied by the carotid plexus, whereas secretomotor innervation is supplied by the glossopharyngeal nerve and delivered to the gland by the auriculotemporal nerve.

The parotid gland receives sensory and autonomic innervation. General sensation is provided by branches of the **great auricular nerve**, from the cervical plexus, as it ramifies over the surface of the gland.

The sympathetic component of the autonomic nervous system reaches the gland via postganglionic sympathetic fibers derived from the carotid plexus; these fibers travel on the external carotid artery and its branches that course through the gland. Sympathetic innervation to the parotid gland mediates vasoconstriction to these vessels.

Parasympathetic innervation is distributed to the gland by the auriculotemporal nerve [a branch of the trigeminal nerve (cranial nerve V)], even though these parasympathetic fibers do not arise within the trigeminal complex. Preganglionic parasympathetic fibers, from the glossopharyngeal nerve (cranial nerve IX), pass from its tympanic branch via the lesser petrosal nerve to the otic ganglion, where they synapse on postganglionic cell bodies. Postganglionic parasympathetic fibers from here then join the auriculotemporal branch of the mandibular division of the trigeminal nerve, to be distributed to the gland effecting secretomotor functions.

CAROTID ARTERIES

Summary Bite. The internal carotid artery ascends in the neck deep to the parotid gland within the carotid sheath in company with the internal jugular vein and the vagus nerve. Several arteries arise from the external carotid artery and pass near or through the parotid gland.

The internal and external carotid arteries arise in the neck from a bifurcation of the common carotid artery at the level of the superior border of the thyroid cartilage (Fig. 11-3).

The internal carotid artery then ascends in the neck, providing no branches before it enters the carotid canal of the petrous portion of the temporal bone. In its ascent deep to the parotid gland, the digastric muscle, and the muscles attached to the styloid process, this artery is contained within the carotid sheath in company with the internal jugular vein and the vagus nerve (cranial nerve X).

The external carotid artery, in contrast, supplies many of the structures of the neck and face. Those branches supplying the neck are described in Chapter 7. Branches originating from the external carotid artery inferior to the parotid bed, such as the lingual and facial arteries, are discussed in appropriate chapters.

Several arteries either originate in or are in close association with the parotid bed and are best described at this point. These are the ascending pharyngeal,

Clinical Considerations

Parotid Secretomotor Innervation

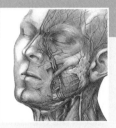

Although secretomotor innervation to the parotid gland is described as being provided from the glossopharyngeal nerve (cranial nerve IX), some evidence suggests that the facial nerve may supply parasympathetic innervation to the parotid gland in addition to that from the glossopharyngeal nerve. This subject is discussed in more detail in Chapter 18.

occipital, posterior auricular, maxillary, and superficial temporal arteries.

The **ascending pharyngeal artery** arises from the external carotid artery near its origin and ascends between the pharynx and the internal carotid artery. Through its several named branches, it supplies some of the prevertebral muscles, a portion of the tympanic cavity, and portions of the soft palate. Pharyngeal branches arise to supply the stylopharyngeus and the pharyngeal constrictor muscles before the ascending pharyngeal artery terminates as two or more meningeal branches that enter the jugular foramen to ascend into the cranium.

The **occipital artery** originates from the posterior aspect of the external carotid artery just before the external carotid dives deep to the posterior belly of the digastric muscle. The occipital artery courses under the cover of the digastric and stylohyoid muscles (Fig. 11-3), supplying both via muscular branches, as it passes posteriorly to groove the mastoid process of the temporal bone. This artery supplies the sternocleidomastoid muscle, auricle, posterior neck musculature, and meninges through its named branches, whereas the terminal branches serve the scalp and its musculature.

The internal and external carotid arteries become separated from their close association in the parotid bed as they pass deep and superficial, respectively, to the styloid process. The superficial position places the external carotid within the substance of the gland and, while there, the posterior auricular artery arises, as do the two terminal arteries of the external carotid, the maxillary and superficial temporal (Fig. 11-3).

The **posterior auricular artery** arises near the apex of the styloid process and, passing through the parotid gland that it supplies, sends branches to the digastric, stylohyoid, and sternocleidomastoid muscles (Fig. 11-2). Named branches include the **stylomastoid artery**, which enters the like-named foramen to supply the tympanic cavity; the **auricular artery**, passing to the posterior aspect of the ear; and the **occipital artery**, which supplies the scalp and occipitalis muscle.

The **maxillary artery** arises from the external carotid artery as it nears the deep aspect of the neck of the mandible (Fig. 11-3); while within the gland, branches named the **deep auricular** and **anterior tympanic** pass posteriorly to the ear and tympanic cavity. The artery then passes anteriorly between the ramus of the mandible and the sphenomandibular ligament, where it exits the substance of the gland to enter the deep face. Its branches and distribution are presented in Chapter 12.

The smaller, terminal **superficial temporal artery** exits the parotid gland to become superficial as it crosses the zygomatic arch posterior to the mandible, in company with the auriculotemporal nerve (Figs. 11-2 and 11-3). While within the parotid gland, the artery sends unnamed branches to the gland, the TMJ, and the masseter muscle.

The **transverse facial artery** also originates within the parotid gland and exits that structure between the zygomatic arch and the parotid duct (Fig. 11-2). Its distribution is discussed in Chapter 8.

Other named branches arising from the superficial temporal artery include the middle temporal; zygomatico-orbital; anterior auricular; and terminal, frontal, and parietal branches. These branches freely anastomose with other arteries distributing to these same areas.

FACIAL NERVE

Summary Bite. The facial nerve exits the cranial vault via the stylomastoid foramen. It then enters the parotid gland where it forms a loop from which arise the five terminal nerves that provide motor innervation to the muscles of facial expression.

The facial nerve is treated in detail in Chapter 18; however, because the nerve is in intimate association with the parotid bed and gland, its relationship and distribution to the structures in this area are discussed here (Figs. 11-1 and 11-2; for more detail see Tables 18-1 and 18-2).

The **facial nerve**, cranial nerve VII, exits from the cranial cavity at the stylomastoid foramen located in the temporal bone just posterior to the styloid process. On exiting, it communicates with the glossopharyngeal and vagus nerves and with the great auricular nerve of the cervical plexus.

The auriculotemporal nerve from the mandibular division of the trigeminal nerve communicates with the facial nerve after it has entered the substance of the parotid gland. Presumably, this communication provides general sensory fibers from the trigeminal nerve to the facial nerve for distribution to the face. Branches arising from the facial nerve as it passes through this area include the posterior auricular, digastric, stylohyoid, and parotid plexus with its terminals.

The **posterior auricular nerve** arises near the stylomastoid foramen and ascends behind the ear. This branch supplies motor innervation to the auricular and occipital muscles. The **digastric** and **stylohoid** branches provide motor innervation to the like-named muscles as each branch arises near that muscle.

Clinical Considerations

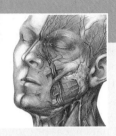

Parotid Tumors

Tumors of the parotid gland may be excised, but extreme care must be exercised during surgery because any damage to the facial nerve will result in at least partial facial paralysis. Total destruction of the facial nerve results in complete facial paralysis (Bell palsy).

On entering the substance of the parotid gland, the facial nerve terminates into two communicating branches, often forming a loop within the gland (Fig. 11-1). The superior of these is the temporofacial branch, whereas the cervicofacial branch is the inferior portion of the nerve.

Arising from this **parotid plexus** are the five major nerve branches emanating from the facial aspect of the parotid gland, ramifying over the superficial face as the temporal, zygomatic, buccal, mandibular, and cervical branches serving the muscles of facial expression with motor innervation. The specific distribution of these branches is described in Chapter 8.

STRUCTURES DEEP TO THE PAROTID BED

Muscles

Summary Bite. Although no muscles reside within the parotid bed, a few are closely associated with that space. These include the masseter, the posterior digastric, and the stylohyoid muscles.

Technically, no muscles reside within the parotid bed. However, several muscles yet to be described are in close association with and/or form the boundaries of the bed and are, therefore, best described here.

The **masseter muscle**, which is attached to the lateral aspect of the ramus of the mandible, is in intimate association with the parotid gland (Figs. 11-1 and 11-2). However, because it is one of the muscles of mastication, a discussion of it is deferred to Chapter 12.

The **digastric muscle**, it will be recalled, serves to form the boundaries of several of the subtriangles in the anterior triangle of the neck. It is composed of

two separate bellies united by an intermediate tendon at the hyoid bone, and also assists in forming the medial boundary of the parotid bed. Its posterior belly, the only portion associated with the parotid bed (Figs. 11-2 and 11-3), arises from the mastoid notch on the temporal bone and passes anteroinferiorly to the hyoid bone. It is about this bone that the intermediate tendon unites the two bellies, as the tendon perforates the stylohyoid muscle near its insertion on the hyoid bone.

The posterior belly of the digastric muscle is innervated by a branch of the facial nerve that enters its deep surface at about midbelly. With its anterior component, the posterior belly functions to fix the hyoid bone. Specifically, the posterior belly pulls the hyoid bone posteriorly. A more thorough discussion of both bellies is presented in Chapter 15 on the submandibular region.

The **stylohyoid muscle**, another muscle forming the medial boundary of the parotid bed, arises from the posterior and lateral aspects of the styloid process of the temporal bone. The origin of this muscle places it anterior to the posterior belly of the digastric (Fig. 11-3). The two muscles are rather closely associated because the stylohyoid also passes anteroinferiorly to insert on the body of the hyoid bone. The muscle is perforated, as described previously, by the digastric tendon.

The stylohyoid muscle is innervated by a branch of the facial nerve, which passes very close by, on its way to the parotid gland. This muscle, not unlike the posterior belly of the digastric, assists in fixing the hyoid bone by pulling it posteriorly and superiorly.

Two other muscles arise from the styloid process in addition to the stylohyoid muscle: the styloglossus and stylopharyngeus muscles. Although a more complete discussion of these two muscles is presented in subsequent chapters, a brief discussion is warranted here.

The **styloglossus muscle** arises from the styloid process and inserts into the side of the tongue. This

Clinical Considerations

Stylohyoid Ligament

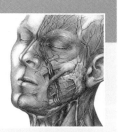

Occasionally, the stylohyoid ligament becomes cartilaginous and/or ossifies and thus appears as a radiopaque structure in a panographic radiograph.

Apparently, this condition has no pathologic consequence.

muscle is innervated by the hypoglossal nerve (cranial nerve XII) and functions to draw the tongue superiorly and posteriorly.

The **stylopharyngeus muscle** arises from the styloid process and inserts into the lateral wall of the pharynx between the superior and medial pharyngeal constrictor muscles. The glossopharyngeal nerve (cranial nerve IX) innervates this muscle, which functions to elevate the pharynx and larynx.

Ligaments

Summary Bite. The stylohyoid ligament, formed by a thickened portion of the parotid fascia, helps to separate the parotid and submandibular glands.

Associated with the stylohyoid muscle and the styloid process is a ligamentous band, the **stylohyoid ligament**, suspended between the tip of the styloid process and the lesser cornu of the hyoid bone. This ligament, formed by a thickening of the deep parotid fascia, assists in separating the parotid and submandibular glands, as does the similarly formed stylomandibular ligament, described as an accessory ligament to the temporomandibular joint (see Chapter 13).

Nerves and Arteries

Summary Bite. Deep to the styloid process are the glossopharyngeal, accessory, and hypoglossal nerves. However, the vagus nerve is within the carotid sheath along with the internal carotid artery and the internal jugular vein.

Immediately deep to the muscles originating on the styloid process are the last four cranial nerves, the internal carotid artery, and the internal jugular vein (Figs. 11-2 and 11-3).

The glossopharyngeal, vagus, and accessory nerves exit the skull through the jugular foramen, whereas the hypoglossal nerve exits the skull via the hypoglossal canal. As these nerves descend to the structures they innervate, they may be observed passing on the lateral surface of the internal carotid artery and internal jugular vein housed, along with the vagus nerve, in the carotid sheath.

Within the carotid sheath, the laterally placed internal jugular vein, originating at the jugular foramen, descends to enter the subclavian vein at the root of the neck. The internal carotid artery ascends within the sheath to enter the carotid canal in the petrous portion of the temporal bone, whereas the vagus nerve descends through the neck on its way to the thorax and abdomen.

Deep Face

Key Terms

Deep Face is that portion of the side of the head located deep to the mandible and zygomatic arch. It contains the origins and insertions of three of the four muscles of mastication.

Depressor of the Jaw is the lateral pterygoid muscle, the muscle of mastication that functions in initiating opening of the jaw.

Elevators of the Jaw are the muscles of mastication, including the masseter, temporalis, and medial pterygoid muscles that function primarily in closing the jaw.

Infratemporal Fossa is the region inferior and deep to the zygomatic arch and the mandible. It contains the origins and insertions of the muscles of

mastication except the masseter. Its contents include branches of the mandibular division of the trigeminal nerve (cranial nerve V), the maxillary artery and its branches, and the pterygoid plexus of veins.

Mandibular Division of the Trigeminal Nerve is the portion of the trigeminal nerve (cranial nerve V) that supplies motor innervation to the muscles of mastication and sensory innervation to the TMJ and the side of the head. Additional branches of the mandibular division that arise in the infratemporal fossa are bound for other regions and will be discussed with those regions.

Maxillary Artery and its branches serve the structures located within the

temporal and infratemporal fossae, including all of the muscles of mastication. Additionally, the maxillary artery serves the external acoustic meatus, tympanum, and TMJ. Other branches of the maxillary artery arise within the deep face but are bound for other anatomical regions and will be discussed with those regions.

Muscles of Mastication are a set of four bilateral muscles whose function is to move the mandible about the temporomandibular joint (TMJ) as it functions in phonation, chewing (masticating), and swallowing. All of these muscles except the masseter muscle originate from either the temporal or infratemporal fossae, and all four muscles insert upon the mandible or about the TMJ.

Pterygoid Venous Plexus lies on and about the pterygoid muscles and extends into spaces within the deep face. This plexus of veins collects venous blood from the deep face and other areas of the superficial face, nasal cavity, orbit, paranasal sinuses, etc. Also, the pterygoid venus plexus is in direct communication with the cavernous sinus, another venous reservoir within the cranial cavity. Because of its vast area of collection and its communications, the pterygoid venous plexus can be a conduit for infection into the cranial vault.

Temporal Fossa is that portion of the side of the head located above the ear and zygomatic arch, and is called the temple. It is outlined and covered by the temporalis muscle.

The region to be described in this chapter is considered the deep face. It encompasses the structures deep to the mandible, including three of the muscles of mastication. The fourth muscle of mastication, the masseter muscle, lies superficial to the mandible, but it is described here for the sake of continuity. Additionally, a newly discovered muscle of the deep face will also be discussed. The normal functioning of this muscle group, a part of the stomatognathic system, is essential for good oral health.

A thorough understanding of this region of anatomy is of paramount importance to the healthcare professional if that person is to comprehend the complexities of the stomatognathic system in normal and pathologic functions. It is imperative that a person diagnosing and treating inadequate anesthesia, malocclusion, the maladies of pain, and the spread of infection in and about the oral cavity "know her or his anatomy."

REGIONAL INNERVATION AND VASCULAR SUPPLY

Located within the deep face are sensory branches of the maxillary and mandibular divisions of the trigeminal nerve which transmit sensory innervation from the teeth and associated structures of the upper and lower jaws, respectively. In addition, the mandibular division provides sensory innervation to the temporomandibular joint, another component of the stomatognathic system.

The motor root of the trigeminal nerve unites with the mandibular division just outside the skull for distribution to the muscles of mastication and the few additional muscles developed within the first pharyngeal arch mesoderm. The vascular supply to this region similarly serves some of the oral cavity and teeth, in addition to supplying the temporomandibular joint, some parts of the ear, and the muscles of mastication.

DESCRIPTIONS AND BOUNDARIES

Temporal Fossa

Summary Bite. The temporal fossa is the region on the side of the head above the external ear canal, which is covered by the temporalis muscle.

The side of the head anterior and superior to the ear is commonly called the temple. The skin, fascia, and portions of the extrinsic muscles of the ear in this region overlie the deeper fan-shaped temporalis muscle attached to the bones of the **temporal fossa** (Fig. 12-1).

Superiorly, this fossa is bounded by the superior temporal line, whereas its inferior boundary is arbitrarily designated to be the zygomatic arch even though the temporalis muscle extends inferiorly below this arch into the infratemporal fossa.

The floor of the temporal fossa is formed by the bones of the side of the head—portions of the frontal, sphenoid, temporal, and parietal bones.

The superior-most extent of the origin of the temporalis muscle and its fascia marks these bones with the inferior and superior temporal lines, respectively. These lines begin at the zygomatic process of the frontal bone and arch posteriorly over the parietal bone before descending to the temporal bone and blending into the zygomatic process of this bone.

Infratemproal Fossa

Summary Bite. The infratemporal fossa lies inferior to the zygomatic arch and deep to the mandible.

The region inferior to the zygomatic arch and deep to the mandible is termed the **infratemporal fossa** (Fig. 12-2 and Table 12-1). This irregular space, posterior to the maxilla which forms its anterior wall, is bounded laterally by the ramus and the coronoid process of the

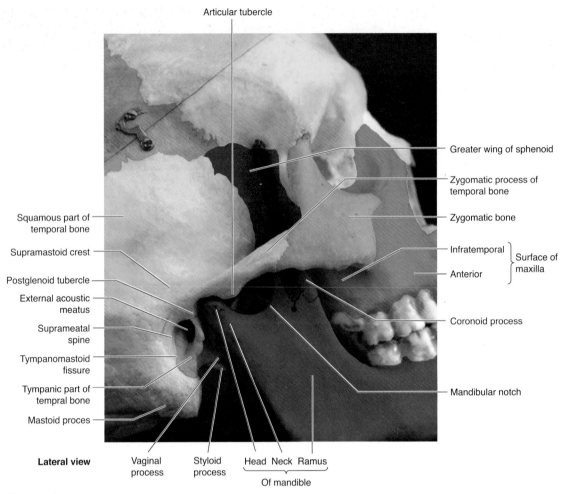

Articular tubercle

Greater wing of sphenoid

Zygomatic process of
temporal bone

Zygomatic bone

Infratemporal — Surface of
maxilla
Anterior

Coronoid process

Mandibular notch

Squamous part of
temporal bone

Supramastoid crest

Postglenoid tubercle

External acoustic
meatus

Suprameatal
spine

Tympanomastoid
fissure

Tympanic part of
tempral bone

Mastoid proces

Lateral view

Vaginal
process

Styloid
process

Head Neck Ramus
Of mandible

Figure 12-1. Temporal fossa.

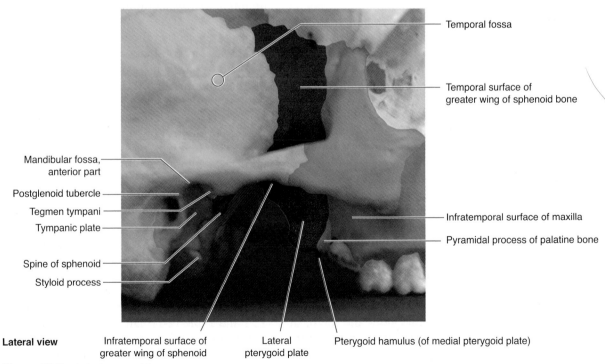

Temporal fossa

Temporal surface of
greater wing of sphenoid bone

Mandibular fossa,
anterior part

Postglenoid tubercle

Tegmen tympani

Tympanic plate

Infratemporal surface of maxilla

Pyramidal process of palatine bone

Spine of sphenoid

Styloid process

Lateral view

Infratemporal surface of
greater wing of sphenoid

Lateral
pterygoid plate

Pterygoid hamulus (of medial pterygoid plate)

Figure 12-2. Infratemporal fossa.

Table 12-1 Boundaries, Communications, and Contents of the Infratemporal Fossa

Region	Boundary	Communications	Contents
Superior	Infratemporal surface of greater wing of sphenoid and infratemporal crest plus small part of temporal	Cranial cavity via foramen ovale, foramen spinosum; temporal fossa	Temporalis muscle (inferior portion) Medial pterygoid muscle Lateral pterygoid muscle Maxillary artery and branches Pterygoid plexus of veins Chorda tympani nerve Otic ganglion Mandibular nerve and branches Posterosuperior alveolar nerve
Inferior	Continuous with submandibular region		
Medial	Lateral pterygoid plate of sphenoid	Pterygopalatine fossa via pterygomaxillary fissure	
Lateral	Ramus and coronoid process of mandible		
Anterior	Posterior aspect of maxilla to the inferior orbital fissure	Orbit via inferior orbital fissure	
Posterior	Continuous with structures about the styloid process		

mandible, whereas its medial extent is the lateral pterygoid plate of the sphenoid bone.

Superiorly, the fossa is limited by the infratemporal surface of the greater wing of the sphenoid bone and the very anteroinferior-most portion of the temporal squama. The bony ridge extending across these two bones, known as the **infratemporal crest**, delineates the superior-most extent of the roof of the fossa. Inferiorly, the infratemporal fossa has no boundary but extends into the neck lateral to the pharynx.

Communications

The infratemporal fossa communicates with the temporal fossa as the temporalis muscle descends from its origin in the temporal fossa to be inserted onto the coronoid process of the mandible (Table 12-1).

Nerves and vessels supplying the temporalis muscle pass from the infratemporal fossa to the temporal fossa to pierce the deep surface of this muscle.

Two foramina open onto its roof on the medial aspect of the infratemporal region of the greater wing of the sphenoid. The larger of the two, the foramen ovale, transmits the mandibular division of the trigeminal nerve exiting from the cranial vault and the accessory meningeal artery proceeding to the cranium.

The smaller foramen, the foramen spinosum, lies between the foramen ovale and the spine of the sphenoid. It transmits the middle meningeal artery and the recurrent meningeal nerve from the fossa into the cranium.

The fossa communicates with the orbit at its most superoanterior aspect via the inferior orbital fissure between the maxilla and the greater wing of the sphe-

noid. Through this fissure pass the maxillary division of the trigeminal nerve, on its way to the floor of the orbit, as well as the zygomatic branch which arises from it.

The cleft between the maxilla and the lateral pterygoid plate is the pterygomaxillary fissure communicating with the pterygopalatine fossa, medially. It is through this fissure that the maxillary artery distributes to the fossa, eventually to reach the nasal cavity via the sphenopalatine foramen.

The posterior superior alveolar nerve, arising from the maxillary nerve as the latter nerve traverses the pterygopalatine fossa, utilizes the pterygomaxillary fissure as an exit on its way to the tuberosity of the maxilla.

MUSCLES AND FASCIA

Muscles of Mastication

Summary Bite. The muscles of mastication and their fascia are located in the temporal and infratemporal fossae.

The muscles of mastication (Table 12-2), all of which are developed in first pharyngeal arch mesoderm, are located within the confines of the deep face, with the exception of the masseter muscle previously described as lateral to the mandible.

These muscles, excepting the masseter, originate on the deep bony aspect of the temporal and infratem-

Table 12-2 Muscles of Mastication

Muscle	Origin	Insertion
Masseter	Superficial: tendinous aponeurosis from zygomatic process of maxilla and anterior two-thirds of inferior border of zygomatic arch Deep: medial aspect and inferior border of posterior one-third of zygomatic arch	Lateral aspect of ramus and angle of mandible as far anteriorly as the last molar tooth, as far superiorly as base of coronoid process
Temporalis	Inferior temporal line and bones of the temporal fossa	As a tendon on coronoid process and anterior border of ramus of mandible as far inferiorly and anteriorly as third molar
Medial (internal) pterygoid	Pterygoid fossa and medial surface of lateral pterygoid plate; one slip from lateral portion of pyramidal process of palatine bone and adjacent maxillary tuberosity	Medial surface of mandibular ramus as far superiorly as the sphenomandibular ligament, inferiorly to mylohyoid groove
Lateral (external) pterygoid	Superior head: greater wing of sphenoid and infratemporal crest Inferior head: lateral surface of lateral pterygoid plate	Superior head: articular capsule of temporo-mandibular joint—the disk and the superior portion of mandibular neck Inferior head: anterior surface of mandibular neck

poral fossae and insert upon the medial aspect of the mandible. The masseter, in contrast, originates on the zygomatic arch and inserts upon the lateral aspect of the mandible (Fig. 12-2).

This group of muscles (the temporalis, medial pterygoid, lateral pterygoid, and masseter) are covered by their epimysia, which become the fascia encircling the masticator compartment. The **masticator compartment** contains the four muscles of mastication and the ramus of the mandible (Fig. 12-3).

Fascia

Summary Bite. The fascia covering the muscles of mastication and the parotid gland are all divisions of the deep fascia. This fascia completely surrounds the muscles of mastication and encircles the ramus of the mandible. It splits to cover the pterygoid muscles, joins again, and then attaches to the stylomandibular ligament, assisting in the formation of the sphenomandibular ligament.

The **temporal fascia** spans from the superior temporal line over the temporalis muscle to attach to the zygomatic arch on both its medial and lateral surfaces.

The **parotideomasseteric fascia**, attached cranially to the zygomatic arch, splits to encompass the parotid gland as it passes on the lateral surface of the masseter muscle to become continuous with the deep cervical fascia about the suprahyoid muscles.

The **masseteric fascia** covers the masseter muscle and encircles the ramus of the mandible, inferi-

orly, where it becomes continuous with the **pterygoid fascia** (Fig. 12-3).

Both the lateral and medial pterygoid muscles are enclosed by the pterygoid fascia. However, the fascia is much thicker covering the inferior aspect of the medial pterygoid muscle, where it becomes continuous with the cervical and masseteric fascia as well as with the stylomandibular ligament.

As the pterygoid fascia reflects over the superior portion of the medial pterygoid muscle, it splits to encompass the lateral pterygoid muscle as well and is attached to the bony origin of that muscle and to the spine of the sphenoid bone. The latter attachment is much thickened, forming the **sphenomandibular ligament** from the spine of the sphenoid bone to the lingula of the mandible (Fig. 13-3). The thickened portion of the pterygoid fascia, located between the two pterygoid muscles spanning between the spine of the sphenoid and the lateral pterygoid plate, is known as the **pterygospinous ligament**. Occasionally this ligament is ossified. When that is the case, a pterygospinous foramen is present between the ligament and the skull for the transmission of branches of the mandibular nerve to the muscles. This fascia possesses an interval, near the neck of the mandible, for the passage of the maxillary vessels to the infratemporal fossa. Lying between the temporalis and over much of the surface of the pterygoid muscles is the **venous pterygoid plexus**, connecting many of the venous tributaries both inside and outside the cranial cavity, face, deep face, orbit, and nasal cavity.

Vascularization	Innervation	Function
Masseteric branch from maxillary artery	Masseteric branch from mandibular division of trigeminal nerve	Powerful elevator of jaw
Anterior and posterior deep temporal arteries from maxillary artery; these anastomose with middle temporal from superficial temporal artery	Anterior and posterior deep temporal nerves of the mandibular division of the trigeminal nerve	Primarily an elevator of mandible; some fibers (post and middle) act as retractor
Branch from maxillary artery	Medial pterygoid nerve from trunk of mandibular division of the trigeminal nerve	Primarily an elevator of mandible
Branch from maxillary artery	Lateral pterygoid nerve from mandibular division of trigeminal nerve	Superior head: mandibular stabilizer Inferior head: jaw depressor and slight protruder; initiates jaw opening

Temporalis Muscle

Summary Bite. The temporalis, a muscle of mastication, originates in the temporal fossa and inserts onto the coronoid process of the mandible.

The **temporalis muscle** is a fan-shaped muscle originating on the bones of the broad temporal fossa (Figs. 12-3 and 12-4). Specifically, the site of origin extends inferiorly from the inferior temporal line over the entire temporal fossa, including parts of the parietal and most of the squama of the temporal bones, and the greater wing of the sphenoid, including its infratemporal crest and the temporal surface of the frontal bone. Occasionally, some fibers arise from the posterior temporal surface of the frontal process of the zygoma. The muscle bundles converge to insert as a tendon on the coronoid process of the mandible and down along its anterior surface and the anterior border of the ramus as far anteriorly as the third molar (Figs. 12-2, 12-3, and 12-4, and Table 12-2). The anterior fibers of this muscle are directed in a vertical plane from origin to insertion, the middle fibers in an oblique plane, and the posterior fibers in an almost horizontal plane.

The muscle is primarily an elevator of the mandible; however, because of the directional alignments of the muscle fibers, the posterior and middle portions of the muscle are reported to act also in retracting the mandible.

The temporalis muscle is innervated by anterior and posterior deep temporal nerves from the mandibular division of the trigeminal nerve. The nerves enter the muscle from its deep aspect in the temporal fossa.

Vascularization is supplied to the temporalis muscle via branches of the superficial temporal and maxillary arteries. Arising from the former is the middle temporal artery, which enters the muscle on its superficial aspect. Anterior and posterior deep temporal arteries, arising from the maxillary artery, accompany the like-named nerves and enter the deep aspect of the muscle, where they anastomose with the middle temporal artery.

Masseter Muscle

Summary Bite. The masseter, the only muscle of mastication located outside the deep face, originates from the zygomatic arch and inserts upon the angle and ramus of the mandible.

The shape of the posterior region of the jaw is due to the quadrangular form of the **masseter muscle** overlying the angle and ramus of the mandible (Figs. 12-1, 12-3, and Table 12-2). The masseter muscle, as previously described, is the only muscle of mastication that lies outside the anatomical confines of the deep face, since it originates on the zygomatic arch and inserts into the lateral surface of the mandible.

This muscle possesses, from its origin, a superficial portion and a smaller, deep portion. The superficial portion arises, via a tendinous aponeurosis, from

Clinical Considerations

Masticator Space Infection

The deep fascia about the mandible splits, forming two laminae around its inferior border. As a consequence, the muscles of mastication (the temporalis, masseter, and medial and lateral pterygoid muscles) are thus enclosed into a compartment termed the masticator space (see Fig. 12-3). The two laminae fuse again at the superior border of temporalis muscle where it originates from the skull. In addition to containing the muscles of mastication, this large space also contains the maxillary artery and many of its branches; the mandibular division of the trigeminal nerve and many of its branches; and much of the buccal fat pad. The masticator space also communicates with many other spaces within the head and neck which may contribute to the spread of infections and or neoplasms from the oral cavity.

Salivary gland tumors, abscesses, hemangiomas, and metastatic extensions of squamous cell carcinoma (especially from the floor of the mouth, tonsilar fossa, and nasopharynx) can extend into the masticator space. Persons suspected of having masticator space infections are very ill and need immediate medical attention.

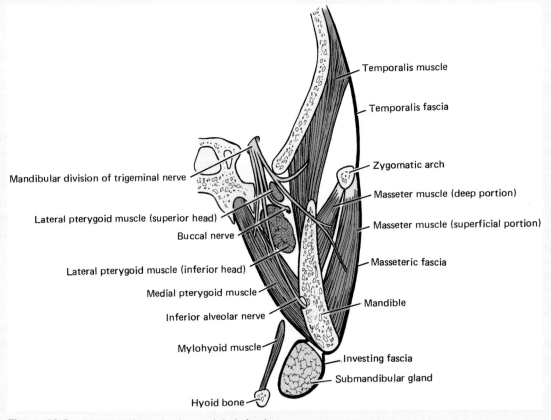

Figure 12-3.   Muscles of mastication and their fascia.

the zygomatic process of the maxilla and the anterior two-thirds of the inferior border of the zygomatic arch.

The smaller, deep portion arises from the inferior border of the posterior one third of the zygomatic arch and from along its entire medial aspect. It is reported that the origin of the superficial portion is limited posteriorly by the zygomaticotemporal suture. The origin of the deep portion is limited posteriorly by the anterior slope of the articular eminence of the zygomatic arch.

The fibers of the superficial and deep portions of the muscle fuse to become inserted on the mandible, broadly covering the angle, along with some of the ramus and the body, as far anteriorly as the region directly below the last molar.

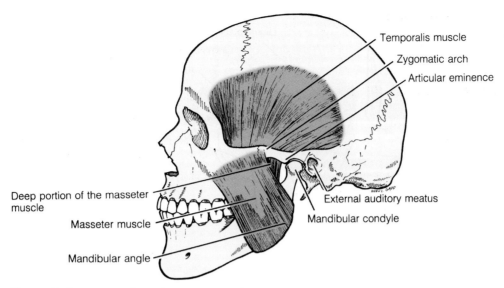

Figure 12-4. Temporalis and masseter muscles.

Some fibers derived from the deeper portion insert as far superiorly as the base of the coronoid process. It is in this region that fibers of the temporalis muscle, arising from the inner surface of the zygomatic arch, may be fused with those of the deep portion of the masseter; in such cases it is termed the **zygomaticomandibularis muscle**.

The masseter muscle functions as a powerful elevator of the jaw. The superficial fibers act to direct a powerful force on the molars, whereas the deep fibers, more vertically directed, effect a retractive force, especially in closing the jaws.

The muscle is innervated by the masseteric nerve derived from the mandibular division of the trigeminal nerve. This motor nerve enters the muscle on its deep aspect adjacent to the mandibular notch, through which it gains access from its origin in the deep face.

Vascular supply to the muscle is provided by the masseteric branch of the maxillary artery. The artery and vein accompany the nerve in its path to the muscle.

Medial Pterygoid Muscle

Summary Bite. The medial pterygoid, the deepest-located muscle of mastication, inserts on the inner aspect of the ramus and angle of the mandible, mirroring the insertions of the masseter.

The **medial (internal) pterygoid muscle**, originating in the deepest aspect of the deep face, inserts onto the medial aspect of the ramus and angle of the mandible. Thus, it is anatomically and functionally a counterpart to the masseter muscle (Figs. 12-2, 12-3, 12-5 through 12-8, and Table 12-2).

The specific sites of origin are the pyramidal process of the palatine bone in the pterygoid fossa and the medial surface of the lateral pterygoid plate. This area of origin is broad in that it extends to the tensor veli palatini muscle.

An additional anterior muscular slip arises from the lateral portion of the pyramidal process and the adjacent region of the maxillary tuberosity. Although the main mass of the muscle lies deep to the lateral pterygoid muscle, the additional anterior slip lies superficial to that muscle.

The medial pterygoid muscle is directed inferiorly, posteriorly, and laterally to be inserted onto the medial surface of the ramus of the mandible. The insertion site lies between the mandibular angle, the mylohyoid groove, and the mandibular foramen.

The sphenomandibular ligament marks the superiormost extent of the insertion. Occasionally, a tendinous inscription denotes the meeting of the fibers of the masseter and medial pterygoid muscles at the inferior border of the angle of the mandible. This arrangement is referred to as the **pterygomasseteric sling**.

The medial pterygoid muscle functions primarily as an elevator of the mandible. Its fibers are directed in an oblique fashion; however, the force is more pronounced in a vertical direction. The insertions of the masseter and medial pterygoid muscles—suspending the angle of the mandible between them—form the **mandibular sling**, about which these muscles act synergistically, utilizing the temporomandibular joint (TMJ) as a guide.

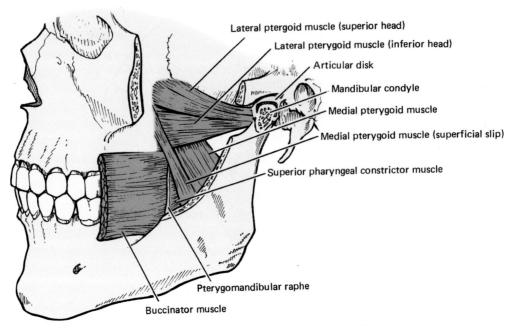

Lateral ptergoid muscle (superior head)

Lateral pterygoid muscle (inferior head)

Articular disk

Mandibular condyle

Medial pterygoid muscle

Medial pterygoid muscle (superficial slip)

Superior pharyngeal constrictor muscle

Pterygomandibular raphe

Buccinator muscle

Figure 12-5. Lateral view of the medial and lateral pterygoid muscles. Note how the heads of the lateral pterygoid muscle insert into the head of the condyle and into the articular disc.

The medial pterygoid muscle receives its motor innervation from a like-named nerve branching from the mandibular division of the trigeminal nerve and entering the deep surface of the muscle. The muscle is vascularized by a branch of the maxillary artery.

Lateral Pterygoid Muscle

Summary Bite. The lateral pterygoid muscle possesses two heads of origin which converge to insert on the neck of the mandible and various structures of the TMJ.

The **lateral (external) pterygoid muscle** is a short muscle, filling the remainder of the infratemporal fossa and covering much of the medial pterygoid muscle. This muscle possesses two heads of origin. The smaller, superior head originates from the infratemporal region of the greater wing of the sphenoid bone as far laterally as the infratemporal crest. The larger, inferior head originates from the lateral surface of the lateral pterygoid plate (Figs. 12-2, 12-3, 12-5 through 12-8, and Table 12-2).

The fibers of the superior head course posteriorly and laterally in an almost horizontal direction from the infratemporal crest. Fibers of the inferior head are

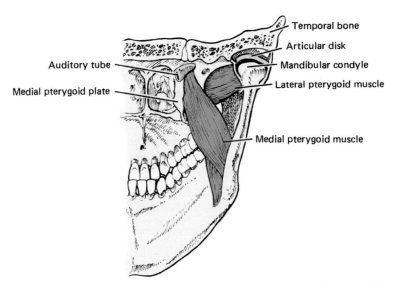

Temporal bone

Articular disk

Mandibular condyle

Auditory tube

Lateral pterygoid muscle

Medial pterygoid plate

Medial pterygoid muscle

Figure 12-6. Medial and lateral pterygoid muscles (posteroinferior view).

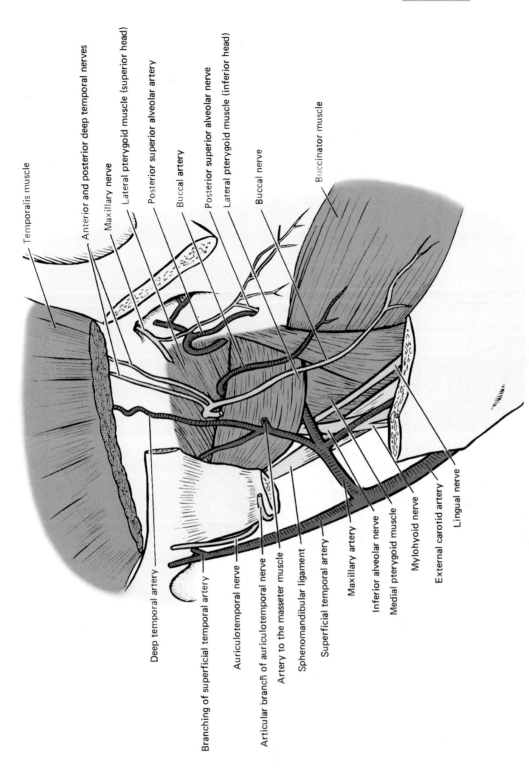

Temporalis muscle

Anterior and posterior deep temporal nerves

Maxillary nerve

Lateral pterygoid muscle (superior head)

Posterior superior alveolar artery

Buccal artery

Posterior superior alveolar nerve

Lateral pterygoid muscle (inferior head)

Buccal nerve

Buccinator muscle

Deep temporal artery

Branching of superficial temporal artery

Auriculotemporal nerve

Articular branch of auriculotemporal nerve

Artery to the masseter muscle

Sphenomandibular ligament

Superficial temporal artery

Maxillary artery

Inferior alveolar nerve

Medial pterygoid muscle

Mylohyoid nerve

External carotid artery

Lingual nerve

Figure 12-7. Deep face. A portion of the zygomatic arch and ramus of the mandible have been cut away to reveal the deep structures. Note the maxillary artery diving beneath the lateral pterygoid muscle.

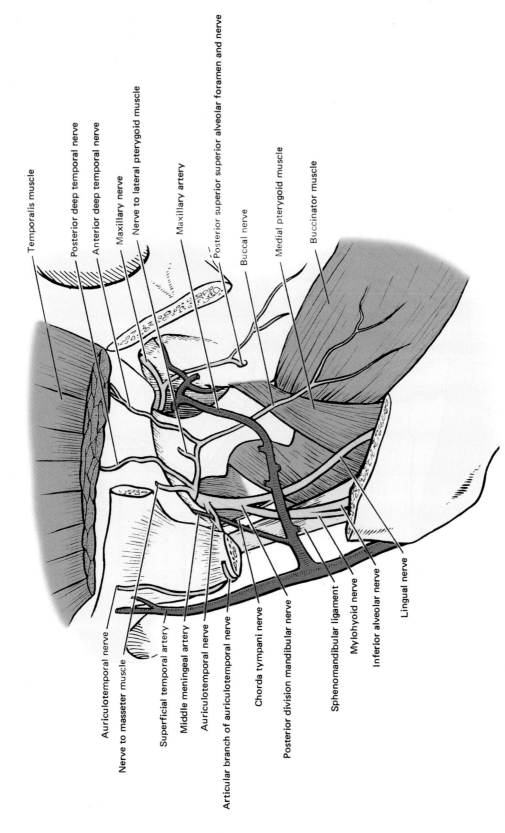

Temporalis muscle

Posterior deep temporal nerve

Anterior deep temporal nerve

Maxillary nerve

Nerve to lateral pterygoid muscle

Maxillary artery

Posterior superior superior alveolar foramen and nerve

Buccal nerve

Medial pterygoid muscle

Buccinator muscle

Auriculotemporal nerve

Nerve to masseter muscle

Superficial temporal artery

Middle meningeal artery

Auriculotemporal nerve

Articular branch of auriculotemporal nerve

Chorda tympani nerve

Posterior division mandibular nerve

Sphenomandibular ligament

Mylohyoid nerve

Inferior alveolar nerve

Lingual nerve

Figure 12-8. Arteries and nerves of the deep face. The lateral pterygoid muscle has been removed to reveal many branches of the mandibular division of the trigeminal nerve.

directed posteriorly, laterally, and slightly superiorly on their way to the mandible.

Though the two heads of origin are separated from each other, their fibers converge as they approach the site of insertion on and about the mandible. The superior head inserts into the articular capsule of the TMJ, the anterior border of the articular disc, and the superior part of the mandibular neck. The inferior head inserts along the anterior surface of the mandibular neck. Recent evidence indicates that the two heads remain separated even at the insertion site, perform different functions, and may be separately innervated.

The lateral pterygoid muscle is described classically as the "jaw opener," which protrudes the mandible and moves the mandible from side to side when functioning unilaterally.

Recent evidence supports the concept that the lateral pterygoid muscle is in fact two separate muscles, with a superior and an inferior head. The superior head, attached to the articular capsule and disc, is reported to function in stabilizing the mandibular condyle, whereas the inferior head is reported to function in pulling the mandible and disc forward and down, effecting jaw opening.

The lateral pterygoid muscle is innervated by a branch entering its deep surface from either the anterior division separately or as a branch of the buccal nerve from the mandibular division of the trigeminal nerve. Vascular supply is provided by a branch from the maxillary artery as it passes either superficial or deep to the muscle. Prolongations of the buccal fat pad fill in the spaces between the muscles of mastication deep to the mandible.

The TMJs are bilateral in that they are formed by the heads of the condyles of the mandible as each articulates with the bilateral temporal bones of the skull at the articular eminence of their zygomatic processes. Interposed between these articulating surfaces is a connective tissue disc that is reinforced by muscle attachment, ligaments, and a strong capsule. The forces that act upon this joint, resulting in opening and closing the mouth as well as side-by-side motions for chewing, are produced by the bilateral muscles of mastication.

The origins and insertion sites of these muscles on the mandible dictate the joint function. Generally, the functions are for opening or closing the jaw; however, subtle variations exist when muscles are acting antagonistically or synergistically with other muscles on one side or the other or on both sides (see Chapter 13).

Sphenomandibularis

Recently an additional muscle, the sphenomandibularis, was discovered in the deep face. Previously this muscle was described to be a part of the temporalis muscle; however, careful dissections have demonstrated it to be a separate entity. The sphenomandibularis muscle originates from the infratemporal surface of the greater wing of the sphenoid and has a tendinous insertion onto the temporal crest of the mandible. The vascular supply of this muscle is derived from small branches of the maxillary artery, in common with vessels destined for the medial pterygoid muscle. Its nerve supply has not as yet been determined.

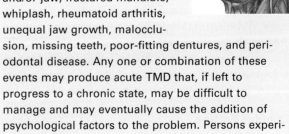

Clinical Considerations

Temporomandibular Disorder

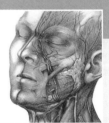

There are instances when the TMJ malfunctions, a term referred to as temporomandibular disorder (TMD). The symptoms are many and include (but are not restricted to) the following: tender, sore jaw muscles (muscles of mastication); pain at opening or closing the jaw; inability to open or close the jaw; pain upon clenching; unusual headaches; clicking or grinding noise when chewing or yawning; and crunching sounds when chewing.

The causes of TMD are not always clear but may include bruxing, grinding the teeth when asleep, clenching during periods of stress, injury to the face and/or jaw, fractured mandible, whiplash, rheumatoid arthritis, unequal jaw growth, malocclusion, missing teeth, poor-fitting dentures, and periodontal disease. Any one or combination of these events may produce acute TMD that, if left to progress to a chronic state, may be difficult to manage and may eventually cause the addition of psychological factors to the problem. Persons experiencing TMD symptoms should consult a dentist or a TMD specialist.

VASCULAR SUPPLY

Summary Bite. Structures of the deep face receive their vascular supply from branches of the maxillary artery.

The vascular supply to the entire region of the deep face is provided by branches of the maxillary artery along with a small contribution from the middle temporal artery to the superior surface of the temporalis muscle.

Maxillary Artery

Summary Bite. The maxillary artery, a terminal of the external carotid artery, courses deep to the mandible and passes through the parotid gland. The artery is described as consisting of three portions and terminates as several branches within the pterygopalatine fossa.

The **maxillary artery** (Table 12-3), the larger of two terminals of the external carotid artery, arises from that artery deep to the neck of the mandible embedded within the substance of the parotid gland.

The artery immediately turns anteriorly, passing between the mandibular ramus and the sphenomandibular ligament on its way to the pterygopalatine fossa, where it subsequently divides into terminal branches (Fig. 12-9). Along its course to that fossa, it provides branches to the ear, TMJ, meninges, muscles of mastication, teeth and supporting structures of the mandible, buccinator muscle, cheek, and mucous membrane of the mouth.

Terminals, branching from the artery while it is within the pterygopalatine fossa, serve the teeth and supporting tissues of the maxilla, the nasal cavity, and the palate. The major terminal enters the floor of the orbit as the infraorbital artery, which eventually exits upon the face.

The following discussion is confined mostly to descriptions of the artery and its branches supplying the structures of the deep face. Excluding a few exceptions, the terminal branches have been or will be detailed in the appropriate chapters.

The maxillary artery is described as consisting of three segments as it courses through the mandibular, pterygoid, and pterygopalatine regions.

Mandibular Portion

Summary Bite. The mandibular portion of the maxillary artery (located deep to the mandible) sends branches to the meninges, to the mandibular teeth, mylohy-

oid muscle, and supporting tissues, and to the lower lips as well as to the chin to anastomose with branches from other sources.

The mandibular portion runs behind the mandible between the ramus and the sphenomandibular ligament. Branches arising from this portion include the deep auricular and anterior tympanic arteries (described in Chapter 21).

Arising also from this portion are the **middle** and **accessory meningeal arteries**. Both of these arteries ascend to enter the skull via the foramen spinosum and foramen ovale, respectively. The distribution of these arteries is described in Chapter 9. Another artery arising from this portion of the maxillary artery is the **inferior alveolar artery**, which gives rise to the **mylohyoid artery** just before entering the mandibular foramen. The mylohyoid artery courses along the mylohyoid groove to the mylohyoid muscle, which it supplies. Within the mandibular canal, the inferior alveolar artery supplies the bone, teeth, and adjacent supporting structures as far anteriorly as the first premolar tooth, where it divides into an incisive branch and a mental branch. The **incisive branch** continues on to vascularize the anterior teeth and supporting structures. The **mental branch** exists the mandible through the mental foramen onto the face to anastomose with the inferior labial and submental arteries vascularizing the area of the chin.

Occasionally, a **lingual artery** may arise from the inferior alveolar artery near its origin from the mandibular portion of the maxillary artery. When present, this artery will descend to assist in vascularizing the mucous membrane of the mouth.

Pterygoid Portion

Summary Bite. The pterygoid portion of the maxillary artery vascularizes the muscles of mastication and the buccinator muscle.

Branches arising from the pterygoid segment of the maxillary artery are responsible for vascularizing the muscles of mastication and the buccinator muscle.

The course of this portion of the artery is not constant, since it may pass either superficial or deep to the lateral pterygoid muscle (see Figs. 12-7 and 12-8).

The **masseteric artery**, arising from this portion of the maxillary artery, passes through the mandibular notch to enter the masseter muscle.

The **anterior and posterior deep temporal arteries** accompany the like-named nerves to enter the deep surface of the temporalis muscle, anastomosing with the middle temporal branch of the superficial temporal artery.

Table 12-3 Maxillary Artery

Portion	Course	Branches	Distribution
Mandibular Portion First Part	Originates deep within parotid gland, coursing behind the mandibular ramus near the condylar process superficial to the sphenomandibular ligament.	Deep auricular artery	Supplies the TMJ, wall of external auditory meatus, and tympanic membrane.
		Anterior tympanic artery	Enters tympanic cavity to supply tympanic membrane and associated structures.
		Inferior alveolar artery	Enters mandibular foramen. Bifurcates into incisive branch supplying mandibular teeth and supporting tissues, and mental branch that exits mandible at the mental foramen to supply chin. The branch arising from the artery just prior to entering the mandibular foramen is the mylohyoid artery, which will supply the mylohyoid muscle.
		Middle and accessory meningeal arteries	Middle and accessory meningeal arteries arise separately or by a common trunk. The middle meningeal artery enters the skull through the foramen spinosum. The accessory meningeal artery enters through foramen ovale. These serve the meninges.
Pterygoid Portion Second Part	May course either superficial or deep to the lateral ptery-goid muscle on way to its way to the pterygopalatine fossa.	Deep temporal arteries	Anterior and posterior deep temporal arteries pass anteriorly and posteriorly as they ascend deep to the temporalis muscle, which they supply.
		Pterygoid arteries	Short branches that provide vascular supplies to the medial and lateral pterygoid muscles.
		Masseteric artery	This artery accompanies the same-named nerve through the mandibular notch to supply the masseter muscle.
		Buccal artery	Accompanies the buccal nerve, passing in close association with the temporalis tendon on its way to arborize on the buccinator muscle, providing a vascular supply to it and associated buccal mucosa of the mouth,
Pterygopalatine Portion Third Part	Courses into the ptery-gopalatine fossa via the pterygomaxillary fissure.	Posterior superior alveolar artery	Branches from the third part as it enters the pterygomaxillary fissure. Travels along the maxillary tuberosity to enter the posterior superior alveolar foramen. Serves the maxillary sinus, molar and premolar teeth, and adjacent gingiva.
		Infraorbital artery	Is the continuation of the maxillary artery, although it may arise in common with the PSA (posterior superior alveolar artery). Enters the floor of the orbit through the infraorbital fissure, then leaves the orbit via the infraorbital canal to exit onto the face at the infraorbital foramen. While in the floor of the orbit, it gives orbital branches serving the inferior oblique muscle and the lacrimal gland. Anterior superior alveolar branches supply the maxillary sinus, canine and incisor teeth, and their associated gingiva. Upon exiting the infraorbital foramen, it supplies branches to some of the regional facial muscles and palpebrae as well as the nasal area and upper lip.

(continued)

Table 12-3   Maxillary Artery (continued)

Portion	Course	Branches	Distribution
		Artery of the pterygoid canal	A small artery that passes through the posterior wall of the pterygopalatine fossa to supply the auditory tube, pharynx, middle ear, and sphenoid sinus.
		Descending palatine artery	Descends in the pterygopalatine canal where it divides into greater and lesser palatine arteries. The greater palatine artery exits onto the palate through the greater palatine foramen to supply the palatine mucosa, gingiva, and glands of the hard palate. It will anastomose with the nasopalatine artery in the incisive canal. The lesser palatine artery exits onto the soft palate at the lesser palatine foramen. It supplies the soft palate and palatine tonsil. It will anastomose with the ascending palatine branch of the facial artery.
		Pharyngeal branch	A small branch passing through the pharyngeal canal to vascularize the auditory tube, pharynx, middle ear, and the sphenoid sinus.
		Sphenopalatine artery	Passes into the nasal fossa via the sphenopalatine foramen to vascularize portions of the nasal chonchae and meatuses via nasal and septal branches. The main and longest branch, the nasopalatine artery, descends into the incisive canal where it will anastomose with branches of the greater palatine artery.

Short pterygoid arteries arise from this portion to vascularize the medial and lateral pterygoid muscles as well as the sphenomandibularis muscle.

The **buccal artery** accompanies the buccal nerve as it passes to and enters the buccinator muscle. Although the buccal nerve does not innervate this muscle, the buccal artery vascularizes it, as well as the adjacent skin and mucous membrane of the mouth. This artery anastomoses with the facial and infraorbital arteries.

Pterygopalatine Portion

Summary Bite. The pterygopalatine portion of the maxillary artery enters the pterygopalatine fossa and terminates in several branches that supply the maxillary molar and premolar teeth, supporting tissues, and the maxillary sinus.

This portion of the maxillary artery enters the pterygopalatine fossa via the pterygomaxillary fissure. As the vessel enters the fossa to terminate into several arteries, the **posterior superior alveolar artery** arises from it and descends over the maxillary tuberosity to enter the posterior superior alveolar foramen with the like-named nerve. This artery vascularizes the molar and premolar teeth, adjacent supporting tissues, and the maxillary sinus.

The remaining arteries of this portion will be described in Chapters 14 and 16.

Pterygoid Plexus and Maxillary Vein

Summary Bite. The pterygoid venous plexus lying on the surfaces of pterygoid muscles and within spaces of the deep face receives tributaries from a number of sources, including all of the venous branches that accompany the named branches of the maxillary artery.

The **pterygoid plexus of veins** is a massive network of venous channels lying on and about the surfaces of the lateral and medial pterygoid muscles and extending into the spaces of the deep face within the infratemporal fossa (Fig. 12-10). The plexus receives venous tributaries from vessels corresponding to the named arteries branching from the maxillary artery. This plexus is in direct or indirect communication with a vast area, including the cranial cavity and cavernous sinus, the nasal cavity, orbit, paranasal sinuses, facial vein, deep facial veins, and angular veins.

The maxillary vein is the short venous trunk that accompanies the maxillary artery as it lies behind the mandible. This vein serves to connect the pterygoid venous plexus with the superficial temporal vein, thus forming the retromandibular vein.

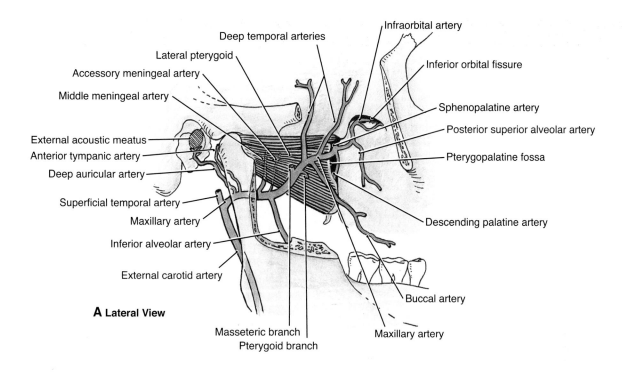

A Lateral View

Infraorbital artery
Deep temporal arteries
Lateral pterygoid
Accessory meningeal artery
Middle meningeal artery
Inferior orbital fissure
Sphenopalatine artery
Posterior superior alveolar artery
External acoustic meatus
Anterior tympanic artery
Pterygopalatine fossa
Deep auricular artery
Superficial temporal artery
Maxillary artery
Inferior alveolar artery
Descending palatine artery
External carotid artery
Buccal artery
Masseteric branch
Pterygoid branch
Maxillary artery

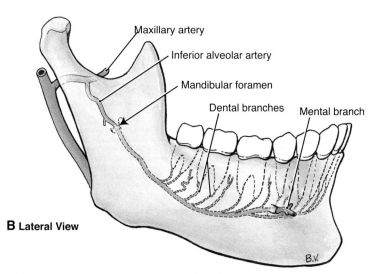

B Lateral View

Maxillary artery
Inferior alveolar artery
Mandibular foramen
Dental branches
Mental branch
B.V.

Figure 12-9.   The maxillary artery and its branches in the deep face.

Clinical Considerations

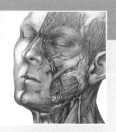

Anesthesia

Improper administration of anesthesia for a maxillary molar tooth may cause the needle to puncture the pterygoid venous plexus, resulting in a hematoma with noticeable swelling. The needle tract may permit the spread of a possibly fatal infection to the cavernous sinus.

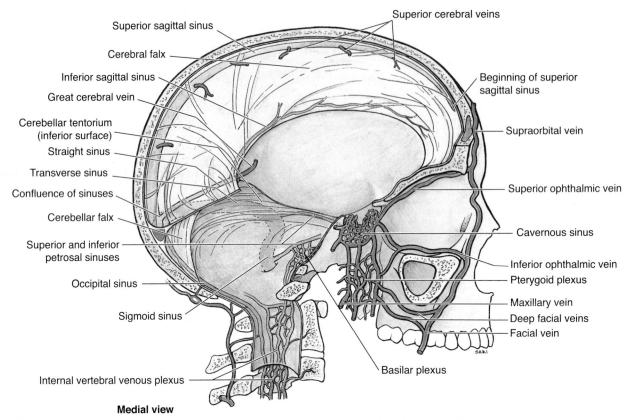

Superior sagittal sinus

Cerebral falx

Inferior sagittal sinus

Great cerebral vein

Cerebellar tentorium (inferior surface)

Straight sinus

Transverse sinus

Confluence of sinuses

Cerebellar falx

Superior and inferior petrosal sinuses

Occipital sinus

Sigmoid sinus

Internal vertebral venous plexus

Superior cerebral veins

Beginning of superior sagittal sinus

Supraorbital vein

Superior ophthalmic vein

Cavernous sinus

Inferior ophthalmic vein

Pterygoid plexus

Maxillary vein

Deep facial veins

Facial vein

Basilar plexus

Medial view

Figure 12-10. Venous sinuses of the dura mater with communications. Note the pterygoid venous plexus and its communications with the deep face, superficial face, and the cavernous sinus.

INNERVATION

Summary Bite. Most of the sensory innervation and all of the motor innervation to the structures of the deep face are supplied by branches of the mandibular division of the trigeminal nerve.

Trigeminal Nerve

Summary Bite. The trigeminal nerve (cranial nerve V) has three divisions: ophthalmic, maxillary, and mandibular. Most of the structures of the deep face are supplied by branches of the mandibular division, with only a small contribution from the maxillary division.

Mandibular Division

Summary Bite. The mandibular division of the trigeminal nerve is the only division that contains both sensory and motor components. The two unite outside the foramen ovale to form the trunk of the mandibular nerve.

The mandibular division of the trigeminal nerve exits the cranium via the foramen ovale. Motor and sensory roots pass individually through the foramen before uniting into a trunk within the infratemporal fossa.

The trunk is very short and it divides into two major divisions. The anterior division is mostly motor with some sensory branches, whereas the posterior division is mainly sensory with some motor branches.

Two branches arise from the trunk: the meningeal branch and the medial pterygoid nerve.

- The **meningeal branch** reenters the cranial cavity through the foramen spinosum in company with the middle meningeal artery. Within the cranial cavity, it provides sensory innervation to the dura mater.
- The **medial pterygoid nerve** arises from the medial aspect of the trunk, passing through the adjacent otic ganglion on its way to the medial pterygoid muscle. Two small branches arise from the medial pterygoid nerve close to its origin and are named:
  - The **nerve to the tensor tympani** and the **nerve to the tensor veli palatini**. The former passes to the auditory tube and on to the same-named muscle in the middle ear cavity. The latter nerve

enters the tensor veli palatini muscle near its origin.

Anterior Division

> **Summary Bite.** The anterior division of the mandibular nerve (mostly motor) innervates all of the muscles of mastication except the medial pterygoid muscle. It also contains sensory nerves to the skin and mucous membranes of the cheek.

The **anterior division of the mandibular nerve** provides motor innervation to all the remaining muscles of mastication (with the possible exception of the sphenomandibularis muscle). This division also contains a sensory component for the skin and mucous membrane of the cheek. Arising from this division are the masseteric, deep temporal, lateral pterygoid, and buccal nerves.

▨ The **masseteric nerve** passes superior to the lateral pterygoid muscle and then laterally to the mandibular notch, sending a twig to the TMJ before gaining access to the deep portions of the masseter muscle.

▨ The **deep temporal nerves**, usually an anterior and posterior (sometimes an intermediate also), ascend between the two heads of the lateral pterygoid muscle to enter the deep surface of the temporalis muscle. Occasionally, these nerves may arise from either the masseteric or buccal nerves.

▨ The **lateral pterygoid nerve** enters the deep surface of the muscle lying over it.

▨ The **buccal nerve** passes between the two heads of the lateral pterygoid muscle and then continues anteriorly beyond the border of the masseter muscle as it forms a plexus on the surface of the buccinator muscle. Here it freely communicates with the facial nerve, sending sensory branches with the facial nerve to supply the skin over the cheek. The nerve then pierces the muscle to provide sensory innervation to the mucous membrane of the cheek and adjacent gingiva.

Posterior Division

> **Summary Bite.** The posterior division of the mandibular nerve possesses only one motor nerve, which serves the mylohyoid muscle and anterior belly of the digastric muscle. Sensory components serve the meninges, the TMJ, mandibular teeth and supporting tissues, skin of the temple region, ear and tympanic membrane, and anterior two thirds of the tongue. It also communicates with the facial and glossopharyngeal nerves.

The **posterior division of the mandibular nerve** is mostly sensory, possessing but one motor nerve—the mylohyoid nerve that supplies innervation to the mylohyoid muscle and the anterior belly of the digastric muscle. Arising from this division are the auriculotemporal, lingual, and inferior alveolar nerves.

▨ The **auriculotemporal nerve** arises from the posterior division of the mandibular nerve, usually as two roots that join after encircling the middle meningeal artery just before that artery enters the foramen spinosum. The auriculotemporal nerve then courses deep to the lateral pterygoid muscle as it passes posteriorly deep to the parotid gland. The nerve then surfaces between the auricula and the temporomandibular joint below the zygomatic arch. It subsequently passes superficial to the zygomatic arch, along with the superficial temporal artery, to be distributed to the side of the head. Near its origin, the auriculotemporal nerve receives communications from the otic ganglion. These are postganglionic parasympathetic fibers to be distributed to the parotid gland via the auriculotemporal nerve (see Table 18-2). As the nerve passes through the gland, these fibers will leave it to provide secretomotor innervation to the gland. The preganglionic fibers are a part of the glossopharyngeal nerve and reach the otic ganglion via the lesser petrosal nerve.

▨ The auriculotemporal nerve communicates also with the facial nerve within the substance of the parotid gland. These sensory fibers are communicated to the facial nerve for further distribution over the face. As the auriculotemporal nerve passes by the ear and the TMJ, it provides the anterior auricular branches to the skin of the anterior portion of the ear and the external acoustic meatus and articular branches to the joint. Superior to the zygomatic arch, the nerve branches into superficial temporal nerves which distribute to the skin of the side of the head.

▨ The **lingual nerve** arises deep to the lateral pterygoid muscle and descends to pass superficially over the medial pterygoid muscle as it courses anteriorly to enter the submandibular region. The lingual nerve is joined by the chorda tympani nerve while it is under the cover of the lateral pterygoid muscle. The chorda tympani nerve, a branch of the facial nerve, makes its appearance in the deep face at the spine of the sphenoid. The nerve carries special sensory fibers for taste and preganglionic parasympathetic fibers destined for the submandibular ganglion (see Table 18-2).

▨ The lingual nerve provides general sensation to the anterior two thirds of the tongue, adjacent areas of the mouth, and the lingual gingiva. Special sensory taste fibers from the chorda tympani are distributed to the anterior two thirds of the tongue by the lingual nerve. Preganglionic parasympathetic fibers leave the nerve at the submandibular ganglion, where they synapse on postganglionic parasympathetic cell bodies whose secretomotor fibers are distributed to the submandibular, sublingual, and minor salivary glands in the floor of the mouth. Details of the pathway followed by the lingual nerve are outlined more precisely in Chapter 15.

■ The **inferior alveolar nerve** originates deep to the lateral pterygoid muscle and lateral to the lingual nerve. This nerve passes between the sphenomandibular ligament and the ramus of the mandible to enter the mandibular foramen. Inside the mandibular canal, the nerve distributes to the mandibular teeth, supporting structures, and gingiva.

   ■ A branch of the inferior alveolar nerve, the **mental nerve**, emerges from the mental foramen to provide sensory innervation to the skin of the chin and lower lip. Incisive branches continue anteriorly in the mandibular canal to innervate the canine and incisor teeth, supporting structures, and gingiva. Just before the inferior alveolar nerve enters the mandibular foramen, it gives off the **mylohyoid nerve**, the only motor component of the posterior division. This motor nerve courses along the groove for the mylohyoid nerve before it enters the mylohyoid muscle. Upon crossing its superficial surface, the nerve also provides motor innervation to the anterior belly of the digastric muscle.

Maxillary Division

Summary Bite. The maxillary division of the trigeminal nerve may be observed in the deep face as it passes through the pterygopalatine fossa. Here a small branch leaves the nerve and courses along the maxillary tuberosity to provide sensory innervation to the mucous membranes of the cheek. A division of this branch enters the posterior superior alveolar foramen to supply the maxillary sinus, gingiva, supporting tissues, and the three molars.

A small contribution from the maxillary division of the trigeminal nerve is observed in the deep face. As the maxillary nerve passes through the pterygopalatine fossa, a small branch arises from it and passes laterally into the deep face via the pterygomaxillary fissure.

This **posterior superior alveolar nerve** descends over the maxillary tuberosity to enter the posterior superior alveolar foramen; some twigs continue on to innervate the gingiva and mucous membranes of the cheek.

Those fibers entering the foramen distribute to the maxillary sinus, teeth, supporting structures, and gingiva as far anteriorly as the first molar, where a dental plexus is formed with the middle and anterior superior alveolar nerves, innervating the remaining maxillary sinus, teeth, supporting structures, and gingiva.

MASTICATION

Summary Bite. The process of ingesting, biting, chewing, and swallowing is a complex process which begins consciously and then blends into a learned, automatic rhythmic activity involving neurological control of the muscles of mastication along with several groups of accessory muscles. Complex neural circuitry, including input from specialized sensory mechanisms within the periodontal ligaments, acts to prevent destruction of the masticatory apparatus.

Although it is not within the scope of this text to detail the precise timing and coordination of events in

Clinical Considerations

Injury to the Mandibular Nerve

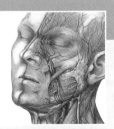

The mandibular nerve division of the trigeminal nerve (cranial nerve V) may be injured due to a number of different events, including trauma to the side of the head or face; fracture of the mandible; fracture of the facial bones; tumors; and meningeal infections. Symptoms of injury may include paralysis of the muscles of mastication on the injured side causing a deviation of the mandible to the opposite side; loss of sensation on the lower face, skin of the temple, chin and lower lip, buccal mucosa, and gingiva of the affected side; and loss of sensation on the anterior two thirds of the tongue and the mandibular teeth on the affected side. The intensity of the symptoms is related to the type and severity of the injury.

the process of mastication, a generalized description is warranted. The reader wishing more detail is referred to the Selected References at the end of this book.

The complex process of mastication involves many muscle groups besides the group commonly known as the "muscles of mastication." The process is initiated consciously; however, the total movements and the rhythmic activity are controlled by complex neural circuitry within the central nervous system. The exact process varies with the individual but, once the pattern is established, it remains fairly constant for that particular person. This is not to imply that the process is static; indeed it is continually altered, since changes within the stomatognathic system are constant and dynamic throughout life.

The process begins with ingestion or the cutting of food by the anterior teeth and continues as the food is maneuvered by the muscles within the cheek and the tongue to position the food between the premolars and molars of the upper and lower arches. The muscles of mastication (masseter, temporalis, medial pterygoid) then act to elevate the mandible, move it from side to side (elevators of contralateral side and ipsilateral medial pterygoid), depress it (lateral pterygoid, digastric, mylohyoid, and geniohyoid), protrude it (external pterygoid), and retrude it (part of temporalis), effecting a grinding action in a coordinated pattern. More information regarding the muscles involved in the exact movement patterns may be found in Chapter 13 on the TMJ.

The forces applied to the bolus of food are carefully monitored by special receptors (proprioception) located within the periodontal ligaments and the muscles themselves, preventing the possible self-destruction of the stomatognathic system.

The process of mastication prepares the food for deglutition by reducing the ingested bolus to less than two centimeters in diameter. Chewing also serves to bring the food in contact with saliva in the mouth and stimulates the secretion of digestive juices within the digestive system.

Temporomandibular Joint

Key Terms

Temporomandibular Disorder (TMD) is the clinical term given to dysfunctions within the stomatognathic system. This is a very broad classification that may include alterations in any one or a combination of the functioning components of the stomatognathic apparatus, which eventually result in TMJ dysfunction syndrome. TMD is considered a musculoskeletal disease.

Temporomandibular Joint (TMJ) is the jaw joint composed of the condylar heads of the mandible and the articular eminence of the temporal bones. The right and left halves of the mandible are mirror images of each other and, because of this arrangement, the right and left heads of the mandible articulate with the right and left temporal bones, respectively. Therefore, the TMJ is considered to be a bilateral joint. Interposed between the articulating surfaces of these two bones is an articular disc contoured to fit over the head of the condyle and into the concavity of the mandibular fossa. The TMJ is operated by four bilateral muscles of mastication assisted by accessory muscles that manipulate the lower jaw in mastication, swallowing, and phonation.

Temporomandibular Joint (TMJ) Articular Coverings include the joint capsule, lateral ligaments, and accessory ligaments on the medial aspect of the joint. The TMJ is entirely enclosed by the joint capsule attached to the temporal bone, and it continues inferiorly where it is attached to the mandibular neck.

The articular disc is attached to the capsule on its medial and lateral surfaces, causing the capsular space to be divided into superior and inferior synovial compartments.

Obliquely oriented ligaments reinforce the capsule. The lateral ligament or temporomandibular ligament restricts mediolateral movement. The sphenomandibular ligament, located on the medial aspect of the TMJ, has been suggested to limit lateral mandibular movement. The other medial ligament, the stylomandibular ligament (a specialization of the deep cervical fascia) may assist in limiting the protrusion of the mandible.

The **temporomandibular joint (TMJ)** is the site of articulation between the mandible and the skull, specifically the area about the **articular eminence of the temporal bone**. This bilateral joint functions to open and close the jaws and to approximate the teeth of the opposing arches during mastication. The articulation consists of parts of the mandible and temporal bones, which are covered by dense, fibrous connective tissue and are surrounded by several ligaments.

Interposed between the two bones is a fibrous articular disc, compartmentalizing the joint into two separate synovial-lined cavities. Several pairs of muscles attached to the mandible produce the movements necessary to suckle, ingest, and masticate food; swallow; yawn; and produce speech.

Interrelationships of the stomatognathic system in occlusion, neuromuscular function, and temporomandibular articulation are of paramount importance to the dental professional because treatment of any component affects the functioning of this entire system.

JOINT ANATOMY

📩 **Summary Bite.** The anatomy of the temporomandibular joint (TMJ) concerns the articular eminence of the temporal bone and the condylar heads of the mandible.

The anatomy of the TMJ structure is depicted in Fig. 13-1A–C, illustrating the relationship between the mandible and the temporal bone as they form the TMJ.

Mandible

📩 **Summary Bite.** The mandible is the only freely moving bone of the skull. It possesses two condylar processes whose condyle articulates with a disc that is pressed against the articular eminence of the temporal bone.

The mandible possesses two articular surfaces, a condyle (head) located on the superior extremity of each of the bilateral condylar processes. Each condyle articulates with a disc that is interposed between it and the temporal bone (Figs. 13-1A–C and 13-2B).

The condyles, which are characteristically "football-shaped," measure about 20 mm through the long mediolateral axis and 10 mm through the anteroposterior axis. The condyles are directed at an oblique angle to each other and to the frontal plane

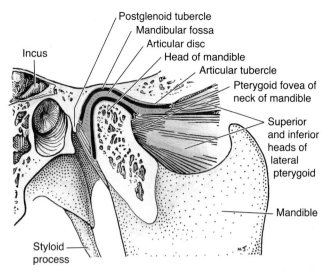

A Sagittal section

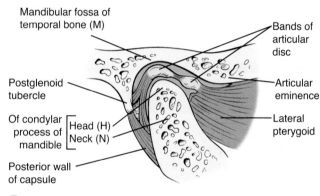

B

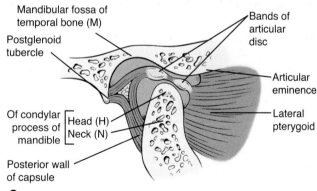

C

Figure 13-1. Sagittal views of the temporomandibular joint (TMJ). **(A)** Anatomy of the temporomandibular articulation. **(B)** Anatomy of the joint with the mouth closed. **(C)** Anatomy of the joint with the mouth open.

so that if the planes of the long axes were continued they would meet at the foramen magnum. The long axis is also at right angles to the ramus of the mandible. Anteriorly, the condyle is strongly convex, whereas posteriorly, the convexity is reduced to

External
auditory
meatus | Temporomandibular
ligament | Articular
tubercle | Coronoid process
of mandible

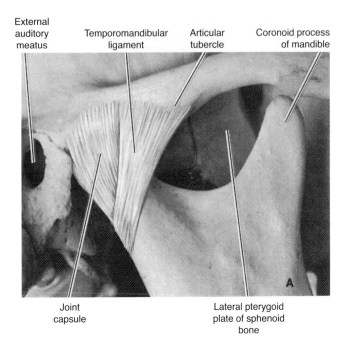

Joint
capsule | Lateral pterygoid
plate of sphenoid
bone

Joint
capsule | Superior synovial
compartment | Articular
disk | Temporomandibular
ligament

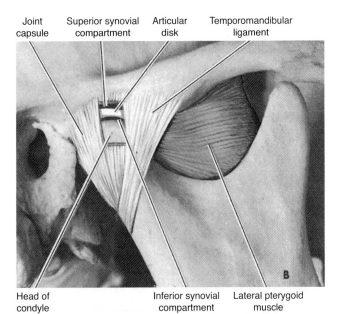

Head of
condyle | Inferior synovial
compartment | Lateral pterygoid
muscle

Figure 13-2. Temporomandibular joint anatomy. **(A)** Note the extent of the capsule model and the differentiated lateral ligament (temporomandibular ligament). **(B)** Observe that the capsule model has been cut away to reveal the disc and its relationship to the articulating surfaces of the joint.

medial and lateral slopes. This resembles (from a lateral view) the profile of an anteriorly tilted clenched fist. It is important to remember, however, that individual variations do exist in the shape, form, and size of the mandibular condyle—variations that may be caused by any one or a combination of factors, including heredity and functional adaptation.

Temporal Bone

Summary Bite. The temporal bone forms the side of the head above the ear, a portion of the zygomatic arch, and the mastoid process.

The site of TMJ articulation on the temporal bone is on the inferior surface of the zygomatic process (Fig. 13-1A). The specific location is situated on the posterior slope of the **articular eminence**. The term "articular eminence," as it applies here, replaced the term "articular tubercle" by those specializing in the study of the temporomandibular articulation. Although the new term has not as yet been adopted universally by anatomists, it will be used in this text because it is the term most often used in the literature regarding the TMJ.

The **articular eminence** is defined as the strongly convex bony elevation on the root of the zygomatic process representing the anterior-most boundary of the articular or mandibular fossa (also referred to as the glenoid fossa). The **articular tubercle** is the bony "knob" on the lateral aspect of the articular eminence, where the fibrous capsule and the temporomandibular ligament attach.

It would appear in the dried skull that, lying immediately anterior to the external auditory meatus, the mandibular condyle articulates within the mandibular fossa between the bony articular eminence and the postglenoid process. However, close observation of the mandibular (glenoid) fossa reveals a rather thin bony roof separating it from the middle cranial fossa. This fact, coupled with the knowledge of the biconcave anatomy of the disc, simply does not support the conclusion that the roof of the mandibular fossa can function as the stress-bearing articulation. Indeed, radiographic evidence indicates that the TMJ articulation occurs against the slope of the articular eminence.

Articular Disc

Summary Bite. The articular disc is a dense, fibrous connective tissue contoured to fit between the articular head of the condyle and the articular eminence of the temporal bone.

The **articular disc** is a compact, dense, and fibrous connective tissue plate that is oval and contoured to fit between the mandibular condyle and the articular eminence of the temporal bone (Figs. 13-1A–C and 13-2B).

The inferior surface of the disc is concavely contoured to fit the convex condyle of the mandible. Superiorly, its surface is concavoconvex. The convex portion conforms to the concave mandibular fossa posteriorly, whereas anteriorly, the disc becomes concave to fit the convex posterior aspect of the articular eminence.

The disc is thickest at its periphery and thinnest at the stress-bearing area of the joint. Peripherally, the disc becomes less dense as it merges into the surrounding capsule.

Posteriorly, the disc is attached to a highly vascular connective tissue known as the retrodiscal tissue. Occasionally, the disc (especially of older individuals) becomes perforated at its center, where it is thinnest.

Articular Coverings

Summary Bite. The articular surfaces of temporal bone and mandibular condyle are covered by a dense, collagenous connective tissue overlying proliferative cells of hyaline cartilage. In adults, the hyaline cartilage is replaced with fibrocartilage covered by a layer of proliferative cells.

The coverings of the articular surfaces of the condyle and the slope of the articular eminence are composed of dense, collagenous connective tissue overlying a thin proliferative layer of cells associated with the underlying hyaline cartilage.

It is reported that the hyaline cartilage of the condyle is present while the individual is still growing, until about 20 years of age, whereas the cartilage covering the articular eminence has a shorter life span. At the termination of growth, this cartilage layer is replaced by compact bone.

In the adult, the compact bone of the condyle is covered by a layer of fibrocartilage that, in turn, is covered by a thin layer of proliferative tissue. Cells of the proliferative layer may become activated to function in remodeling of the joint as a result of changes in function, wear, and tooth movement. Superficial to the proliferative layer is a relatively thick layer of dense, irregular collagenous connective tissue whose deeper layers house fibroblasts.

Although the articular structures are avascular, they are bathed in synovial fluid, which provides lubrication and nourishment for the cellular coverings.

Peripheral regions of the disc are very vascular, whereas the central, stress-bearing portion is devoid of blood vessels.

Capsule

Summary Bite. A dense, irregular collagenous connective tissue capsule encloses the articulating surfaces of the TMJ. The capsule is attached to the temporal bone and the neck of the mandible. The position of the disc within the capsule forms a superior compartment above the disc and an inferior compartment below the disc. Each compartment is lined with synovial membrane.

The TMJ capsule, composed of dense, irregular collagenous connective tissue, encloses the entire articulating region of the temporal bone, disc, and mandibular condyle, sealing the joint space (Figs. 13-2A,B and 13-3).

Superiorly, the capsule is attached to the temporal bone about the circumference of the mandibular fossa and, anteriorly, around the articular eminence. Inferiorly, the capsule is attached to the mandibular neck. The placement of the disc between the two articulating bones and its peripheral attachments to the walls of the capsule causes the capsule space to be divided into separate compartments.

The larger, superior compartment between the disc and temporal bone (Figs. 13-1A and 13-2B) permits some freedom of movement between the disc and articular eminence.

Anteriorly, the capsule and disc are tightly fused, permitting the insertion of some fibers of the lateral pterygoid muscle into the disc. Medially and laterally, the capsule and disc are attached to the condyle margins, thus necessitating associated simultaneous movement of the condyle and disc.

The inferior compartment encloses the entire neck of the mandible and is more firmly attached to the disc. This attachment prohibits excessive movement between the disc and condyle.

Innervation and Vascularization

Summary Bite. The joint and joint capsule are heavily endowed with sensory nerves derived from the mandibular division of the trigeminal nerve (cranial nerve V).

The joint capsule is richly endowed with sensory endings from the mandibular division of the trigeminal nerve, most of which are supplied from articular branches of the auriculotemporal nerve (see Fig. 12-8). Additional articular branches supplying the joint are derived from the masseteric branch of the mandibular division of the trigeminal nerve. Vascular supply to the joint is provided by branches of the superficial temporal and maxillary arteries as they approximate the joint.

Ligaments

Summary Bite. The temporomandibular joint is reinforced by collateral ligaments on the medial and lateral aspects. The temporomandibular ligament is the large obliquely oriented lateral ligament reinforcing the joint. Two accessory ligaments reinforce the medial aspect of the joint.

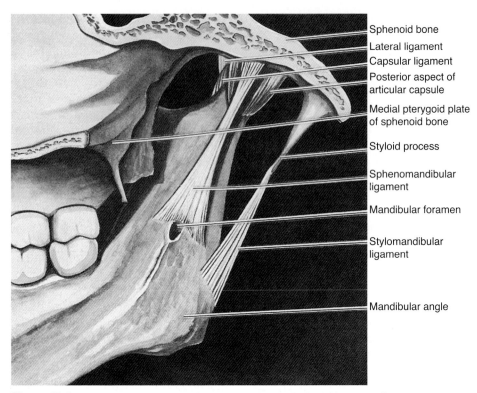

Sphenoid bone
Lateral ligament
Capsular ligament
Posterior aspect of
articular capsule
Medial pterygoid plate
of sphenoid bone

Styloid process

Sphenomandibular
ligament

Mandibular foramen

Stylomandibular
ligament

Mandibular angle

Figure 13-3. Accessory ligaments of the temporomandibular joint drawn from a medial view.

Two collateral ligaments (discal ligaments) serve to anchor the medial and lateral borders of the articular disc to the poles of the condyle. Reinforcements of the joint capsule along its lateral margin by obliquely oriented bundles of collagenous fibers are responsible for naming this pronounced lateral portion of the capsule, the **lateral ligament or temporomandibular ligament** (Fig. 13-2A,B).

The **temporomandibular ligament** possesses two separate bands of fibers, whose directions are oblique to each other. The superficial layer, which is more extensive, arises as a broad band from the lateral surface of the articular eminence at the articular tubercle. The ligament narrows as it passes obliquely inferior and posterior to be inserted on the posterolateral aspect of the mandibular neck just inferior to the lateral pole of the condyle.

The smaller, medially situated portion of the lateral ligament arises from the crest of the eminence to pass almost horizontally to insert into the lateral aspect of the condyle. The lateral ligaments permit free movement in the anteroinferior plane but check mediolateral movements of the joint.

The superficial portion of the temporomandibular ligament prevents lateral movement, whereas the deeper horizontal portion prevents posterior displacement of the condyle.

A similar arrangement does not exist on the medial side of the condyle with the capsular ligament. This difference can be understood by recognizing that the bilateral TMJs are connected through the mandible and, therefore, the articulations function as a single unit rather than independently.

Two additional ligaments are considered accessory to the temporomandibular articulation (Fig. 13-3). The **sphenomandibular ligament**, a remnant of the Meckel cartilage, is a flat band that spans the space between the spine of the sphenoid bone and the lingula at the mandibular foramen. The **stylomandibular ligament**, the other accessory ligament, is a specialization of the deep cervical fascia. This ligament extends as a thin band from the apex of the styloid process of the temporal bone to the posterior border of the angle and ramus of the mandible.

Although the precise functions of these two accessory ligaments are not fully understood as they relate to the temporomandibular articulation, it has been suggested that the sphenomandibular ligament assists in limiting lateral mandibular movement, whereas the stylomandibular ligament apparently assists in limiting the anterior extent of protrusion of the mandible.

TYPES OF MOVEMENT

Summary Bite. The anatomy of the TMJ dictates that there are only two possible movements of this joint, namely, ginglymus (hinge) movement and arthrodial (gliding) movement.

The joint just described is composed essentially of two convex structures opposed to each other, with an intermediate articular disc placed between them. Considering the anatomy of the disc, it becomes clear that movement within the TMJ is basically of two types.

Ginglymus (hinge) movement is possible between the condyles of the mandible and the inferior surface of the disc. The other movement possible within the joint is an **arthrodial (gliding)** motion. This becomes possible as the superior surface of the articular disc slides down at the articular eminence. Therefore, the TMJ is considered a ginglymoarthrodial joint.

The mandibular/disc movement is **rotatory**, and that of the disc/temporal bone is **translatory**. Functionally, movements of the joint are translated as mandibular locations away from the resting position, such as opening, closing, protrusion, retrusion, and lateral rotation.

▨ The **resting position** is defined as having the patient's head in the anatomic position (in an upright posture). This places the masticatory musculature at rest, permitting a small free-way space to exist between the teeth of the upper and lower jaws but having the upper and lower lips touching. It is in this attitude that the mandibular condyles are positioned so that the anterosuperior articulating surfaces are opposite the posterior slopes of the articular eminence of the temporal bone, with the disc between the two bones.

▨ **Opening the jaws** involves the **translatory (gliding) movement** of the disc and condyle down the slope of the articular eminence coupled with **rotatory (hinge) movement** of the mandibular condyles against the disc.

The translatory phase effects a slight anteroinferior movement as the mandibular condyle slides down the eminence.

The hinge action phase (condyles rotating) produces a center of suspension in the ramus. Thus, the posterior portion of the angle of the mandible moves slightly posterior, and the mandibular body moves inferiorly to open the jaw. The lateral ptery-

goid muscles initiate the action, followed by the digastric, geniohyoid, and mylohyoid muscles depressing the mandible. This assumes that the hyoid bone has been fixed by the infrahyoid musculature.

The lateral pterygoid muscles are always in a state of tonus and are able to stabilize the condyle against gravity, thus maintaining the free-way space for long periods of time without tiring. However, falling asleep while sitting in an upright position relaxes this muscle tone, and the mandible opens in response to gravity.

▨ **Closing the jaws** is more involved. First, the mandible is protruded as the condyles and disc slide down and forward on the articular eminence.

This is followed by fixing the condyles and elevating the mandible, coupled with depression/retraction.

The lateral pterygoid muscles, assisted by the medial pterygoid muscles, protrude the mandible, whereas the masseter and temporalis muscles elevate it. Retrusion is performed by the deep portion of the masseter and some fibers of the temporalis muscles.

▨ **Mandibular protrusion**, or jutting the mandible forward, is accomplished by contracting the lateral pterygoids, which causes the disc and condyles to slide forward and down the articular eminence.

▨ **Mandibular retrusion**, in contrast, returns the mandible to a position posterior to the resting position. This action is accomplished by portions of the temporalis muscles.

▨ **Mandibular lateral rotation** (i.e., a lateral rotatory motion on one side) is accomplished by the condyle and disc of the opposite side sliding inferiorly and anteriorly on the articular eminence while moving medially.

The result of this active process effects a passive lateral rotation on the opposite side. The lateral pterygoid muscle of the side opposite the lateral rotation effects the movement.

It must be pointed out that the entire masticatory and accessory musculatures are involved in producing any one or combinations of these movements. Space limitations do not permit an extensive discussion of the muscles involved in the entire masticatory process.

Generally, the information presented here is in agreement with published research regarding muscle function for specific and separate actions of the TMJ. The process of ingesting and masticating food is an intricate one, involving the entire stomatognathic complex under the control of the voluntary and involuntary nervous system.

Clinical Considerations

Temporomandibular Disorders (TMD)

Alterations in any one or a combination of the functioning components of the stomatognathic system (i.e., teeth, periodontal ligament, TMJ, or muscles of mastication) eventually result in TMJ dysfunction syndrome. These dysfunctions are clinically referred to as **TMD**, the term now used to describe a number of clinical manifestations in the masticatory system involving muscles and the joint (or both) and involving pain of nondental origin. Although the term is not ideal, it is considered to be a subclassification of musculoskeletal disease. Changes in the free-way dimensions (usually 2 to 4 mm) of the rest position imposed by occlusal changes, disease, muscle spasms, nervous tension, restorative prostheses, and so on may develop into temporomandibular disorders.

Crepitus
Crepitus (clicking) is one of the most common complaints of patients with TMD and, for the most part, it is believed to evolve from a delay in the anterior disc movements on opening and/or closing the mouth. Unless the condition worsens or becomes socially irritating, it is usually left untreated.

Dislocation of the TMJ
Dislocation of the mandible from its articulation with the temporal bone may occur in an anterior direction only as

the condyles slide down unchecked along the slope of the articular eminence to pass anteriorly into the infratemporal fossa. When this occurs, the jaw remains open and the person is unable to close it. This condition may result from a side blow to the chin, a fractured mandible, or spasm of the lateral pterygoid muscles causing an excessive contraction, as in taking an exceptionally large bite of food or from deep yawning (Fig. 13-4).

Intense blows to the chin (e.g., from a fall) may fracture the neck of the mandible. When this happens, great care must be taken during the surgical procedure to prevent damage to the facial nerve and the auriculotemporal nerve, both being in close association with the joint.

Failure to protect the facial nerve may lead to a drooping face on the damaged side with loss of facial muscle tone (Bell palsy). Damage to the auriculotemporal nerve, particularly its articular branches, may lead to instability of the TMJ.

Arthritis of the TMJ
Temporomandibular disorders, especially those that are chronic, may give rise to arthritic changes in the joint and create lasting inflammation of the TMJ. These arthritic changes may eventually lead to crepitus and may affect occlusion.

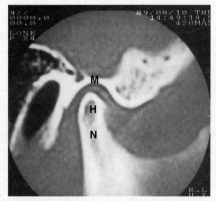

A
Sagittal CT

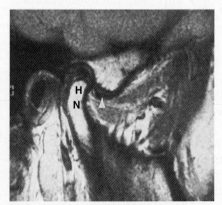

B
Sagittal MRI

Figure 13-4.   Temporomandibular joint scans. **(A)** Magnetic resonance image of a sagittal section through a normal closed temporomandibular joint. **(B)** Magnetic resonance image of a coronal section through a normal temporomandibular joint.

Clinical Considerations

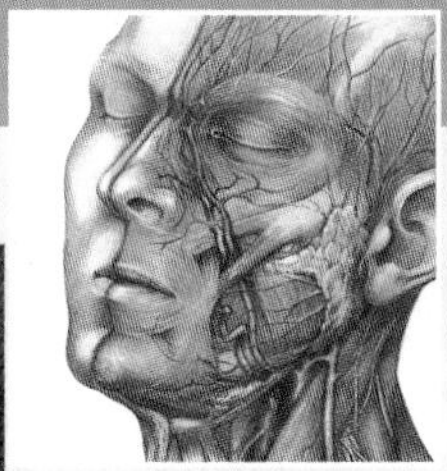

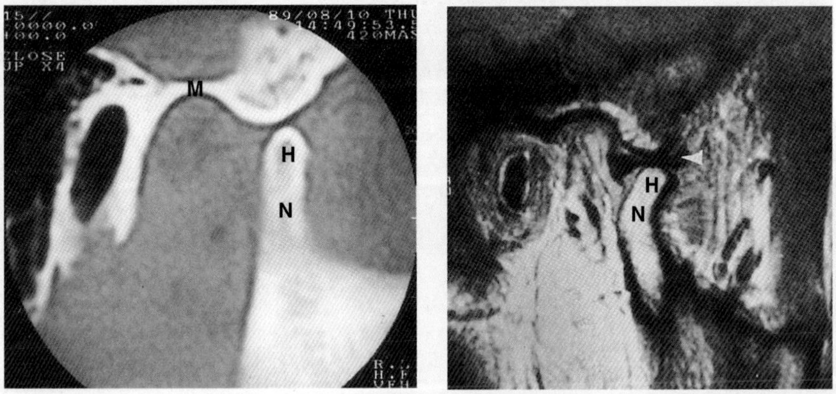

Sagittal CT

Sagittal MRI

Figure 13-4. *(continued)* **(C)** Magnetic resonance image of an open temporomandibular joint with a "click." **(D)** Tomographic scan of an open temporomandibular joint.

Table 13-1   Muscles Acting on the Temporomandibular Joint

Muscle	Opening	Closing	Protrusion	Retrusion	Lateral Shift
Muscles of mastication					
Masseter		+	+	√	
Temporalis		+ A, M, P		+ M, P	√ + P (Ipsilateral)
Medial pterygoid		+	+	√	√
Lateral pterygoid	+		+		+
Suprahyoid muscles					
Digastric	√	√	√	√	√
Mylohyoid	√	√	√	√	√
Geniohyoid	√	√	√	√	√
Stylohyoid"					

+ = major activity; √ = minor activity; A = anterior; M = middle; P = posterior
The stylohyoid, although not connected to the mandible, assists in fixing the hyoid bone.

It should be clear from this brief description that the double TMJ is not controlled by one or a pair of muscles at any one time. Rather, the actions of all of the muscles affecting movement are synchronized and these muscles function in unison as prime movers, synergists, antagonists, fixers, sling balancers, and so on. Considerable disagreement exists concerning the actions of certain muscles in producing the various movements at the temporomandibular articulation. The major difficulties in resolving this dilemma arise from the duality of the joint, its interrelated multiple movements, its complex movements from particular points in space, and associated organs and musculatures in and about the oral apparatus.

A table of muscular activity affecting TMJ function is presented in this chapter. This table is grossly oversimplified and attempts to present merely a synopsis of muscle function in a general manner (Table 13-1). The reader seeking more information on the subject of the TMJ is referred to material cited in the Selected Readings at the end of this book.

Pterygopalatine Fossa, Nasal Cavity, and Paranasal Sinuses

14

Key Terms

Maxillary Nerve is a purely sensory division of the trigeminal nerve (cranial nerve V). It leaves the cranial fossa to enter the pterygopalatine fossa. Its continuation enters the floor of the orbit and exits the orbit via the infraorbital foramen onto the face and side of the nose. Along its route, its branches provide sensory fibers to the face, paranasal sinuses, tonsil, palate, maxillary teeth and supporting tissues, nasopharynx, and auditory tube. Additionally, the maxillary nerve delivers secretomotor fibers derived from the facial nerve (cranial nerve VII) from the pterygopalatine ganglion to the lacrimal

gland and mucosal glands of the nasal fossa, palate, and pharynx.

Paranasal Sinuses are hollow cavities within the maxillae, frontal, ethmoid, and sphenoid bones. These sinuses, lined with respiratory mucosa, are in communication with the nasal fossa via small ostia. The function of the paranasal sinuses is not clear. The mucus produced within the sinuses drains, via the ostia, into the nasal cavity. However, during nasal congestion, the ostia may be closed so that the sinus(es) may be filled and unable to drain, thus increasing

pressure that may be related to sinusitis, sinus headache, and sinus infection.

    The maxillary sinus is the largest sinus and, because of the location of its ostium (high on the medial wall), it is difficult to drain and is frequently a source of sinusitis and congestion. Also, the roots of the molar teeth bulge into the floor of the sinus and may create problems for dental treatment.

Pterygopalatine Fossa is that pyramid-shaped space surrounded by the sphenoid, maxilla, and palatine bones. Housed within this space are the terminals of the maxillary artery, the maxillary division (V₂) of the trigeminal nerve, and the pterygopalatine ganglion (a parasympathetic ganglion of the facial nerve). Branches of these structures and their communications serve the region about the nasal cavity, paranasal sinuses, the maxilla, palate, dentition and supporting structures of the maxillary arch, and parts of the face and cheek.

Pterygopalatine Ganglion is housed in the pterygopalatine fossa. It is a parasympathetic ganglion of the autonomic nervous system. Preganglionic parasympathetic nerve fibers originating in the facial nerve (cranial nerve VII) synapse in the ganglion with postganglionic cell bodies whose secretomotor fibers join the maxillary division (V₂) of the trigeminal nerve and its branches to distribute to the lacrimal gland, and mucosal glands of the nasal fossa, palate, and pharynx.

PTERYGOPALATINE FOSSA

Summary Bite. The pterygopalatine fossa is a small, open space where the maxilla, sphenoid, and palatine bones approximate each other. It is a place where nerves, ganglia, and vessels converge to communictate with other regions of the skull.

The pterygopalatine fossa—a small, pyramid-shaped space—is situated between the maxilla, sphenoid, and palatine bones. It communicates via canals, fissures, and foramina with various regions of the skull. The contents of the pterygopalatine fossa include the terminal portion of the maxillary artery; the pterygopalatine ganglion; the maxillary division of the trigeminal nerve; and branches of these structures. The osteology of this region is detailed in Chapter 6, where its communications with other regions are noted.

Maxillary Artery

Summary Bite. The third portion of the maxillary artery leaves the deep face and enters the pterygopalatine fossa via the pterygomaxillary fissure. Branches of the pterygopalatine artery serve structures in the orbit as well as the maxilla and teeth, palate, pharynx, paranasal sinuses, nasal cavity, and auditory tube.

The third, or **pterygopalatine portion**, of the maxillary artery enters the pterygopalatine fossa from the infratemporal fossa via the pterygomaxillary fissure (Fig. 14-1; see Chapter 21). Branches of the pterygopalatine portion of the maxillary artery are the posterosuperior alveolar, infraorbital, greater palatine, pharyngeal, and sphenopalatine arteries as well as the artery of the pterygoid canal.

▪ The **posterior superior alveolar artery** branches from the maxillary artery as that vessel enters the pterygomaxillary fissure. It travels on the maxillary tuberosity and enters the posterior superior alveolar foramen accompanied by the like-named nerve. The vessel ramifies within the maxilla to vascularize the maxillary sinus, molars, and premolars as well as the neighboring gingiva.

▪ The **infraorbital artery**, a continuation of the maxillary artery, enters the orbit through the inferior orbital fissure, lies in the infraorbital groove, leaves the orbit via the infraorbital canal, and enters the face by way of the infraorbital foramen. Branches of the infraorbital artery are the **orbital branches**, serving the lacrimal gland and the inferior oblique and inferior rectus muscles; the **anterior superior alveolar branches**, which vascularize the anterior teeth and the maxillary sinus; and the facial branches, discussed in Chapter 8.

▪ The **greater palatine artery** and its branch, the **lesser palatine artery**, pass through the pterygopalatine canal and gain entrance to the palate via the **greater palatine** and **lesser palatine foramina**, respectively, to vascularize the hard and soft palates as well as associated structures. The **pharyngeal branch** passes dorsally, through the **pharyngeal canal**, to vascularize the auditory tube, sphenoidal sinus, and portions of the pharynx. The **sphenopalatine artery** leaves the pterygopalatine fossa via the **sphenopalatine foramen** on its medial wall to enter the nasal fossa. The distribution of this vessel and its branches is discussed later in this chapter. The small **artery** of the **pterygoid canal** passes through the posterior wall of the pterygopalatine fossa via the pterygoid canal. It supplies part of the auditory tube, pharynx, middle ear, and sphenoidal sinus.

Maxillary Nerve

Summary Bite. The maxillary nerve (V₂), a purely sensory nerve, enters the pterygopalatine fossa where it gives rise to nerves that serve the orbit, the hard and soft palate, maxillary molars and supporting tissues, portions of the nasal cavity, anterior maxillary teeth and supporting tissues, and nasopharynx. It also communicates

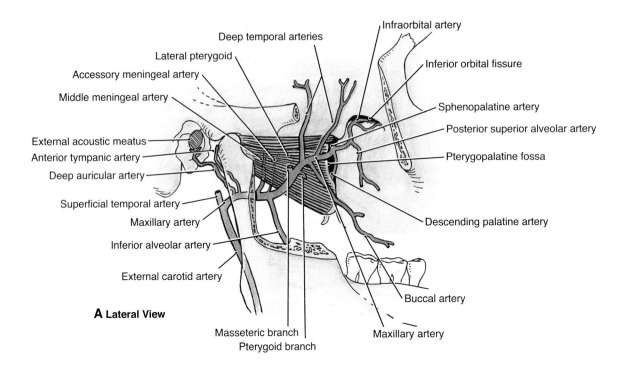

A Lateral View

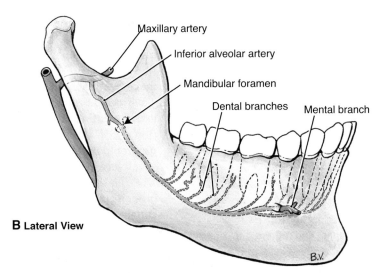

B Lateral View

Figure 14-1. Maxillary artery and its distribution in the deep face.

with the pterygopalatine ganglion (a parasympathetic ganglion associated with the facial nerve [cranial nerve VII] while in the pterygopalatine fossa).

The **maxillary division** of the **trigeminal nerve** enters the pterygopalatine fossa at its posterior boundary via the **foramen rotundum** (Fig. 14-2; see Table 18-3). While in the fossa, it gives off the **zygomatic nerve**, which, passing into the orbit through the inferior orbital fissure, will bifurcate to form the zygomaticotemporal and zygomaticofacial nerves.

The **posterior superior alveolar nerves** also branch from the maxillary nerve, exit the fossa via the pterygomaxillary fissure, and enter the maxillary tuberosity to serve the maxillary sinus, molars, and adjacent gingiva and cheek. The maxillary nerve then enters the orbit by way of the inferior orbital fissure and is referred to as the **infraorbital nerve**.

While in the pterygopalatine fossa, the maxillary nerve communicates with the **pterygopalatine ganglion** via two small trunks, the **pterygopalatine**

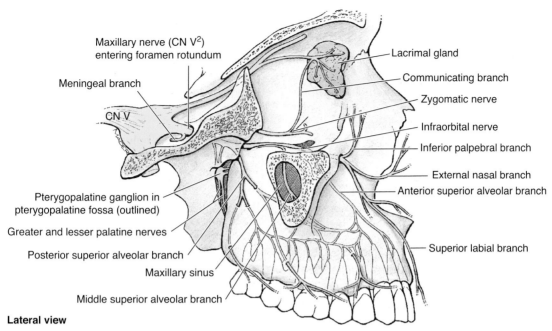

Lateral view

Figure 14-2. The maxillary division of the trigeminal nerve.

nerves (Figs. 14-2 and 14-3); however, these nerves do not bear a functional relationship with the ganglion. Postganglionic parasympathetic fibers derived from the ganglion ride along and distribute with branches of the maxillary division of the trigeminal nerve. These branches, which appear to arise from the ganglion, are described here and, in more detail, in Chapter 18.

Orbital branches are slender nerves that supply the periosteum of the orbit and the mucoperiosteum of the ethmoidal and sphenoidal sinuses. The **greater palatine nerve** and its branches, the **lesser palatine** and **posterior inferior nasal branches** (Fig. 14-3), descend through the pterygopalatine canal to supply regions of the palate, gingiva, tonsil, and lateral wall of the nasal fossa.

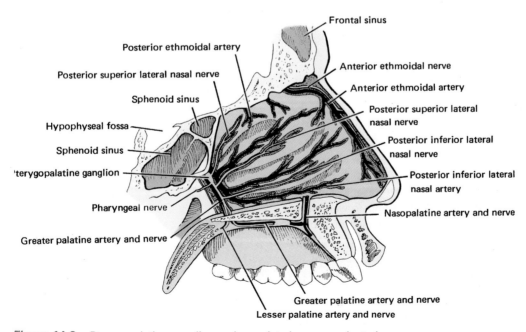

Figure 14-3. Pterygopalatine ganglion and associated nerves and arteries.

Posterior superior nasal branches leave the pterygopalatine fossa via the sphenopalatine foramen to serve the posterior aspect of the nasal fossa and part of the ethmoidal sinus. Its **nasopalatine branch** grooves the vomer bone in its path to the incisive foramen of the anterior hard palate, which it supplies (Fig. 14-3). The **pharyngeal nerve** traverses the **pharyngeal canal** to innervate part of the nasopharynx.

Pterygopalatine Ganglion

Summary Bite. The pterygopalatine ganglion is a parasympathetic ganglion of the facial nerve (cranial nerve VII). Preganglionic parasympathetic fibers enter the ganglion where they synapse on postganglionic cell bodies. Postganglionic parasympathetic fibers are communicated to the maxillary nerve for distribution to the lacrimal gland, mucosal glands of the nasal fossa, palate, and pharynx.

The pterygopalatine ganglion seems to be functionally associated with the maxillary division of the trigeminal nerve because it is suspended by the pterygopalatine nerves within the fossa. It is, however, a parasympathetic ganglion of the facial nerve (cranial nerve VII) (Figs. 14-2 and 14-3, and Table 18-2).

This ganglion receives its parasympathetic preganglionic root by way of the pterygoid canal, which opens onto the posterior wall of the fossa. The preganglionic parasympathetic fibers synapse with postganglionic parasympathetic cell bodies within the ganglion. Postsynaptic parasympathetic fibers leave the ganglion and distribute with branches of the maxillary division of cranial nerve V. These fibers are secretomotor in function. They provide parasympathetic flow to the lacrimal gland and mucosal glands of the nasal fossa, palate, and pharynx.

EXTERNAL NOSE

General Morphology

Summary Bite. The base of the nose, located between the two orbits and projecting forward from there to overhang the upper lip, is composed of a bony skeleton that is continuous with a cartilaginous skeleton anteriorly. The entire nose is covered by skin.

The external nose is triangular. The base of the nose is located between the two orbits, and its distal portion overhangs the upper lip. Its skeleton is both bony and cartilaginous and is covered by integument. The skin is movable over the bony and superior part of the

cartilaginous support but is intimately attached to the cartilage composing the bulb of the nose (Fig. 14-4).

The region of the nose between the two orbits is known as the **root**, from which the bony bridge extends along the dorsum, inferiorly, to terminate in the movable bulbous apex. The inferior surface of the apex contains the two oval openings, the **nares**, leading into the internal nose. The two nares are separated by a midline **columna** (columella), the inferior part of the cartilaginous nasal septum.

The lateral aspect of the naris is formed by the **ala**, or wing, of the nose. The skin of the nose follows the contours of the nares and enters the internal nose for a short distance to form a junction with the mucous membrane lining the cavity.

Short, thick, bristlelike hairs, **vibrissae**, protrude from skin rich in sebaceous glands to strain particulate matter from the inhaled air.

Nasal Skeleton

Summary Bite. Nasal bones, located at the root of the nose, articulate with bones of the face. The remainder of the nose is composed of a framework of several cartilages, the principal one being the median nasal septum.

The skeleton of the nose is both bony and cartilaginous. The bony root is composed of the nasal bones, which articulate with each other, the maxillae, frontal, and ethmoid bones (Fig. 14-4).

The cartilaginous framework of the external nose is composed of five large, principal cartilages and a variable number of smaller cartilages. The principal cartilages are the median nasal septal and the paired lateral nasal and greater alar cartilages. The smaller

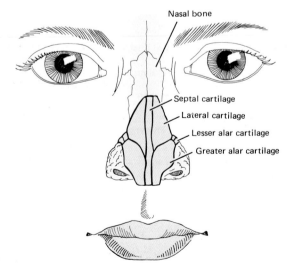

Nasal bone

Septal cartilage

Lateral cartilage

Lesser alar cartilage

Greater alar cartilage

Figure 14-4. Skeleton of the nose.

ones are the vomeronasal, lesser alar, and accessory cartilages.

The **median nasal septal cartilage** is a quadrangular plate of hyaline cartilage that articulates with the nasal bone and the lateral and greater alar cartilages superoanteriorly; the perpendicular plate of the ethmoid bone posteriorly; and the vomer, anterior nasal spine, and vomeronasal cartilage inferiorly. It separates the nasal cavity into right and left halves (see Figs. 6-3 and 6-4). The **lateral nasal cartilage** forms the part of the dorsum of the nose. It is a triangular plate of hyaline cartilage whose base articulates with the nasal and maxillary bones superolaterally, the median septal cartilage medially, and the lesser and greater alar cartilages inferiorly. The **greater alar cartilage** is a C-shaped hyaline cartilage forming the lateral and medial walls of the nostril of the same side so that the nares present a constant opening. It is connected to the lesser alar and lateral nasal cartilages superiorly and the median nasal septal cartilage medially and inferiorly.

The muscles, vascular supply, and nerve supply of the nose are discussed in Chapter 8.

INTERNAL NOSE

The internal nose is the nasal cavity and the structures surrounding it. The osteology of this region is described in Chapter 6.

NASAL CAVITY

 Summary Bite. The nasal cavity is divided into right and left nasal fossae by the median nasal septum. The

anterior aperature of each fossa is the naris, whereas the posterior aperature is the choana. Each nasal fossa possesses four outpocketings called paranasal sinuses.

The **median nasal septum**, consisting of bony and cartilaginous components, subdivides the **nasal cavity** into a right and a left **nasal fossa** (see Figs. 6-3 and 6-4). Each nasal fossa has anterior and posterior apertures, the **naris** and **choana**, respectively. In addition, each possesses four outpocketings termed the **paranasal or accessory sinuses**, a medial and a lateral wall, a floor, and a roof. The entrance into the nasal fossa immediately superior to the naris is a bilateral area of that cavity ringed by the greater alar cartilage termed the **vestibule**. The vestibule is lined by skin possessing vibrissae and sebaceous glands. The superior-most portion of the nasal fossa, specialized for olfaction, is the olfactory region, whereas the larger, inferior portion is the respiratory region.

Medial Wall

The medial wall of the nasal fossa—the median nasal septum—is composed of the vomer, the perpendicular plate of the ethmoid, and the median nasal septal cartilage. The entire median nasal septum is covered by mucoperiosteum. Frequently, this septum deviates to one side, infringing on the nasal fossa of that side. Associated with the anteroinferior aspect of the septum is the vestigial vomeronasal organ (the Jacobson organ) lying on the vomeronasal cartilage. This structure, olfactory in nature, is well-developed in some lower animals.

Lateral Wall

The lateral wall of the nasal fossa differs from the medial wall. Instead of being relatively smooth, it presents three scrolled laminae of bone that jut medially

Clinical Considerations

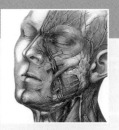

Epistaxis (Nosebleed)

Bleeding from the nose subsequent to injury of the nose is a common occurrence and is usually relatively easy to control. Normally, the source of blood flow is the **Kiesselbach area**—the anteroinferior region of the nasal septum where the septal branch of the superior labial, anterior ethmoidal, nasopalatine, and greater palatine arteries anastomose. The bleeding is controlled by pressure or by packing the nose with cotton. Occasionally, bleeding is from higher up in the nose where control may require more heroic action. When the injury is from a direct blow, the cribiform plate of the ethmoid bone may fractured.

Clinical Considerations

Deviated Nasal Septum

The nasal septum can be deviated from birth but, more often, it is from an injury in childhood or during adulthood, especially those associated with contact sports. A slight deviation may be unnoticeable or it may be observed as a lateral bend in the nose when observed from a frontal view. When severe, the nasal septum may be displaced to one side so that it is in contact with the lateral nasal wall, thus reducing respiratory cability, causing infection, inflammation, and sinusitis, indicating the necessity for surgical treatment.

into the nasal fossa. These **turbinate bones**, covered by mucoperiosteum, are referred to as the **superior, middle**, and **inferior nasal conchae** (Fig. 14-5).

Inferior and lateral, under the cover of the projecting concha, is the correspondingly named meatus. Superior to the **superior meatus**, just anterior to the body of the sphenoid bone, is the **sphenoethmoidal recess** containing the **ostium** (opening) **of the sphe-** **noidal sinus**. A region of another sinus, the posterior ethmoidal air cells, opens below the superior concha into the anterior region of the superior meatus.

The middle nasal concha overlies and covers the lateral wall of the **middle meatus**. A marked, rounded projection is formed on this wall by the middle ethmoidal air cells of the ethmoidal air sinus. This rounded projection is known as the **ethmoidal bulla**,

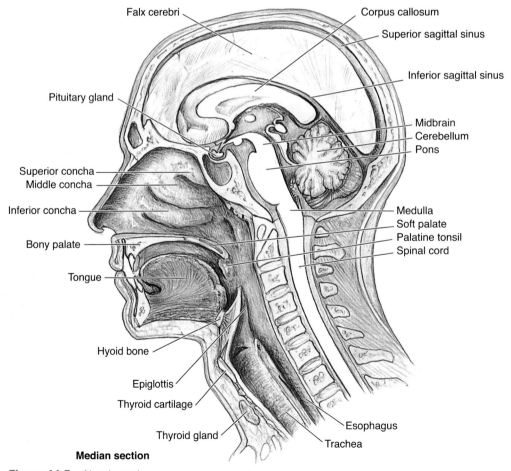

Falx cerebri
Corpus callosum
Superior sagittal sinus
Inferior sagittal sinus
Pituitary gland
Midbrain
Cerebellum
Pons
Superior concha
Middle concha
Inferior concha
Medulla
Soft palate
Palatine tonsil
Spinal cord
Bony palate
Tongue
Hyoid bone
Epiglottis
Thyroid cartilage
Esophagus
Thyroid gland
Trachea

Median section

Figure 14-5. Nasal concha.

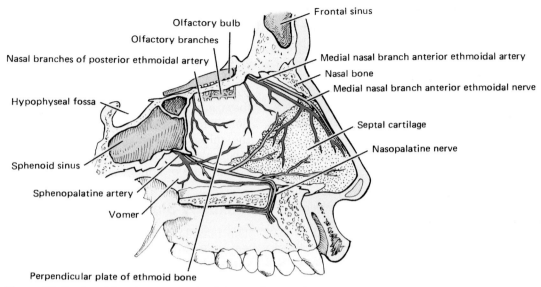

Figure 14-6. Arterial and nerve supply of the median nasal septum.

inferior to which is a thin, arched ledge of bone, the **uncinate process of the ethmoid**. Located between the bulla and the uncinate process is an arch-shaped opening, the **semilunar hiatus**, connecting the ethmoidal infundibulum with the middle meatus. The anterior ethmoidal air cells, the maxillary sinus, and, frequently, the frontonasal duct from the frontal sinus open into the ethmoidal infundibulum.

The inferior nasal concha, usually the largest of the three conchae, is a separate bone, whereas the middle and superior conchae are projections of the ethmoid bone. The inferior concha overhangs the inferior meatus, whose inferior extent is formed by the floor of the nasal cavity. The **nasolacrimal duct** opens into the anterosuperior aspect of the inferior meatus.

Floor and Roof

The floor of the nasal fossa is formed by the horizontal process of the palatine bone and the palatine process of the maxilla. The **incisive canal**, transmitting the nasopalatine nerve and vessels, perforates the mucous membrane of the anteromedial aspect of the floor adjacent to the septum, leading into the **incisive foramen** (Fig. 14-6). The contained nerves and vessels serve the anterior hard palate.

The roof of the nasal fossa is concave cranially, and its bony vault is composed of the cribriform plate of the ethmoid bone as well as parts of the sphenoid, palatine, vomer, frontal, and nasal bones.

The mucous membrane lining the nasal fossa may be classified into two categories: a pink to red,

Clinical Considerations

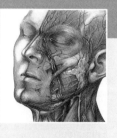

Nose and Nasal Passages

The nose usually is not affected by anomalous development, with the exception of incomplete fusion of the lateral nasal process with the maxillary process resulting in cleft lip and oblique facial clefts, as discussed in Chapter 5 in the section on the development of the head and neck. Occasionally, one or both nasal passages are blocked or are completely absent. This condition is known as **congenital atresia** of the nose. The oc- clusion may involve the anterior nares, the nasal fossae, and/or the choanae.

Frequently, a slight depression may be noted at the tip of the nose. This may be an indication of a very mild form of **bifid nose**, which in certain individuals may be severe enough to involve the entire bulb of the nose.

richly vascularized respiratory mucosa lining most of the nasal fossa and moistening the inhaled air, and a yellowish-brown olfactory mucosa, responsible for olfaction, located superiorly.

PARANASAL SINUSES

Summary Bite. Paranasal sinuses are hollow cavities lined with respiratory mucosa within the maxillae, frontal, ethmoid, and sphenoid bones. These sinuses are in communication with the nasal fossa via small ostia.

The maxillae, frontal, ethmoid, and sphenoid bones contain hollow cavities, the paranasal sinuses, lined by respiratory mucosa (Fig. 14-7). These cavities, as described earlier, communicate with the nasal fossae via small ostia. The function of these sinuses is not known, although it has been suggested that they act as resonators during speech and decrease the weight of the head. The latter explanation is not reasonable because the weight of bone marrow and cancellous bone that would occupy this space is negligible. The capacity of these sinuses as resonators during speech is also questionable because they are present in animals that seldom vocalize. Furthermore, in humans, blocked or fluid-filled sinuses do not impair speech production to any great extent.

The sinuses develop postnatally, although the anlagen of the sphenoidal, maxillary, and ethmoidal sinuses are present at birth. The mucous membrane lining the sinuses is continuous with that of the nasal fossae via the various ostia of the sinuses into the fossa. These openings and the chambers with which they are associated are listed in Table 14-1.

The ostia, although already small on the dry skull, are reduced even further in size in the living individual, so much so that they are minute. Hence, communication between the sinuses and the nasal fossa is readily impeded during respiratory congestion. Three of the four sinuses are bilateral. Although the sphenoidal sinus, located in the midline, is not bilateral, it is divided into two halves by an interposed plate of bone.

Maxillary Sinus

The maxillary sinus, the largest of the paranasal sinuses, is positioned lateral to the nasal cavity, inferior to the orbit, and often extends into the zygomatic process of the maxilla (Fig. 14-7).

The floor of the sinus is intimately related to the maxillary first and second molars, whose roots not only form considerable bulges but also may perforate the osseous floor of the sinus. Moreover, if the sinus is large, the third molar and second premolar may also be involved with its floor.

The superomedial wall of the sinus consistently communicates with the ethmoidal infundibulum by way of the **maxillary ostium**, and inconsistently communicates with the middle meatus via the accessory maxillary ostium.

Frontal Sinus

The frontal sinus pneumatizes the forehead and is incompletely subdivided into two or more compartments

Table 14-1 Openings of the Paranasal Sinuses

Sinus	Opening	Location	Constancy
Maxillary	Maxillary ostium	Middle meatus via ethmoidal infundibulum	Constant
	Accessory maxillary ostium	Middle meatus	Inconstant
Frontal	Frontonasal duct	Frontal recess of middle meatus	Constant
	Frontal ostium	Middle meatus via the ethmoidal infundibulum	Inconstant
Ethmoidal			
Posterior air cells	Ostia of the posterior ethmoidal air cells	Superior meatus	Constant
Middle air cells	Ostia of the middle ethmoidal air cells	Middle meatus	Constant
Anterior air cells	Ostia of the anterior ethmoidal air cells	Middle meatus via ethmoidal infundibulum or via frontal recess	Inconstant
Sphenoidal	Sphenoidal ostium	Sphenoethmoidal recess	Constant

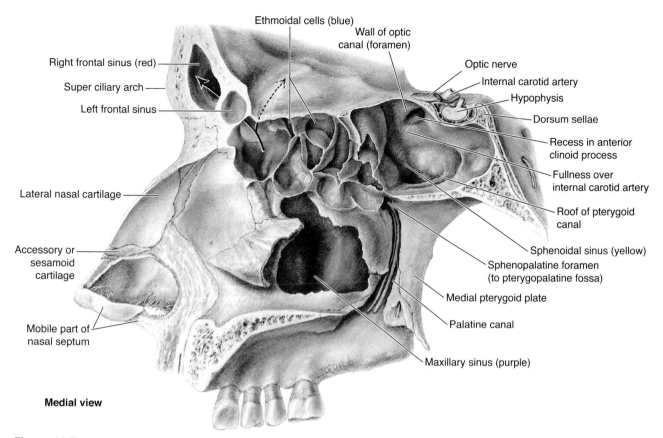

Figure 14-7. Paranasal sinuses (medial view).

(Fig. 14-7). The right and left frontal sinuses are separated from each other by the frontal septum, which usually deviates to one side, resulting in asymmetry of the two sinuses. The frontal sinus drains into the frontal recess of the middle meatus by way of the frontonasal duct, or into the ethmoidal infundibulum via the same duct.

Ethmoidal Sinus

The ethmoidal sinus is composed of three sets of ethmoidal air cells: the anterior, middle, and posterior (Fig. 14-7). These thin-walled, bony, honeycombed spaces collectively form the ethmoidal labyrinth located between the orbits and the nasal fossae. The

Clinical Considerations

Maxillary Molars and the Maxillary Sinus

The roots of the maxillary molars bulge into the floor of the maxillary sinus but normally do not perforate the mucus membrane of the sinus. Extreme care must be given when extracting the maxillary molars because a fractured root may be driven into the maxillary sinus, forming a communication between the oral cavity and the maxillary sinus and thus increasing the chance of sinus infection.

Maxillary sinus inflammation can be confused with toothache in the molar region because the posterior superior alveolar nerve of the maxillary division of the trigeminal nerve serves both the maxillary sinus and the molar teeth with sensory innervation.

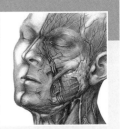

Clinical Considerations

Cerebrospinal Rhinorrhea

During fracture of the ethmoid bone, cerebrospinal fluid may leak into the nasal fossa and out through the external nares. This condition, **cerebrospinal rhinorrhea**, may lead to meningitis, with possibly fatal consequences.

---

posterior air cells drain into the superior meatus; the middle cells into the middle meatus just above the bulla ethmoidalis; and the anterior air cells into the ethmoidal infundibulum and thence into the middle meatus via the semilunar hiatus.

Sphenoidal Sinus

The sphenoidal sinus hollows out the body of the sphenoid bone and is separated into two asymmetrical halves by a plate of bone, the sphenoidal septum, which usually deviates to one side (Fig. 14-7). The sphenoidal sinus drains into the sphenoethmoidal recess of the nasal fossa through the sphenoidal ostium.

VASCULAR AND NERVE SUPPLY OF THE NASAL CAVITY AND PARANASAL SINUSES

Vascular Supply

⇒ **Summary Bite.** Branches of the facial, ophthalmic, and maxillary arteries vascularize the nasal cavity and paranasal sinuses.

The vascular supply of the nasal fossa is derived from several sources: branches of the facial, ophthalmic, and maxillary arteries. The vestibule receives septal branches from the facial artery. The ophthalmic artery supplies anterior and posterior ethmoidal branches to regions of the superior and middle conchae and meatuses, to the middle nasal septum, and to the frontal and ethmoidal sinuses.

The maxillary artery provides several branches to the nasal fossa. The greater palatine branches serve the anterior floor and posterior aspect of the nasal fossa. The sphenopalatine branch, entering via the sphenopalatine foramen, vascularizes portions of

the nasal conchae and meatuses via its **posterior lateral nasal branches** as well as the posterior segment of the median nasal septum by its **posterior septal branches**. Terminal branches of these vessels form a rich anastomotic vascular plexus in the mucoperiosteum. The maxillary artery provides vascularization of the four paranasal sinuses (Table 14-2) via the **posterior lateral nasal branch** of the sphenopalatine artery. In addition, the anterior and posterior superior alveolar arteries serve the maxillary sinus, whereas the pharyngeal artery and the artery of the pterygoid canal supply the sphenoidal sinus.

The ophthalmic artery, via its **anterior and posterior ethmoidal branches**, assists in vascularizing the frontal, ethmoidal, and sphenoidal sinuses.

Venous drainage of the nose and paranasal sinuses is by way of the anterior and posterior ethmoidal veins into the ophthalmic vein, the sphenopalatine vein into the pterygoid plexus of veins, and the vein of the foramen cecum into the superior sagittal sinus. Because these venous elements usually do not possess valves, infection may be propagated throughout the entire system, affecting the dural venous sinuses—especially the cavernous sinus—and resulting in serious and, perhaps, life-threatening complications.

Nerve Supply

⇒ **Summary Bite.** Ophthalmic (V_1) and maxillary (V_2) divisions of the trigeminal nerve provide general sensation to the respiratory mucosa. Olfaction (smell) is provided by cranial nerve I. Secretomotor fibers from the facial nerve (cranial nerve VII) are communicated from the pterygopalatine ganglion to the maxillary division (V_2) for delivery to the mucoperiosteum.

General sensory innervation to the respiratory mucosa is derived from the trigeminal nerve, in particular from its ophthalmic and maxillary divisions. The olfactory epithelium receives its special visceral afferent fibers for smell from the olfactory nerves (cranial

Table 14-2 Vascular and Sensory Nerve Supply of the Paranasal Sinuses

Sinus	Arteries	Veins	Nerves

Maxillary	Maxillary
	  Sphenopalatine
	    Posterior lateral nasal
	  Greater palatine
	  Posterior superior alveolar
	  Infraorbital
	    Anterior superior alveolar
		Sphenopalatine, greater palatine anterior, middle and posterior superior alveolar	Maxillary division
			  Infraorbital
			    Anterior superior alveolar
			    Middle superior alveolar
			    Posterior superior alveolar

Frontal	Ophthalmic
	  Anterior ethmoidal
	Maxillary
	  Sphenopalatine
	    Posterior lateral nasal
		Anastomosis of supraorbitals and superior ophthalmic	Opththalmic division
			  Frontal
			  Nasociliary
			    Anterior ethmoidal

Ethmoidal	Ophthalmic
	  Anterior ethmoidal
	  Posterior ethmoidal
	Maxillary
	  Sphenopalatine
	    Posterior lateral nasal
		Anterior ethmoidal
		Posterior ethmoidal
		Sphenopalatine
			Opthalmic division
			  Nasociliary
			    Anterior ethmoidal
			    Posterior ethmoidal
			Maxillary division
			  Orbital branch
			    Posterior superior nasal

Sphenoidal	Ophthalmic
	  Posterior ethmoidal
	Maxillary
	  Artery of the pterygoid canal
	  Pharyngeal branch
	  Sphenopalatine
	    Posterior lateral nasal
		Posterior ethmoidal
		Sphenopalatine
			Ophthalmic division
			  Nasociliary
			    Posterior ethmoidal
			Maxillary division
			  Orbital branch

Clinical Considerations

Paranasal Sinuses

Sinusitis, or inflammation of the mucosa of the paranasal sinuses, results in swelling of the mucoperiosteum, which blocks the ostia of the sinuses. This irritation causes accumulation of mucus in the sinuses, resulting in increased pressure and displacement of the air normally located therein. This pressure causes "sinus headaches" of varied intensity, and, if untreated, the infection may spread to the inner ear and the middle ear as well as to other areas.

Infection of the frontal sinus, if left untreated, may result in frontal bone osteomyelitis because venous drainage of this sinus is intimately related to diploic veins and indirectly related with those of the dura and scalp.

The ethmoidal air cells are in close relationship with the orbit, with only a paper-thin lamina of bone separating these structures. Hence, in cases of severe infection, this bony separation may be perforated and the infection may involve the orbit, resulting in orbital cellulitis.

The maxillary sinus is prone to infection because it is intimately associated with the first and second maxillary molars. Dental involvement may result from abscess, from carious lesions, or from tooth extractions with part of the floor of the maxillary sinus being removed in the process. Knowledge of the anatomy of the sinuses and roentgenographic analysis of the involved area should be a prerequisite to maxillary tooth extraction.

nerve I), axons of which pass via perforations in the overlying cribriform plate of the ethmoid bone to the olfactory bulb. Secretomotor fibers derived from the facial nerve (cranial nerve VII) reach the mucoperiosteum via communications carried by branches of the maxillary division of the trigeminal nerve.

The paranasal sinuses also receive sensory innervation via the ophthalmic and maxillary divisions of the trigeminal nerve (Table 14-2). The frontal sinus receives its sensory innervation via branches of the frontal and nasociliary nerves of the ophthalmic division of the trigeminal nerve.

The ethmoidal sinuses are served by ethmoidal branches of the nasociliary nerve and by orbital and nasal branches of the maxillary division of the trigeminal nerve. The sphenoidal sinus is served by ethmoidal branches of the nasociliary nerve and orbital branches of the maxillary division. The maxillary sinus receives its innervation solely from the maxillary division, specifically from the superior alveolar nerves.

Submandibular Region and Floor of Mouth

15

Key Terms

Major Salivary Glands are six in number (three pairs). These are the parotid, submandibular, and sublingual glands. Because the parotid gland is not located in this region, it is not studied here. The submandibular gland is located primarily in the submandibular triangle, whereas the sublingual gland is located in the floor of the oral cavity, beneath the tongue.

Submandibular Region or **Suprahyoid Region** includes the region from the inferior border of the mandible to the hyoid bone. This includes some of the structures of the floor of the oral cavity, including those muscles that originate on the mandible and insert on the hyoid bone as well as those that originate on the hyoid bone and insert into the tongue.

    The submandibular or suprahyoid region lies between the hyoid bone and the mandible in the anterior triangle of the neck. However, it is more often studied with the head because it is a transition zone between these two regions and because the structures contained therein function in association with the jaws and the floor of the mouth.

Suprahyoid Muscle Group Functions include those muscles that originate or insert on the hyoid bone and function on structures in the region. These would include, among some others, all of the muscles whose name ends in "hyoid"

(i.e., stylohyoid, mylohyoid, geniohyoid) and the anterior and posterior bellies of the digastric muscle.

Tongue Muscles include both intrinsic extrinsic muscles. The intrinsic tongue muscles, located within the tongue, include longitudinal, transverse, and vertical groups. These three groups function to alter the shape of the tongue when necessary for mastication, phonation, and deglutition. The extrinsic muscles whose names end in "glossus" originate from several anatomic sites and insert into the tongue to intermingle with other tongue muscles. The intrinsic muscles and three of the extrinsic muscles are innervated by the hypoglossal nerve (cranial nerve XII).

CONTENTS AND BOUNDARIES

Summary Bite. The submandibular region and floor of the mouth are contained mostly within the submandibular triangle and the space spanning across the midline between them. Contained within this region are the suprahyoid muscles as well as the muscles of the tongue. Two of the major salivary glands are also contained in this region.

Muscles contained within the submandibular region and the floor of the mouth and/or forming its boundaries include the anterior and posterior bellies of the digastric, stylohyoid, mylohyoid, and geniohyoid muscles. Both intrinsic and extrinsic tongue musculatures, namely, the styloglossus, genioglossus, and hyoglossus muscles, also occupy the region. Strictly described, the middle pharyngeal constrictor muscle also may be included because it originates from the hyoid bone. The platysma, a muscle immediately deep to the skin, overlies this region.

Cutaneous sensation to the area is provided by branches of the cervical plexus. Additionally, branches of several cranial nerves, including the trigeminal (cranial nerve V), facial (cranial nerve VII), and hypoglossal (cranial nerve XII) nerves, provide sensory, special sensory, motor, and secretomotor innervation to the structures within this region.

The major vascular supply to the region is provided by branches of the lingual artery but branches of the facial and maxillary arteries also contribute to its vascularization. Venous drainage is accomplished by like-named veins and the anterior jugular vein.

Two of the three major salivary glands, the submandibular and sublingual glands, occupy the submandibular and sublingual regions, respectively. These two glands receive postganglionic parasympathetic innervation from the submandibular ganglion located in the vicinity of the submandibular gland.

The submandibular region is bounded superiorly by the inferior rim of the mandible and inferiorly by the anterior and posterior bellies of the digastric muscle, as these two bellies converge onto the hyoid bone to form the submandibular triangle.

The mylohyoid muscle, spanning between the two sides of the mandible, is attached inferiorly to the anterior aspect of the hyoid bone. Its superior surface underlies the tongue, thus forming the floor of the mouth, whereas its inferior surface forms the floor of the submandibular triangle.

Attached to much of the posterior aspect of the hyoid bone is the hyoglossus muscle ascending into the tongue. The interval between the mylohyoid and hyoglossus muscles permits the passage of neurovascular and lymphatic elements into and out of the floor of the oral cavity.

MUSCLES AND FASCIA

Summary Bite. Muscles contained within the submandibular region include the suprahyoid muscles and those attaching either to the mandible or to the hyoid bone. The tongue muscles are also included in this region, with the exception of the palatoglossal muscle, which originates from the palate and is innervated by the trigeminal instead of the hypoglossal nerve. The mylohyoid muscle forms the floor of this region.

Muscles constituting the submandibular region and the floor of the oral cavity include the suprahyoid muscles of the anterior triangle of the neck and those attaching either to the mandible or hyoid bone forming the floor of the mouth and/or the tongue. Both intrinsic and extrinsic muscles of the tongue are generally described with this region, the exception being the palatoglossus muscle, which originates from the palate and is thus more appropriately described with muscles of that region.

The suprahyoid structures are enclosed in the investing fascia of the neck. This fascia is attached to the hyoid bone and extends superiorly, attaching to the inferior border of the mandible. Enclosing the anterior belly of the digastric muscle, the investing fascia continues posteriorly and laterally to encase the submandibular gland. The deeper layers of this fascia envelop the muscles of the submandibular region, including those of the tongue. Fusing with the deep fascia of the posterior digastric muscle, the investing fascia assists in forming the stylomandibular ligament. The fascial compartment containing these structures reaches the floor of the mouth, the sublingual gland, and the tongue. Clefts between the fascial layers posteriorly, at the border of the mylohyoid muscle, into the lateral pharyngeal cleft and into the cleft around the submandibular gland.

Suprahyoid Muscles

Digastric Muscle

Summary Bite. The digastric muscle consists of two heads that originate from different locations; however, both insert onto the hyoid bone via an intermediate tendon. These two heads, along with the inferior border of the mandible, form the boundary of the submandibular triangle.

Table 15-1 Suprahyoid Muscles and Extrinsic Muscles of the Tongue

Muscle	Origin	Insertion	Innervation	Action
Posterior belly of digastric	Mastoid notch of temporal bone	Intermediate tendon	Facial nerve	*Posterior belly:* draws hyoid bone posteriorly
Anterior belly of digastric	Digastric fossa of mandible	Intermediate tendon	Mandibular division of trigeminal	*Anterior belly:* draws hyoid bone anteriorly *Both bellies:* elevates hyoid bone and open mandible when hyoid bone is fixed
Stylohyoid	Styloid process (posterior and lateral surfaces)	Body of hyoid bone	Facial nerve	Draws the hyoid bone superiorly and posteriorly; also assists in fixing the hyoid bone
Mylohyoid	Mylohyoid line of the mandible	Median raphe (anterior fibers) and the body of the hyoid bone (posterior fibers)	Mylohyoid nerve (mandibular division of trigeminal nerve)	Depresses mandible (when hyoid bone is fixed); elevates the hyoid bone (when the mandible is fixed)
Geniohyoid	Inferior mental spine of the mandible	Body of the hyoid bone	CI (transported by the hypoglossal nerve)	Draws hyoid bone anteriorly
Genioglossus	Superior mental spine of the mandible	From the tip to the back of the tongue (also body of the hyoid bone)	Hypoglossal nerve	Protrudes the tongue and depresses the tip of the tongue
Hyoglossus	Body and greater cornu of the hyoid bone	Body of the tongue	Hypoglossal nerve	Depresses the tongue
Styloglossus	Styloid process (anterior surface) and stylomandibular ligament	Body of the tongue to the tip of the tongue	Hypoglossal nerve	Retracts the tongue and elevates its tip
Palatoglossus	Fascia and lateral aspect of soft palate	Side of the tongue	Pharyngeal plexus	Elevates root of the tongue and constricts the fauces

The **digastric muscle** consists of two portions: a **posterior belly**, which arises from the mastoid notch of the temporal bone, and an **anterior belly**, arising from the digastric fossa of the anterior lower border of the mandible. Both of these muscle bellies descend to the hyoid bone to be inserted by an intermediate tendon (Table 15-1).

A fibrous loop surrounds the tendon as well as the body and the greater cornu of the hyoid bone. At the loop, the tendon perforates the stylohyoid muscle at its attachment on the hyoid bone.

The combined function of the two bellies of the digastric is to elevate the hyoid bone and also to assist in opening the mouth when the hyoid bone is fixed by the infrahyoid muscles. Acting independently, the anterior belly draws the hyoid anteriorly, whereas the posterior belly draws it posteriorly.

Embryologically, the digastric muscle is really two separate muscles, each derived from different pharyngeal arches. The anterior belly originates from the mandibular arch (pharyngeal arch I) and is innervated by a branch of the mylohyoid nerve from the mandibular division of the trigeminal nerve. The posterior belly develops in the hyoid arch (pharyngeal arch II) and is innervated by a branch of the facial nerve that enters its deep surface at midbelly.

The posterior belly of the digastric muscle is vascularized by the posterior auricular artery, with contributions from the suprahyoid branch of the lingual artery and muscular branches of the occipital artery. The anterior belly is vascularized by the submental branch of the facial artery.

Stylohyoid Muscle

Summary Bite. The stylohyoid muscle originates from the styloid process of the temporal bone and descends to the hyoid bone in association with the posterior belly of the digastric muscle, which perforates it close to the insertion.

The **stylohyoid muscle** arises from the posterior and lateral surfaces of the styloid process of the temporal bone (Fig. 15-1 and Table 15-1). As this muscle descends to insert on the body of the hyoid bone, it is in close association with the posterior belly of the digastric muscle, which perforates it close to its insertion.

The stylohyoid muscle functions to draw the hyoid bone superiorly and posteriorly, in addition to assisting in fixing it. Motor innervation to this muscle is provided by a branch of the facial nerve that enters its midbelly. Vascular supply is provided by posterior auricular and occipital branches of the external carotid artery. Additional vascular elements may reach the muscle via the suprahyoid branch of the lingual artery and from muscular branches of the facial artery.

Mylohyoid Muscle

Summary Bite. The mylohyoid muscle originates from the mylohyoid line on each half of the mandible and inserts upon itself in the median raphe to form the floor of the oral cavity.

The **mylohyoid muscle** forms the floor of the mouth as it unites in the midline with its counterpart from the opposite side of the mandible. This muscle arises from the entire length of the mylohyoid line of the mandible, from the symphysis menti to the region opposite the last molar tooth (Fig. 15-2 and Table 15-1). Anteriorly, the fibers of each side insert into a median raphe, whereas the more posteriorly oriented fibers insert into the body of the hyoid bone.

The mylohyoid muscle assists in depressing the mandible when the hyoid bone is fixed. When the mandible is fixed, the muscle elevates the hyoid bone, and consequently the tongue, for swallowing.

The mylohyoid nerve from the inferior alveolar branch of the mandibular division of the trigeminal nerve innervates this muscle as the nerve approaches its inferolateral border. Vascular supply is provided by the anastomoses from the submental branch of the facial artery and the sublingual branch of the lingual artery.

Geniohyoid Muscle

Summary Bite. The geniohyoid muscle originates superior to the mylohyoid muscle from the inferior mental spine of the mandible and inserts upon the hyoid bone.

Immediately superior to the mylohyoid muscle is the **geniohyoid muscle**, originating from the inferior mental spine (genial tubercle) of the mandible before descending to the anterior surface of the body of the hyoid bone (Figs. 15-1 and 15-2, and Table 15-1). At its insertion, the geniohyoid is in contact with its counterpart from the opposite side of the mandible.

The geniohyoid muscle functions to draw the hyoid bone anteriorly and, in so doing, draws the tongue as well because some of the extrinsic muscles of the tongue are attached to the hyoid bone.

The geniohyoid muscle is innervated by fibers of the first cervical nerve, which are transported to it via the hypoglossal nerve. Vascularization is provided by the sublingual branch of the lingual artery.

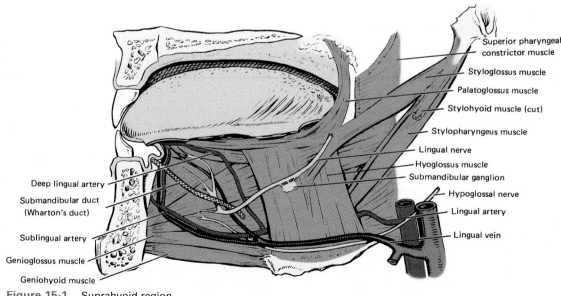

Figure 15-1. Suprahyoid region.

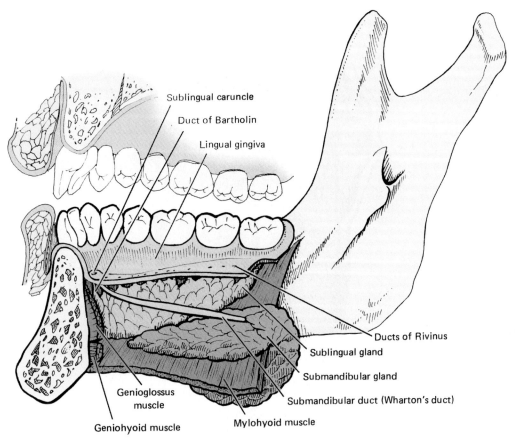

Sublingual caruncle

Duct of Bartholin

Lingual gingiva

Ducts of Rivinus

Sublingual gland

Submandibular gland

Submandibular duct (Wharton's duct)

Genioglossus muscle

Geniohyoid muscle

Mylohyoid muscle

Figure 15-2. Submandibular and sublingual glands.

Group Actions

Summary Bite. The suprahyoid muscles all originate from various areas superior to the hyoid bone, but all insert upon the hyoid bone, hence their names end in "hyoid." As a group, these muscles assist in fixing the hyoid bone for swallowing and for retracting the mandible. They function in concert with the infrahyoid muscles of the neck.

The suprahyoid muscles, all of which attach to the hyoid bone and another structure superior to it, function as a group to assist in swallowing by lifting the hyoid bone, the floor of the mouth, and the tongue. As food passes down the esophagus, the stylohyoid and posterior digastric muscles retract the hyoid bone to prevent regurgitation. This muscle group may also assist in fixing the hyoid bone and in retracting the mandible when the hyoid bone is fixed by the infrahyoid muscles.

Tongue Muscles

Summary Bite. Intrinsic muscles of the tongue are confined within the tongue, whereas the extrinsic muscles originate from various places and insert into the tongue.

The tongue muscles are composed of two groups: intrinsic tongue muscles and extrinsic tongue muscles (Figs. 15-1, 15-3, 15-4, and Table 15-1).

The **intrinsic muscles** of the tongue are confined within the tongue itself and are described as longitudinal, transverse, and vertical muscles. The longitudinal muscle group is subdivided into a superior and an inferior group.

The intrinsic muscles function generally to alter the shape of the tongue as necessary in mastication, deglutition, and phonation. The varying shapes of the tongue can be predicted by relating the fiber orientations of the intrinsic muscles as named.

The four **extrinsic muscles** of the tongue originate outside it: the genioglossus, hyoglossus, styloglossus, and palatoglossus muscles. The palatoglossus muscle, as was stated at the beginning of the chapter, is described in Chapter 16 rather than here because it originates from the palatal region.

Genioglossus Muscle

Summary Bite. The genioglossus muscle originates from the superior mental spine and inserts into the internal aspect of the inferior surface of the tongue.

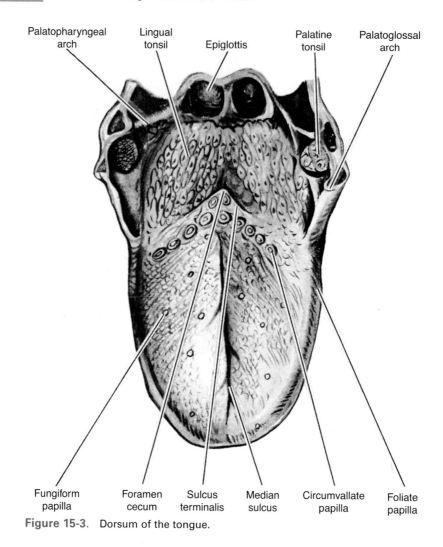

Palatopharyngeal arch

Lingual tonsil

Epiglottis

Palatine tonsil

Palatoglossal arch

Fungiform papilla

Foramen cecum

Sulcus terminalis

Median sulcus

Circumvallate papilla

Foliate papilla

Figure 15-3. Dorsum of the tongue.

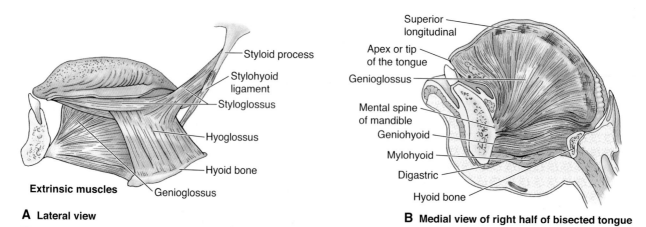

Styloid process

Stylohyoid ligament

Styloglossus

Hyoglossus

Hyoid bone

Extrinsic muscles

Genioglossus

A Lateral view

Superior longitudinal

Apex or tip of the tongue

Genioglossus

Mental spine of mandible

Geniohyoid

Mylohyoid

Digastric

Hyoid bone

B Medial view of right half of bisected tongue

Figure 15-4. Muscles of the tongue. **(A)** Lateral view. **(B)** Medial view of the right half of bisected tongue.

The **genioglossus muscle** arises from the superior mental spine (genial tubercle) of the mandible directly above the geniohyoid muscle (Figs. 15-1, 15-4A and B, and Table 15-1). From here, the muscle fans out to enter the entire length of the inferior surface of the tongue. The most anterior fibers curve upward to insert into the tip of the tongue. The posterior fibers pass to the base of the tongue, whereas some of the most inferior fibers are attached to the body of the hyoid bone. The genioglossus muscle acts to protrude the tongue, whereas the most anterior fibers depress the tongue tip.

Hyoglossus Muscle

Summary Bite. The hyoglossus muscle originates from the hyoid bone and passes vertically to insert into the tongue.

The **hyoglossus muscle** originates from the side of the body and greater cornu of the hyoid bone, passing vertically to enter the tongue, where the fibers intermingle with those of the styloglossus muscle (Figs. 15-1, 15-4A and B, and Table 15-1).

A separate slip of muscle, referred to by some as the **chondroglossus muscle** because it is separated from the hyoglossus by a small interval, is considered a part of the hyoglossus in this text. The hyoglossus functions as the major depressor of the tongue.

Styloglossus Muscle

Summary Bite. The styloglossus muscle originates from the styloid process of the temporal bone and inserts into the tongue on its lateral surface to intermingle with fibers of the hyoglossus muscle.

The **styloglossus muscle** arises from the anterior surface of the styloid process of the temporal bone and the stylomandibular ligament (Figs. 15-1 and 15-4A, and Table 15-1). It then descends anteriorly and medially to enter the tongue from the lateral aspect, as it turns horizontally. Most fibers of the styloglossus muscle continue on to the tip of the tongue. Some of the posterior fibers decussate with those of the hyoglossus muscle. This muscle functions to retract the tongue, whereas the more anterior fibers elevate the tip.

Innervation and Vascularization

Summary Bite. All of the muscles (extrinsic as well as intrinsic) of the tongue, with the exception of one, are innervated by the hypoglossal nerve (cranial nerve XII). The palatoglossal muscle, which originates from the palate, is innervated by the pharyngeal plexus. Vascular supply is provided by branches of the lingual artery, again except for the palatoglossal muscle, which is vascularized by arteries of the palate.

All of the tongue musculature is innervated by the hypoglossal nerve, with the exception of the palatoglossus, which is innervated by the pharyngeal plexus (Figs. 15-5 and 15-6).

The vascular supply to the muscles of the tongue is provided primarily by the deep lingual artery, the terminal branch of the lingual artery (Figs. 15-7 and 15-8). The exception, again, is the palatoglossus, which is served by the arteries of the palate.

Group Actions

Summary Bite. The intrinsic tongue muscles generally function to alter the shape of the tongue, whereas

---

Clinical Considerations

Lingual Cancer

Cancer of the tongue is the most common cancer of the oral cavity (36.2%). About 95% of the cancers located on the tongue and floor of the mouth are squamous cell carcinomas that are correlated with a history of high use of alcohol and tobacco. Two thirds of the tongue cancers occur on the lateral surfaces of the middle third of the tongue, whereas one third are located on the ventrolateral or the anterior undersurface of the tongue. Malignancies in the posterior portion of the tongue metastasize to deep cervical lymph nodes early on, whereas those on the anterior part of the tongue do not metastasize to the deep cervical lymph nodes until later in the disease. Thus, because the deep cervical lymph nodes drain into the internal jugular vein, it is extremely important that the disease be identified and treated as early as possible to prevent metastases into structures within the neck.

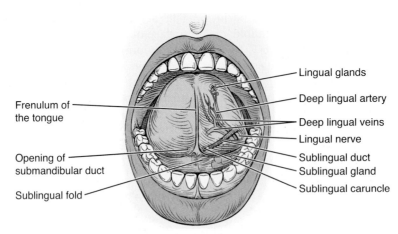

Lingual glands

Deep lingual artery

Deep lingual veins

Lingual nerve

Sublingual duct

Sublingual gland

Sublingual caruncle

Frenulum of
the tongue

Opening of
submandibular duct

Sublingual fold

Figure 15-5. Inferior surface of the tongue and floor of the mouth. Mucosa has been removed from the left side.

the extrinsic tongue muscles generally function to direct the movement of the tongue (e.g., retract, protrude). All tongue movements are the result of coordinated contractions of several intrinsic and extrinsic muscles.

Complex movements of the tongue are accomplished by intricate and coordinated contractions of both intrinsic and extrinsic muscles of the tongue. Generally,

"movements" other than those that basically alter the shape of the tongue are the result of contractions of the extrinsic muscles, although one group seldom functions alone.

The overlapping, intermingling, and decussating nature of the intrinsic and extrinsic muscle groups permit the fine coordinated effort so necessary in speech.

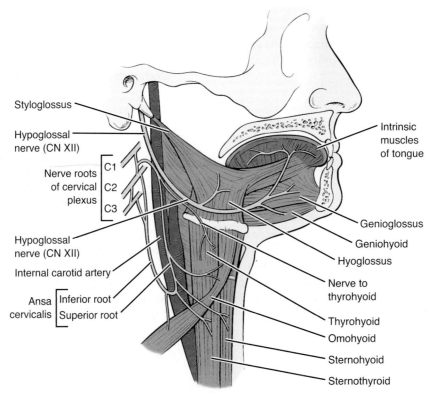

Styloglossus

Hypoglossal
nerve (CN XII)

Nerve roots
of cervical
plexus   C1
C2
C3

Hypoglossal
nerve (CN XII)

Internal carotid artery

Ansa   Inferior root
cervicalis   Superior root

Intrinsic
muscles
of tongue

Genioglossus

Geniohyoid

Hyoglossus

Nerve to
thyrohyoid

Thyrohyoid

Omohyoid

Sternohyoid

Sternothyroid

Figure 15-6. Hypoglossal nerve. Notice its association with the ansa cervicalis.

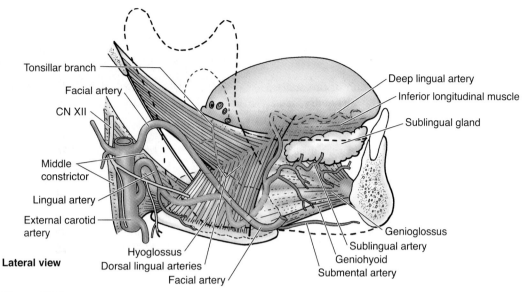

Figure 15-7. Blood supply of the tongue.

SALIVARY GLANDS

Summary Bite. Two of the three major salivary glands, the submandibular and sublingual glands, are located in this region. Both empty their secretions into the floor of the mouth.

Two of the three major salivary glands are located within the submandibular region or in the floor of the mouth: the submandibular and sublingual glands. The third major salivary gland, the parotid gland, is located on the side of the face and in the retromandibular space. It has been described in Chapter 11.

Most of the submandibular gland is located superficially in the submandibular triangle, with only a small portion extending into the floor of the mouth. The entire sublingual gland, however, is housed in the floor of the mouth.

Submandibular Gland

Summary Bite. The submandibular gland is located mostly within the submandibular triangle and in the

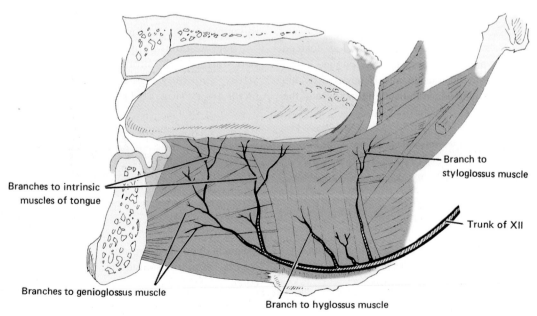

Figure 15-8. Hypoglossal nerve.

submandibular recess, a region situated on the medial surface of the mandible. The submandibular duct extends to the sublingual caruncula, where its contents are emptied into the mouth.

The submandibular gland occupies much of the space within the submandibular triangle. Superficially, it is covered by skin, platysma, and the superficial layer of the deep cervical fascia. The superior extent of the gland is recessed under the cover of the mandible in the submandibular fossa. Inferiorly, the gland extends to the hyoid bone, overlapping the intermediate tendon of the digastric muscle. The gland extends anteriorly to the anterior belly of the digastric muscle and posteriorly as far as the stylomandibular ligament.

The deep surface of the gland lies on the hyoglossus, stylohyoid, styloglossus, and mylohyoid muscles. Usually, a fingerlike projection extends into the sublingual space on the superior surface of the mylohyoid muscle.

It is from this deep process that the **submandibular duct (the Wharton duct)** emerges to pass anteriorly between the mylohyoid, hyoglossus, and genioglossus muscles, then between the last-named muscle and the sublingual gland to open onto the **sublingual caruncula**, just lateral to the base of the lingual frenulum (Fig. 15-9).

The facial artery vascularizes the submandibular gland as that artery passes through the gland's posterior portion on its way to the superficial face (Fig. 15-7). The artery ascends across the lateral border of the mandible just anterior to the masseter muscle. The sublingual branch of the lingual artery also provides additional vascular supply to the gland. Venous drainage follows the named arterial channels.

Sublingual Gland

Summary Bite. The sublingual gland is located beneath the anterior aspect of the tongue. It lies superior to the mylohyoid muscle and is covered by the sublingual fold. The gland lies in the sublingual fossa of the

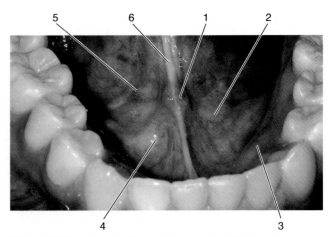

Figure 15-9. Anterior floor of the mouth. (1) Lingual caruncle; (2) Sublingual sulcus; (3) Mandibular torus; (4) Sublingual fold; (5) Sublingual vein; (6) Lingual frenum.

mandible and is bordered medially by the genioglossus muscle. Saliva is delivered by tiny excretory ducts onto the floor of the mouth, although some ducts join to form a sublingual duct that empties into the submandibular duct.

The sublingual gland, the smallest of the three major salivary glands, is housed in the floor of the mouth between the sublingual fold (mucous membrane of the oral cavity) superiorly and the mylohyoid muscle inferiorly. This almond-shaped gland lies between the genioglossus muscle medially and the sublingual fossa of the mandible laterally. Posteriorly, it is in contact with the submandibular gland.

Ducts from the sublingual gland may open into the oral cavity as tiny excretory ducts (ducts of Rivinus) on the surface of the plica sublingualis located in the sublingual sulcus. Some ducts may unite to form the **sublingual duct (duct of Bartholin)**, opening into the submandibular duct (Fig. 15-9).

The vascular supply to this gland is derived from two sources: the sublingual artery from the lingual artery and the submental artery, a branch of the facial artery (Fig. 15-7).

Clinical Considerations

Sialography

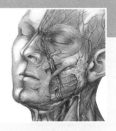

Sometimes the ducts of the parotid and submandibular glands become obstructed. After injecting the duct with a contrast medium, a sialogram (a special type of radiograph) may be taken to visualize the contents of the duct.

Autonomic Innervation

> **Summary Bite.** Secretomotor innervation to the salivary glands originates in the facial nerve (cranial nerve VII) and is transmitted to the submandibular ganglion via the chorda tympani. Postganglionic fibers are transmitted to the glands via the lingual nerve, a branch of the trigeminal nerve (cranial nerve V₃). Vasomotor innervation originates in the carotid plexus and is delivered via the facial artery.

Autonomic innervation to the submandibular and sublingual glands is provided by secretomotor fibers originating in the facial nerve. These fibers are transmitted to the submandibular ganglion via the chorda tympani branch of the facial nerve and on to the lingual nerve of the trigeminal nerve.

Sympathetic innervation (vasomotor) is provided from the superior cervical ganglion via the carotid plexus, whose nerve fibers are transmitted to these two glands by the facial artery. A more complete description of the autonomic system's relationships with these two glands is detailed in Chapter 18.

Innervation

Two cranial nerves may be observed coursing through the submandibular region. The trigeminal nerve is represented by two branches from the mandibular division. The other cranial nerve is the hypoglossal nerve serving the tongue musculature (Fig. 15-1).

Trigeminal Nerve

> **Summary Bite.** The mandibular division of the trigeminal nerve (cranial nerve V₃) innervates muscles of the first pharyngeal arch. Autonomic fibers to the salivary glands and taste sensation to the anterior two thirds of the tongue (both from cranial nerve VII) travel on the lingual nerve to reach their destinations. The lingual nerve also provides general sensation to the anterior two thirds of the tongue, gingiva, and adjacent mucosa.

The trigeminal nerve is represented by branches of its mandibular division in the vicinity of the submandibular region (Fig. 15-10; see Tables 18-1 through 18-3). Arising from the inferior alveolar nerve, just before that nerve enters the mandibular foramen, is the **mylohyoid nerve**. This nerve courses inferiorly in a groove on the deep surface of the mandibular ramus to reach the mylohyoid muscle, which it supplies with motor innervation. A small branch continues along the superficial surface of the mylohyoid muscle to supply motor innervation to the anterior belly of the digastric muscle.

The **lingual nerve** arises from the posterior division of the mandibular division of the trigeminal nerve within the infratemporal fossa. Here it is joined by the **chorda tympani**, a branch of the facial nerve, carrying special sensory fibers for taste and preganglionic parasympathetic fibers for the submandibular ganglion (Fig. 15-10).

The lingual nerve courses anteriorly between the mandible and medial pterygoid muscle, obliquely across the styloglossus muscle, and then into the submandibular region. It next passes between the submandibular gland and the hyoglossus muscle and over the submandibular duct to the tip of the tongue, where it provides general sensation to the anterior two thirds of the tongue as well as the adjacent mucosa and gingiva.

Special sensory fibers transmitted to the lingual nerve from the chorda tympani are distributed to all the taste buds on the anterior two thirds of the tongue, with the exception of the taste buds of the circumvallate papilla, which are supplied by the glossopharyngeal nerve.

The **submandibular ganglion**, suspended from the lingual nerve by short filaments, lies on the hyoglossus muscle in the vicinity of the posterior margin of the mylohyoid muscle. In this position, this parasympathetic ganglion is in close association with the submandibular gland (Fig. 15-1).

Preganglionic parasympathetic fibers from the chorda tympani leave the lingual nerve and enter the ganglion to synapse on postganglionic cell bodies. Postganglionic fibers exit the ganglion some to enter the submandibular gland, and some to reenter the lingual nerve for distribution to the sublingual gland and minor salivary glands of the oral cavity, providing them with secretomotor innervation.

Hypoglossal Nerve

> **Summary Bite.** The hypoglossal nerve (cranial nerve XII) provides motor innervation to all of the muscles of the tongue, with the exception of the palatoglossus muscle.

The hypoglossal nerve exits the cranial cavity through the hypoglossal canal to make its way to the tongue musculature. In its course, it passes anteriorly across the external carotid and lingual arteries, remaining above the hyoid bone and lying deep to the posterior digastric and stylohyoid muscles. It continues forward along the genioglossus muscle to the tip of the tongue, providing motor innervation to all of the muscles of the tongue, except the palatoglossus, as described previously (Figs. 15-1, 15-6, and 15-8).

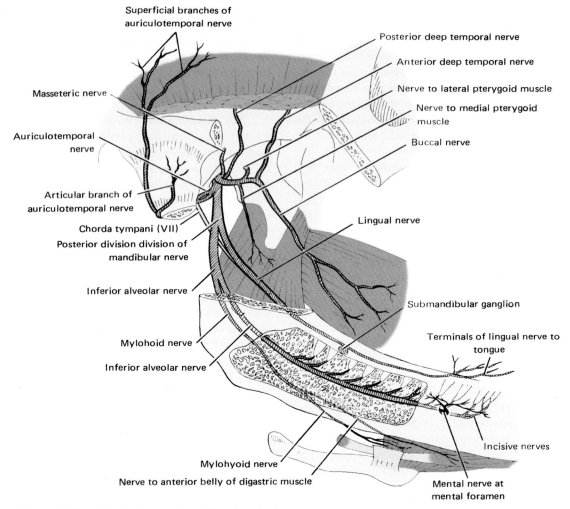

Figure 15-10. Mandibular division of the trigeminal nerve.

Clinical Considerations

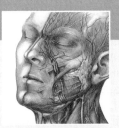

Hypoglossal Nerve Injury

Difficult third molar extractions and/or fractures of the mandible may damage the hypoglossal nerve (cranial nerve XII), causing paralysis of the tongue on the affected side. When the mouth is opened and the tongue is protruded, the genioglossus of the unaffected side will cause the tongue to deviate to the affected side. If the damage is prolonged, the tongue muscles will atrophy.

Near the posterior border of the hyoglossus muscle, branches communicated to the hypoglossal nerve from the first cervical nerve leave the hypoglossal nerve to pass to the thyrohyoid and geniohyoid muscles, providing them with motor innervation.

Nerves to the posterior one third and root of the tongue are derived from branches of the glossopharyngeal and vagus nerves, respectively. Discussion of their contributions to innervation of the tongue is in Chapter 18.

Vascular Supply

> **Summary Bite.** Branches of the lingual and facial arteries provide vascular supply to the submandibular region and floor of the mouth.

Vascular supply to the submandibular region and the floor of the mouth is provided mainly by the lingual and facial arteries (Fig. 15-7).

Other contributions of minor importance provide vascular supply to those structures originating outside the region or located on its periphery, including the occipital and posterior auricular arteries, serving the posterior digastric and stylohyoid muscles, and the mylohyoid artery from the inferior alveolar branch of the mandibular portion of the maxillary artery, serving the mylohyoid muscle.

Lingual Artery

> **Summary Bite.** The lingual artery arises from the external carotid artery and passes deep into the submandibular triangle to enter the tongue, coursing to its tip. On its way, it provides several branches that supply the suprahyoid structures and the substance of the tongue.

The lingual artery arises from the external carotid artery, usually near the greater cornu of the hyoid bone. Sometimes, however, it arises in common with the facial artery, and that common vessel is known as the linguofacial trunk.

The lingual artery passes deep to the posterior digastric, stylohyoid, and hyoglossus muscles to ascend to the tongue, turning anteriorly as it courses to its tip (Fig. 15-7). During its passage, it gives off the following branches: suprahyoid, dorsal lingual, sublingual, and deep lingual arteries.

- The **suprahyoid artery** arises near the hyoid bone and, while staying cranial to it, supplies most of the muscles attaching to the hyoid bone.
- The **dorsal lingual artery** arises deep to the hyoglossus muscle and ascends to the posterior dorsum of the tongue to supply the palatoglossal arch, mucous membrane of the tongue, palatine tonsil, and some of the soft palate; it freely anastomoses with other vessels in the area.
- The **sublingual artery** arises at the anterior margin of the hyoglossus muscle to course between the genioglossus and mylohyoid muscles on its way to the sublingual gland, which it supplies along with other nearby muscles in addition to the mucous membrane of the floor of the mouth and gingiva. This artery anastomoses with the submental branch of the facial artery by branches piercing the mylohyoid muscle.
- The **deep lingual artery** is the terminal of the lingual artery lying immediately deep to the mucous membrane of the inferior surface of the tongue (Fig. 15-5). It lies lateral to the genioglossus muscle and is accompanied by the lingual nerve. Anastomosis is accomplished with its counterpart of the opposite side at the tip of the tongue.

Facial Artery

> **Summary Bite.** The facial artery arises from the external carotid artery to ascend to the submandibular triangle to supply the submandibular gland. Before crossing the mandible to enter the face, it provides several branches to structures in the neck and to suprahyoid structures.

Clinical Considerations

Sublingual Artery Damage

The sublingual artery, occasionally injured during dental procedures, may present problems to the surgeon attempting to ligate its source because it may arise from the submental branch of the facial artery rather than from the lingual artery.

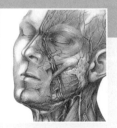

The facial artery, as detailed in Chapter 7, arises from the external carotid artery just cranial to the lingual artery (Fig. 15-7). At first, it ascends deep to the posterior belly of the digastric and stylohyoid muscles and passes through the substance of the submandibular gland before crossing the lateral border of the mandible to enter the face.

Four named branches arise from this artery as it courses through the neck: the ascending palatine, tonsillar, glandular, and submental arteries. These arteries are described in Chapters 7 and 16.

Particularly important to this description are the glandular and submental branches.

■ **Glandular branches** arise from the facial artery as it courses through the submandibular gland, which these branches supply. Postganglionic sympathetic fibers enter the gland via these branches of the facial artery as it courses through it.

■ The **submental artery** arises near the anterior border of the masseter muscle, after the facial artery has exited the submandibular gland but before it ascends to enter the face. The submental artery courses on the mylohyoid muscle, which it serves, in addition to providing branches to the anterior belly of the digastric muscle. A deep branch perforates the mylohyoid muscle to anastomose with the sublingual and mylohyoid arteries. At the symphysis menti, a branch of the artery ascends craniad onto the face to anastomose with the inferior labial artery.

Veins

Summary Bite. Several veins drain the tongue and sublingual area, including the deep lingual vein that is visible on the ventral surface of the tongue. These veins drain into the facial vein or directly into the internal jugular vein.

The tongue and sublingual area are drained by several dorsal lingual veins and a large **deep lingual** vein visible on the ventral surface of the tongue (Fig. 15-5). These veins may empty directly into the internal jugular vein or may drain into the **facial vein**, along with the submental and sublingual veins.

Lymphatics

Summary Bite. A considerable amount of lymph drains into the submandibular/sublingual area. Lymph from the tongue is drained through several nodes. Submandibular nodes drain the nose, lips, gingival, and part of the tongue. Efferents from these and from the submental nodes pass through the jugulodiagastric lymph node (the principal node of the tongue), which is located close to the bifurcation of the common carotid artery.

Several lymphatic channels drain the submandibular/sublingual area (see Fig. 20-2). The lymph vessels of the tongue drain into the submandibular region, with nodes located along the posterior digastric and omohyoid muscles. One node of particular importance, the **jugulodigastric lymph node** (known as the **principal node of the tongue**), lies in close association with the bifurcation of the common carotid artery.

Submandibular nodes, located beneath the mandible in the submandibular triangle, drain that area, including the nose, upper lip, lower lip, gingiva, and the part of the tongue.

Efferents from the submental and submandibular nodes pass into the jugulo-omohyoid lymph node of the deep cervical nodes and eventually into the jugular trunk before emptying into the subclavian vein. The lymphatic system is detailed in Chapter 20.

Palate, Pharynx, and Larynx

16

Key Terms

Palate forms the roof of the oral cavity and separates it from the nasal cavity. The anterior palate contains a bony shelf and is immovable, whereas the posterior soft palate is a flexible muscular structure that seals off the nasal pharynx from the oral pharynx during the process of swallowing.

Pharyngeal Plexus is the neural complex that provides sensory and motor innervation to the structures about the oropharyngeal isthmus, including the palate, nasal pharynx, and oral pharynx. The pharyngeal plexus is located on the posterior wall of the pharynx and receives contributions from the glossopharyngeal nerve (cranial nerve IX), serving the sensory modality; the vagus nerve (cranial nerve X), serving the motor modality; and postganglionic sympathetic nerves from the superior cervical ganglion that supply vasomotor innervation.

Pharynx is a fibromuscular tube that extends from the base of the skull to become continuous with the esophagus at the level of the cricoid cartilage. The pharynx is divided into three regions: nasal pharynx, oral pharynx, and laryngeal pharynx. The posterior pharyngeal wall is composed of three layers of pharyngeal constrictor muscles that partially overlap to appear as partly telescoped.

The pharynx is a passageway for the respiratory and digestive systems, which are separated in the laryngeal pharynx.

Tonsils The palatine tonsils are located in a sinus between the palatoglossal and palatopharyngeal arches. They form a part of a tonsilar ring (the Waldeyer ring) of lymphoid tissue that guards the oropharyngeal entrance. The other components of this ring include a mass of lymphoid tissue, the pharyngeal tonsil located in the posterior wall of nasopharynx, as well as another mass of lymphoid tissue known as the lingual tonsil.

PHARYNGEAL PLEXUS

Innervation of the muscles of the palate, pharynx, and larynx seems confusing because the terminology describing their nerve supply is delineated differently in the various textbooks of anatomy. Two of the muscles, the tensor veli palatini and the stylopharyngeus muscle, are easily detailed because they are innervated by the trigeminal nerve and the glossopharyngeal nerve, respectively. All of the remaining muscles of the palate, pharynx, and larynx receive their innervation either directly by named branches of the vagus nerve or by those branches that the vagus nerve supplies to the pharyngeal plexus. This plexus of nerve fibers, located on the posterior pharyngeal wall at the level of the middle pharyngeal constrictor muscle, consists of pharyngeal branches provided by the glossopharyngeal and vagus nerves, as well as branches from the superior cervical sympathetic ganglion. Glossopharyngeal contributions to the pharyngeal plexus are sensory, the vagal branches are motor, and the sympathetic fibers are vasomotor.

An additional complication must be resolved to clarify the components of the pharyngeal plexus. The cranial portion (motor root) of the accessory nerve and the motor components of the vagus and glossopharyngeal nerves all arise from a singular nucleus in the brain, the nucleus ambiguus.

The motor root of the accessory nerve joins the vagus nerve within the cranial vault, and the three cranial nerves (glossopharyngeal, vagus, and accessory nerves) exit the skull together via the jugular foramen. Because of these complications, some authors specify the pharyngeal plexus, others the vagus nerve, and still others the cranial portion of the accessory nerve as the motor supply of the muscles of the palate, pharynx, and larynx.

For purposes of the present text, with the noted exception of the tensor veli palatini and the stylopharyngeus muscles, *all muscles of the palate, pharynx, and larynx are said to be innervated by named branches of the vagus nerve or via its contributions to the pharyngeal plexus.* This is with the understanding that the motor fibers to these muscles are contributed to the vagus nerve from the cranial root of the accessory nerve.

PALATE

 Summary Bite. The palate forms the roof of the mouth, separating the nasal from the oral cavity. The

anterior portion is bony and is called the hard palate, whereas the posterior portion is without bone and is called the soft palate.

The palate forms the roof of the mouth and the floor of the nasal cavities. It consists of two regions, one containing a bony shelf, the immovable hard palate, and the other, a more posteriorly located, muscular, movable soft palate.

Hard Palate

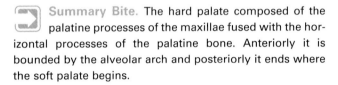 **Summary Bite.** The hard palate composed of the palatine processes of the maxillae fused with the horizontal processes of the palatine bone. Anteriorly it is bounded by the alveolar arch and posteriorly it ends where the soft palate begins.

The hard palate is a bony plate composed of the palatine processes of the maxillae and the horizontal processes of the palatine bones fused in the midline with their counterparts of the opposite side (Fig. 16-1).

Anteriorly and laterally, it is bounded by the alveolar arches, and posteriorly its boundary is demarcated by the beginning of the soft palate. The bone is covered by a specialized mucoperiosteum on both its oral and nasal surfaces. The posterior border of the hard palate possesses the palatine aponeurosis for attachment of the muscles of the soft palate.

The oral aspect of the hard palate may be divided into several regions according to the composition of its soft tissues. Hence, the median raphe region, along the palatal midline, the anterolateral adipose region, and the posterolateral glandular region are recognized as regions of the hard palate (Fig. 16-1).

Soft Palate

Summary Bite. The soft palate is a muscular structure suspended between the oral pharynx and nasal pharynx. Since it is flexible, it may be elevated to isolate the oral cavity from the nasal pharynx.

The soft palate is a muscular structure, encased in a mucous membrane, suspended between the oral pharynx and the nasal pharynx. Its sides are attached to the lateral pharyngeal walls. The anterior portion of the soft palate, near its junction with the hard palate, is almost immobile, whereas its posterior-most extent, the uvula, is capable of great excursion (Fig. 16-1).

Lateral to the uvula is the **palatoglossal arch (palatoglossal fold)**, containing the palatoglossal muscle, forming the **anterior pillar** of the **oropharyngeal isthmus (fauces)**, extending into the side of the tongue.

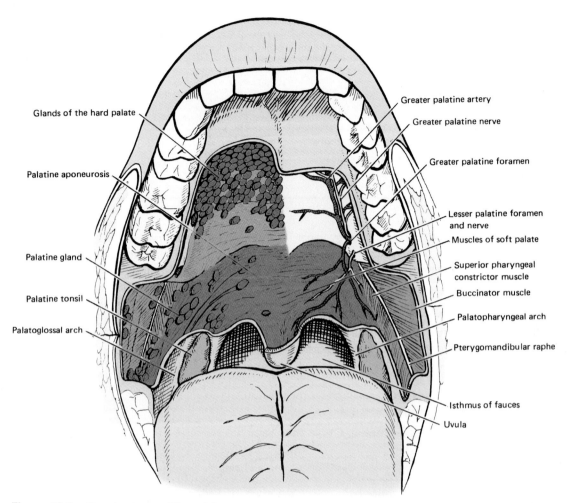

Figure 16-1. The structures of the palate.

Glands of the hard palate

Palatine aponeurosis

Palatine gland

Palatine tonsil

Palatoglossal arch

Greater palatine artery

Greater palatine nerve

Greater palatine foramen

Lesser palatine foramen and nerve

Muscles of soft palate

Superior pharyngeal constrictor muscle

Buccinator muscle

Palatopharyngeal arch

Pterygomandibular raphe

Isthmus of fauces

Uvula

Arising posteriorly is the **palatopharyngeal arch**, containing the **palatopharyngeus muscle**, forming the **posterior pillar of the oropharyngeal isthmus** extending into the lateral pharyngeal wall. The palatine tonsils are located between the two fauces in the tonsillar sinus (Fig. 16-1).

Muscles of the Soft Palate

Summary Bite. Five muscles are associated with the soft palate. These include muscles that originate outside of the soft palate proper and insert into it and other muscles that originate in the soft palate and insert into the

Clinical Considerations

Cleft Palate

Congenital defects of the palate, such as the various degrees of cleft palate, are discussed in Chapter 5.

Hard Palate

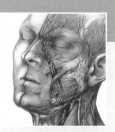

Osseous protrusions, palatal tori, may be observed on the hard palate. These tori, usually bilateral, are asymptomatic, although they can interfere with fitting of maxillary dentures. They may need to be excised surgically before the taking of impressions.

Clinical Considerations

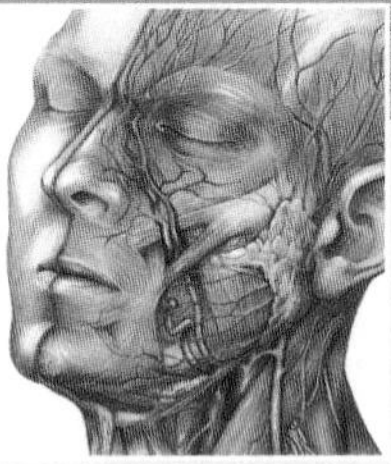

Soft Palate

The soft palate is a movable structure and must be avoided by the posterior aspect of a maxillary denture because its muscular action will break the palatal seal and dislodge the prosthesis.

The posterior aspect of the soft palate is sensitive to touch and may induce vomiting on tactile stimulation.

tongue and/or pharyngeal wall. All are innervated by vagal contributions to the pharyngeal plexus except the tensor veli palatine, which in innervated by the mandibular division of the trigeminal nerve.

The muscles of the soft palate are the levator veli palatini, tensor veli palatini, musculus uvulae, palatoglossus, and palatopharyngeus (Figs. 16-1 and 16-2 and Table 16-1).

Levator Veli Palatini

The **levator veli palatini** is a thick, pencil-shaped muscle that is intimately associated with the lateral aspect of the choana. It has three regions of origin, one tendinous and two fleshy. The tendinous origin is the inferior aspect of the petrous portion of the temporal bone on the proximal aspect of the apex just anteromedial to the entrance into the carotid canal.

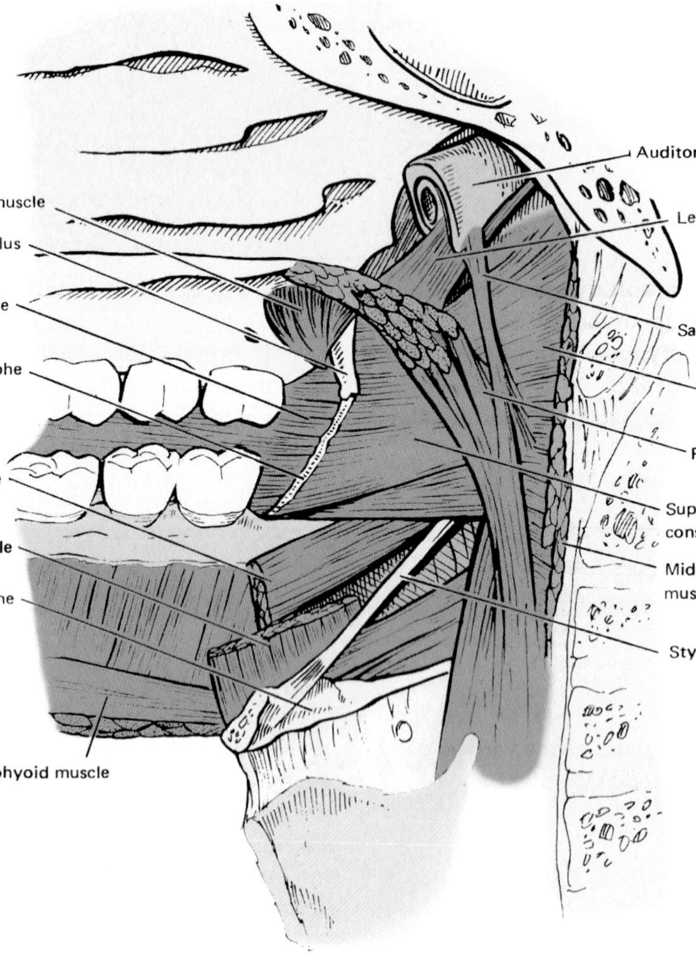
Auditory tube
Tensor veli palatini muscle
Levator veli palatini muscle
Pterygoid hamulus
Buccinator muscle
Salpingopharyngeus muscle
Pterygomandibular raphe
Superior pharyngeal constrictor muscle
Palatopharyngeus muscle
Styloglossus muscle
Superior pharyngeal constrictor muscle
Hyoglossus muscle
Middle pharyngeal constrictor muscle
Hyoid bone
Stylohyoid ligament
Geniohyoid muscle

Figure 16-2. Medial view of a sagittal section of the oropharynx.

Table 16-1   Muscles of the Palate and Pharynx

Name	Origin	Insertion	Innervation	Action
Levator veli palatini	Petrous temporal, tympanic temporal, auditory tube	Palatal aponeurosis	Pharyngeal plexus	Elevates the soft palate; opens auditory tube (?)
Tensor veli palatini	Scaphoid fossa, spine of sphenoid, auditory tube	Palatine aponeurosis	Mandibular division of the trigeminal	Tenses the soft palate, opens auditory tube (?)
Musculus uvulae	Posterior nasal spine, palatine aponeurosis	Uvula	Pharyngeal plexus	Elevates and retracts the uvula
Palatoglossus	Fascia and muscles, lateral aspect of soft palate	Side of the tongue	Pharyngeal plexus	Elevates root of tongue and constricts fauces
Palatopharyngeus	Soft palate	Thyroid cartilage and muscular wall of pharynx	Pharyngeal plexus	Constricts oropharyngeal isthmus and elevates larynx
Stylopharyngeus	Styloid process	Muscular wall of the pharynx, thyroid cartilage	Glossopharyngeal	Elevates the larynx and pharynx
Salpingo-pharyngeus	Auditory tube	Muscular wall of the pharynx	Pharyngeal plexus	Elevates pharynx; opens auditory tube (?)
Superior pharyngeal constrictor	Medial pterygoid plate and hamulus; pterygo-mandibular raphe; mylohyoid line of mandible; alveolar process of mandible; root of tongue	Pharyngeal raphe; pharyngeal tubercle	Pharyngeal plexus	Constricts the pharynx
Middle pharyngeal constrictor	Lesser and greater cornua of hyoid bone; stylohyoid ligament	Pharyngeal raphe	Pharyngeal plexus	Constricts the pharynx
Inferior pharyngeal constrictor	Cricoid cartilage; thyroid cartilage	Pharyngeal raphe	Pharyngeal plexus and external and recurrent laryngeal branches of vagus	Constricts the pharynx and acts as a pharyngoesophageal sphincter

The fleshy origins are from the tympanic part of the temporal bone and from the cartilage of the auditory tube. The muscle fibers are directed medially, between the salpingopharyngeus and tensor veli palatini muscles, to insert into the palatal aponeurosis, passing between the two layers of the palatopharyngeus muscle.

As the levator inserts into the soft palate, its muscle fibers interdigitate with those of its counterpart from the other side. This muscle is innervated by the vagus nerve via its contributions to the pharyngeal plexus. The levator veli palatini, as its name implies, elevates the soft palate.

Tensor Veli Palatini

The **tensor veli palatini**, a pyramid-shaped muscle, is situated anterior to the levator veli palatini and medial to the medial pterygoid muscle. It originates in the scaphoid fossa, on the spine of the sphenoid bone, and the cartilaginous portion of the auditory tube. The fibers collect into a tendinous cord that wraps medially around the hamulus of the medial pterygoid plate to insert into the palatine aponeurosis.

The tensor veli palatini is innervated by a branch of the nerve to the medial pterygoid, arising from the mandibular division of the trigeminal nerve. This muscle acts to flatten and tense the soft palate.

Musculus Uvulae

The **musculus uvulae** is a small, thin muscle lying between the two layers of the palatine aponeurosis. The muscle originates on the posterior nasal spine of the palatine bone and from the palatine aponeurosis to insert in common with its counterpart from the opposite side, forming the substance of the uvula.

The musculus uvulae is innervated by the vagus nerve via its contributions to branches of the pharyngeal plexus. It acts to retract and elevate the uvula.

Palatoglossus

The **palatoglossus muscle**, a small, longitudinally disposed muscle, is overlaid by a mucous membrane, thus forming the palatoglossal arch. It is a thin, cylindrical muscle originating in the fascia and musculature of the lateral aspect of the soft palate. It inserts by interdigitating with the intrinsic muscles of the tongue in its lateral margin.

Motor innervation to the muscle is derived from the vagus nerve via its contributions to branches of the pharyngeal plexus. The palatoglossus acts to elevate the posterior one third of the tongue and, acting with its counterpart on the other side, constricts the fauces.

Palatopharyngeus

The **palatopharyngeus muscle** and its mucosal covering form the palatopharyngeal arch. It is a long, thin, cylindrical muscle arising by two fleshy slips from the side of the soft palate, with the levator veli palatini and the musculus uvulae being interposed between the two origins. The muscle inserts, along with fibers of the stylopharyngeus muscle, into the posterior aspect of the thyroid cartilage and also into the muscular coat of the pharynx.

The palatopharyngeus receives its motor fibers from the vagus nerve via its contributions to branches of the pharyngeal plexus. This muscle functions to elevate the pharynx and larynx and to assist in closing the oropharyngeal isthmus.

Vascular and Sensory Nerve Supply

Vascular Supply

Summary Bite. The major vascular supply to the palate is provided by the greater and lesser palatine arteries (branches of the maxillary artery), whereas minor contributions are from the ascending palatine branch of the facial artery and the ascending pharyngeal branch of the external carotid artery.

The vascular supply of the palate is derived chiefly from the greater and lesser palatine branches of the maxillary artery, the ascending palatine branch of the facial artery, and the ascending pharyngeal artery from the external carotid artery (Fig. 16-1).

The greater and lesser palatine arteries descend in the pterygopalatine canal to enter the palate via the greater and lesser palatine foramina, respectively.

The **greater palatine artery** passes anteriorly on the lateral aspect of the hard palate to supply the palatal mucosa, gingiva, and glands, and then proceeds to anastomose with the nasopalatine artery in the incisive canal.

The **lesser palatine artery** vascularizes the soft palate and tonsil and then anastomoses with the ascending palatine branch of the facial artery. The lesser palatine bifurcates, and one branch travels along the surface of the levator veli palatini muscle to vascularize the soft palate. The other branch perforates the superior constrictor muscle to serve the auditory tube and the tonsil.

The **ascending pharyngeal artery** from the external carotid artery travels along the lateral external surface of the superior constrictor muscle, reaches the levator veli palatini muscle, and gives off a palatine branch to serve the tonsil, auditory tube, and soft palate.

Venous drainage is by similarly named veins that are tributaries of the pterygoid and tonsillar plexus.

Sensory Nerve Supply

Summary Bite. The major sensory nerve supply to the palate is provided by the greater and lesser palatine branches of the maxillary division of the trigeminal nerve as well as from its nasopalatine nerve.

Sensory nerve supply of the palate is derived chiefly from the greater and lesser palatine branches of the maxillary division of the trigeminal nerve, which also carry sensory fibers from the facial nerve via the greater petrosal nerve. Additional sensory supply is derived from the nasopalatine nerve of the posterosuperior nasal branch of the maxillary division of the trigeminal nerve and the tonsillar branches of the glossopharyngeal nerve.

Palatine Tonsil

Summary Bite. The palatine tonsil is a lymphoid mass that lies within a sinus between the palatoglossal and palatopharyngeal arches. It is a part of the Waldeyer ring, which guards the oropharyngeal entrance. The tonsil is richly vascularized and receives its nerve supply by the tonsillar branches from the glossopharyngeal nerve.

The **palatine tonsil**, located in the tonsillar sinus between the palatoglossal and palatopharyngeal arches, is an almond-shaped mass of lymphoid tissue covered

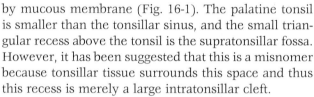

Clinical Considerations

Palatine Tonsils

The palatine tonsils of a child are much larger than those of an adult. They are prone to infection because they tend to accumulate debris in the tonsillar crypts. Frequent tonsillitis may indicate the need for tonsillectomy, a relatively minor surgical procedure in children. However, the proximity of the tonsils to the common carotid artery and the rich vascular supply of the tonsils necessitate extreme care in the procedure. Moreover, the glossopharyngeal nerve as well as an unusually tortuous internal carotid artery may also be vulnerable to injury.

by mucous membrane (Fig. 16-1). The palatine tonsil is smaller than the tonsillar sinus, and the small triangular recess above the tonsil is the supratonsillar fossa. However, it has been suggested that this is a misnomer because tonsillar tissue surrounds this space and thus this recess is merely a large intratonsillar cleft.

The medial surface of the tonsil is visible when the tongue is depressed, and presents tonsillar crypts that may invade nearly the entire depth of the tonsil. The lateral or deep surface is covered by a fibrous capsule, separating the tonsil from the pharyngeal musculature. The palatine tonsil forms a part of the **tonsillar circle (the Waldeyer ring)**, which guards the oropharyngeal entrance.

Arterial supply to the palatine tonsil is derived from branches of four arteries. The facial artery via its tonsillar branch is the chief vascular supplier of the tonsil, but this artery also makes a minor contribution via its ascending palatine branch. Other minor vessels serving the palatine tonsil are the palatine branch of the ascending pharyngeal, the lesser palatine branch of the maxillary artery, and the tonsillar twig from the dorsal lingual branch of the lingual artery.

Venous drainage is by way of the tonsillar plexus of veins on the deep aspect of the tonsil, a tributary of the pharyngeal venous plexus, and the facial vein.

Sensory innervation to the palatine tonsil is from the glossopharyngeal nerve and the lesser palatine branches of the maxillary division of the trigeminal nerve. Contributions are also derived from the greater petrosal branch of the facial nerve via the trigeminal nerve.

PHARYNX

Summary Bite. The pharynx extends from the base of the skull to become continuous with the esophagus.

It is divided into the nasal, oral, and laryngeal parts. The basic muscular wall is composed of the constrictor muscles that resemble a telescoped fibromuscular tube.

The pharynx is a fibromuscular tube, 12 to 14 cm long, extending from the base of the skull to become continuous with the esophagus. It is broadest at its cranial extent and narrowest at its esophageal junction.

- Superiorly, it is attached to the basilar part of the occipital bone and the body of the sphenoid bone.
- Laterally, it is fixed to the medial pterygoid plate, pterygomandibular raphe, alveolar process of the mandible, lateral aspect of the tongue, hyoid bone, and thyroid and cricoid cartilages.
- Posteriorly, the pharynx approximates the bodies of the first six cervical vertebrae, being separated from them by the prevertebral fascia.
- Anteriorly, the pharynx has no complete wall; instead, it opens into the nasal, oral, and laryngeal cavities.

Consequently, the pharynx is conveniently divided into nasal, oral, and laryngeal parts.

Nasal Pharynx

Summary Bite. The nasal pharynx is the superior-most portion of the pharynx. It communicates with the oral pharynx via the pharyngeal isthmus, which can be sealed by the soft palate. It also communicates with the auditory tube. The posterior wall contains the pharyngeal tonsil.

The nasal pharynx is the superior-most and broadest region of the pharynx. Its walls are rigid and present, on the two lateral aspects, several elevations. Anteriorly, it begins at the paired choanae; inferiorly, it is limited by the soft palate (Figs. 16-2 through 16-5).

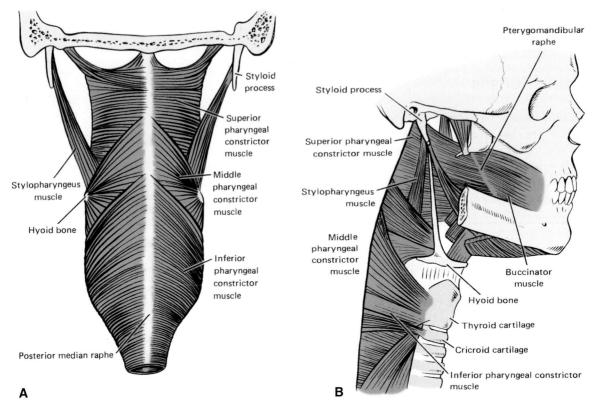

Figure 16-3. Muscles of the pharynx. **(A)** Posterior view. **(B)** Lateral view.

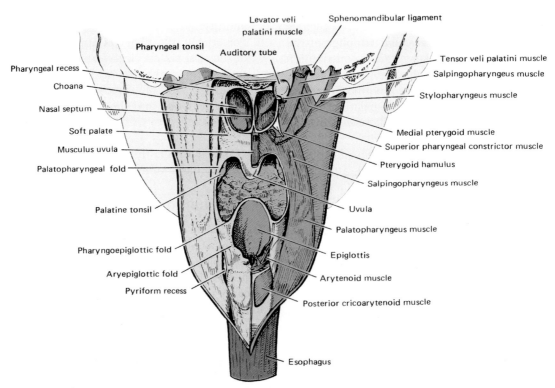

Figure 16-4. Posterior view of the palate, pharynx, and larynx.

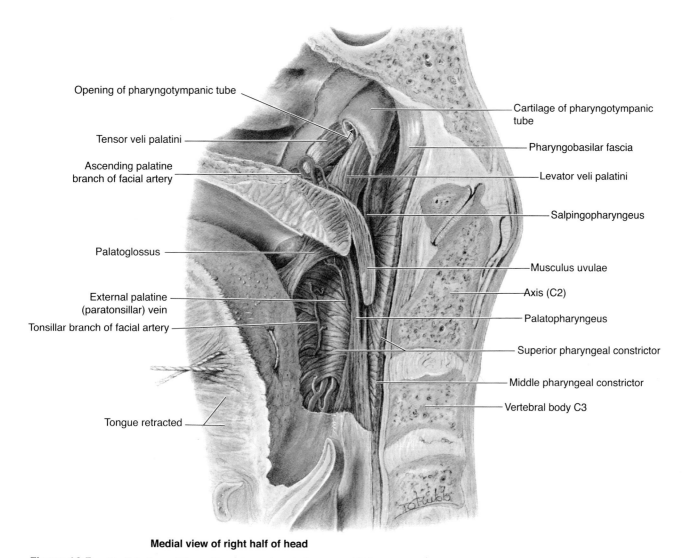

Opening of pharyngotympanic tube

Tensor veli palatini

Ascending palatine
branch of facial artery

Palatoglossus

External palatine
(paratonsillar) vein

Tonsillar branch of facial artery

Tongue retracted

Cartilage of pharyngotympanic
tube

Pharyngobasilar fascia

Levator veli palatini

Salpingopharyngeus

Musculus uvulae

Axis (C2)

Palatopharyngeus

Superior pharyngeal constrictor

Middle pharyngeal constrictor

Vertebral body C3

Medial view of right half of head

Figure 16-5. Medial view of the soft palate and oral pharyngeal isthmus.

During respiration, the soft palate is flaccid and the nasal pharynx communicates with the oral pharynx through the **pharyngeal isthmus**, a space between the posterior wall of the pharynx and the free border of the soft palate.

During deglutition, the soft palate is elevated and contacts the posterior wall of the pharynx, blocking the communication between the nasal and oral cavities.

The lateral wall of the nasal pharynx presents an opening, the **ostium of the auditory tube**, which is located inferoposterior to the inferior nasal concha. This ostium is located on the medial end of the cartilaginous auditory tube, which, protruding into the nasal pharynx, forms an elevation called the **torus tubarium**.

Behind the torus is the **pharyngeal recess**, a mucosa-lined space extending to the base of the skull. Two folds extend from the torus: the smaller salpingopalatal fold covers the levator veli palatini muscle, extending

from below the ostium of the internal auditory tube to the root of the soft palate, and the larger salpingopharyngeal fold covers the salpingopharyngeus muscle, extending from the posteroinferior aspect of the torus and passing inferiorly, becoming indistinguishable as the muscle merges with the muscles of the pharynx.

The posterior wall of the nasopharynx contains a mass of lymphatic tissue, the **pharyngeal tonsil**.

Oral Pharynx

Summary Bite. The oral pharynx extends from the soft palate to the epiglottis and contains the palatine tonsil.

The oral pharynx is relatively uncomplicated, being that portion of the chamber that leads into the laryngeal pharynx. It extends from the soft palate to the

Clinical Considerations

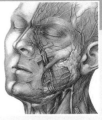

Adenoids

Adenoids is the term that commonly refers to the pathologic state when the pharyngeal tonsil becomes hypertrophied due to infection. Excessive hypertrophy partially (or completely) blocks the posterior choanae, necessitating mouth breathing and causing nasal speech and loud snoring during sleep. Persistent inflammation and infection of the pharyngeal tonsil may lead to spreading of the infection into the internal auditory tube, resulting in otitis media, with subsequent temporary or permanent hearing loss. The infection may eventually reach the mastoid air cells. Although in the past this was a relatively common disease (treated with mastoidectomy), the advent of antibiotics has done much to control and subdue it.

---

cranial aspect of the epiglottis, which is positioned at the level of the hyoid bone.

Anteriorly, the oral pharynx begins at the oral cavity via the **oropharyngeal isthmus**. The lateral wall of the oral pharynx presents the palatine tonsil between the palatoglossal and palatopharyngeal arches (Figs.16-1 through 16-5).

Laryngeal Pharynx

> **Summary Bite** The laryngeal pharynx begins at the epiglottis and becomes continuous with the esophagus at the inferior border of the cricoid cartilage.

The laryngeal pharynx, the inferior-most region of the pharynx, extends from the epiglottis, at the level of the hyoid bone, to the esophagus, at the level of the inferior border of the cricoid cartilage (Figs. 16-4 and 16-5).

Anteriorly, it begins at the larynx, whose aperture appears to be guarded by the epiglottis—a movable, flaplike structure. The **epiglottis** is connected to the midline and side of the pharyngeal root of the tongue by the **median** and **lateral glossoepiglottic folds**, respectively. The resultant fossa on either side of the median glossoepiglottic fold is known as the **epiglottic vallecula**.

Inferior to the laryngeal opening, the anterior wall of the laryngeal pharynx consists of the posterior, mucosa-lined aspect of the arytenoid and cricoid cartilages. The mucosal **aryepiglottic fold** connecting the epiglottis to the arytenoid cartilage constitutes the lateral boundary of the opening of the larynx. Lateral to this fold is a fossa, the **pinform recess**, whose lateral border is the thyroid cartilage with its thyrohyoid membrane.

The internal laryngeal nerve and its branches pass just deep to the mucosal floor of this recess.

Pharyngeal Wall

> **Summary Bite** The pharyngeal wall consists of an inner-most mucous layer, a middle fibrous and muscular layer, and the outer fibrous layer. Lying deep to the mucosa is the pharyngobasilar fascia attached to the base of the skull. It also attaches at various bony or cartilaginous structures along its path. Finally, it attaches to the pharyngeal raphe, a longitudinal fibrous band on the posterior wall of the pharynx.

Clinical Considerations

Pharynx

The laryngopharynx, specifically the piriform recess, is a common site for lodging of sharp objects, such as chicken and fish bones. The presence of foreign material in this region causes gagging, and the person is unable to remove the irritant. Care must be exercised in working in the piriform recess, for deep to the mucous membrane is the internal laryngeal nerve, which may be damaged during probing procedures.

The pharyngeal wall is composed of three layers: an inner-most mucous layer, a middle fibrous and muscular layer, and an outer fibrous layer. The mucosa lining the pharynx is continuous with the mucosa of the chambers into which the pharynx opens. Hence, it is either a respiratory or an oral type of mucosa.

Just deep to the mucosa is the **pharyngobasilar fascia**, a layer of fibrous connective tissue that is especially thick craniad but dwindles as it progresses caudally. The cranial portion of the pharyngobasilar fascia has no muscular covering. It is attached to the base of the skull at various points: at the basilar portion of the occipital bone, anterior to the pharyngeal tubercle; at the petrous temporal bone; and at the medial pterygoid plate. Further anteriorly, it is attached to structures in the neck, thyroid cartilage, hyoid bone, stylohyoid ligament, and pterygomandibular raphe. A region of this fascia is attached posteriorly to a strong, longitudinally oriented, fibrous band of connective tissue, the **pharyngeal raphe**, which extends from the pharyngeal tubercle of the occipital bone almost to the caudal border of the pharynx.

The constrictor muscles of the pharynx insert into the pharyngeal raphe. The muscular layer of the pharynx is positioned between the pharyngobasilar fascia and the thin, outer-most layer of the pharynx, the **buccopharyngeal fascia**. Cranially, in the region devoid of the superior constrictor, this fascia fuses with the pharyngobasilar fascia.

Nerves and vessels traveling along the pharynx course in the buccopharyngeal fascia.

Muscles of the Pharynx

Summary Bite. In addition to the superior, middle, and inferior pharyngeal constrictor muscles of the pharynx, additional accessory muscles originate from other areas and insert into the pharynx.

The musculature of the pharynx is composed of the superior, middle, and inferior pharyngeal constrictors as well as the stylopharyngeus, salpingopharyngeus, and palatopharyngeus muscles (the last muscle is discussed earlier in this chapter; Figs. 16-2 through 16-5, and Table 16-1).

The constrictor muscles partly overlap each other and may be visualized as three sleeves partially telescoped inside one another from superior to inferior.

Superior Pharyngeal Constrictor
The **superior pharyngeal constrictor** is a thin, quadrilateral muscle whose fibers originate from the pterygoid hamulus and an adjoining region of the medial pterygoid plate, the pterygomandibular raphe, the posterior quarter of the mylohyoid line, the alveolar

process of the mandible, and the lateral aspect of the root of the tongue.

The muscle fibers curve posteriorly to insert into the pharyngeal raphe and pharyngeal tubercle. A thin slip of this muscle, couched on the internal surface of its cranial portion, passes lateral to the levator veli palatini muscle. It arises from the palatal aponeurosis and merges with the fibers of the main muscle mass of the superior constrictor. This muscle slip, the **palatopharyngeal sphincter**, produces a ridge, the **bar of Passavant**, on the posterior pharyngeal wall, which is contacted by the elevated soft palate during deglutition, effectively separating the nasal pharynx from the oral pharynx.

The superior constrictor, innervated by the vagus nerve via its contributions to branches of the pharyngeal plexus, acts to constrict the pharynx.

Middle Pharyngeal Constrictor
The **middle pharyngeal constrictor**, a fan-shaped muscular sheet, originates on the lesser and greater cornua of the hyoid bone and the stylohyoid ligament. The cranial fibers pass superficial to the superior constrictor muscle, thus covering part of it; the inferior fibers pass deep to the inferior constrictor muscle. The middle constrictor inserts into the median raphe.

The middle pharyngeal constrictor is innervated by the vagus nerve via its contributions to branches of the pharyngeal plexus and acts to constrict the pharynx.

Inferior Pharyngeal Constrictor
The **inferior pharyngeal constrictor**, the caudal-most of the three constrictors, envelops the lower part of the middle constrictor. It arises from the lateral aspect of the cricoid cartilage, from the oblique line of the thyroid cartilage and the area behind it, to insert into the pharyngeal raphe. The caudal-most fibers of the inferior constrictor are continuous with the cranial-most, circular inner muscle fibers of the esophagus.

The inferior constrictor receives its motor nerve supply from the vagus nerve via its contributions to branches of the pharyngeal plexus and from the external and recurrent laryngeal branches of the vagus nerve.

Functionally, the inferior constrictor may be considered to have two parts: the superior thyropharyngeal and the inferior cricopharyngeal. The former constricts the pharynx, and the latter acts as a pharyngoesophageal sphincter, preventing reflux of esophageal contents into the pharynx.

Stylopharyngeus
The **stylopharyngeus muscle**, a long, thin, cylinder-shaped muscle, arises from the styloid process of the

temporal bone and passes inferomedially between the middle and superior pharyngeal constrictor muscles to insert in common with the palatopharyngeus muscle on the dorsal aspect of the thyroid cartilage.

The stylopharyngeus is the only muscle to receive its motor innervation from the glossopharyngeal nerve. It acts to elevate the larynx and pharynx.

Salpingopharyngeus

The **salpingopharyngeus muscle** is a thin, fusiform muscle arising from the inferior aspect of the cartilaginous auditory tube at its terminal end in the nasopharynx. The salpingopharyngeus passes inferiorly, deep to the pharyngeal mucosa, to insert into the muscular wall of the pharynx by interdigitating with the fibers of the palatopharyngeus muscle.

The salpingopharyngeus is innervated by the vagus nerve via its contributions to branches of the pharyngeal plexus. It functions in elevating the pharynx and may assist in opening the auditory tube during deglutition.

Vascular and Sensory Nerve Supply of the Pharynx

Vascular Supply

> **Summary Bite.** Pharyngeal branches from the external carotid artery, the maxillary artery, and branches of the facial artery supply the pharynx. The caudal portion of the pharynx is supplied by the superior and inferior thyroid arteries.

Arterial supply of the cranial portion of the pharynx is derived chiefly from the ascending pharyngeal branch of the external carotid artery, the pharyngeal branches of the maxillary artery, and the ascending palatine and tonsillar branches of the facial artery.

The superior thyroid and, to a lesser extent, the inferior thyroid arteries supply the caudal portion of the pharynx.

Venous drainage is via a plexus of veins, the **pharyngeal plexus**, located between the prevertebral fascia and the constrictor muscles. This plexus is drained by the pterygoid plexus of veins and the internal jugular and facial veins.

Sensory Nerve Supply

> **Summary Bite** Sensory nerves to the naso- and oropharynx are branches of the maxillary division of the trigeminal and glossopharyngeal nerves, whereas the sensory supply to the remainder of the pharynx is supplied by the glossopharyngeal and vagus nerves.

Sensory innervation of the nasopharynx and part of the oropharynx is via branches of the maxillary division of the trigeminal and glossopharyngeal nerves.

The remainder of the pharynx is supplied by branches of the glossopharyngeal and vagus nerves. In addition, as indicated previously, overlapping innervation in the region of the fauces is provided by the facial nerve via its greater petrosal branch.

ESOPHAGUS

> **Summary Bite.** The esophagus serves as a passageway for food from the pharynx to the stomach. The trachea lies anterior to it, and the groove between these two structures is a passageway for the recurrent laryngeal nerve.

The esophagus is a 25-cm long muscular tube whose main function is to serve as a passageway for food from the pharynx to the stomach (Fig. 16-4).

Along its length, the esophagus resides in the neck, thorax, and abdomen. It is situated somewhat anterior to the bodies of the vertebrae, until it pierces the diaphragm to enter the abdomen. The lumen of the esophagus is normally closed in its cervical and abdominal portions, whereas the thoracic portion is usually partially patent and contains air.

The esophagus is in close association with various important structures along its descent through the neck and thorax, but only its cervical relations will be considered here.

It begins at the level of the sixth cervical vertebra, as a continuation of the pharynx, near the inferior border of the cricoid cartilage, where the esophagus lies on the prevertebral fascia over the longus colli muscle. The trachea lies directly anterior to the esophagus, thus creating a tracheoesophageal groove in which the recurrent laryngeal nerve makes its ascent.

Lateral to the esophagus is the carotid sheath, with its neurovascular contents. The thyroid gland, specifically its lateral lobes, is also in close association with the lateral aspect of the esophagus. Although the microscopic anatomy of the esophagus is not pertinent to the study of its gross morphology, mention should be made of the fact that the external muscular layers are composed of skeletal muscle in the cervical portion of the esophagus, smooth muscle in the lower thoracic and abdominal regions, and a combination of the two in the upper and middle thoracic regions.

Vascular supply of the cervical portion of the esophagus is via the inferior thyroid arteries and veins, and its nerve supply is derived from the recurrent laryngeal nerve, a branch of the vagus nerve, and the cervical sympathetic trunk.

Clinical Considerations

Esophageal Defects

A relatively common type of developmental defect of the esophagus is the tracheoesophageal fistula, which usually occurs just cranial to or at the bifurcation of the trachea. This anomaly is less common in females than in males. The fistula provides esophageal (and occasionally gastric) contents with free access to the respiratory system. This defect is the result of abnormal partitioning of the esophagus and trachea by the tracheoesophageal septum during embryonic development.

LARYNX

Summary Bite. The larynx is continuous with the laryngeal pharynx and the trachea. It is composed of several cartilages, intrinsic muscles, membranes, and ligaments that, acting in concert, control the inspiration and expiration of air between the laryngeal pharynx and the trachea. It also functions as the organ of phonation and modulation of sound.

The larynx, or voice box, is continuous with the -laryngeal pharynx cranially and with the trachea caudally (Figs. 16-3, 16-4, 16-6, and 16-7).

It is a passageway for inspired and expired air; a sphincter preventing the entry of solids or liquids into the respiratory system caudal to itself; and an organ of phonation permitting the production and modulation of sound.

It is composed of a series of cartilages, muscles, membranes, and ligaments that, acting in concert,

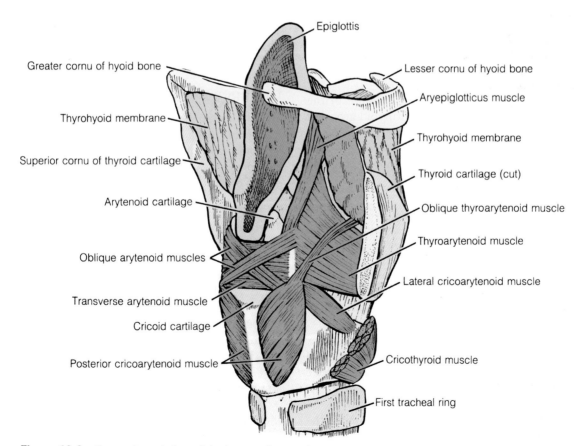

Figure 16-6. Posterolateral view of the laryngeal musculature.

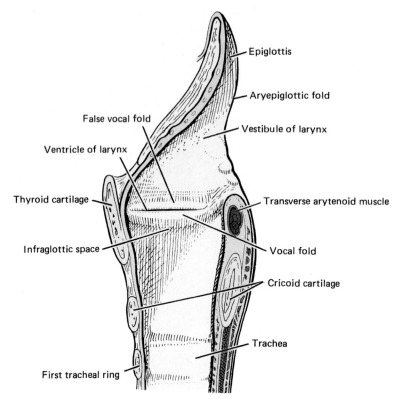

Figure 16-7. Sagittal section of the larynx.

accomplish these functions. It is interesting to note that the larynx of the male and female are the same size before puberty; however, in adults the male larynx is larger than that of the female.

The larynx lies anteriorly in the midline of the neck and is covered by skin, the infrahyoid group of muscles, and associated fascia. The great vessels of the neck pass posterolateral to it. It is lined by a mucous membrane, which is continuous with and similar to those of the pharynx and trachea. This membrane is modified in places to form two pairs of folds, the cranially positioned ventricular fold (false vocal folds) and the caudally placed vocal folds (true vocal folds), the latter overlying the vocalis muscles and being responsible for the formation of sound (Fig. 16-7).

It is convenient to describe the **cavity of the larynx** as consisting of three compartments: the vestibule, the ventricle, and the infraglottic cavity.

- The **vestibule** extends from the **superior laryngeal aperture** (aditus) to the **rima glottidis** (the space between the two true vocal folds and the two arytenoid cartilages).
- The **ventricle** is a space lying directly between the ventricular and vocal cords, being lateral outpocketings of the vestibule.

- The **infraglottic cavity** is the space between the rima glottidis and the beginning of the tracheal cavity.

Laryngeal Cartilages

Summary Bite. Nine cartilages make up the framework of the larynx: the unpaired thyroid, cricoid, and epiglottic cartilages and the paired arytenoid, cuneiform, and corniculate cartilages. Most of these cartilages serve as origins or insertion sites for the intrinsic muscles.

Thyroid Cartilage

The **thyroid cartilage** is composed of two quadrilateral plates, the right and left **laminae**, which fuse to form the **laryngeal prominence** (Adam's apple) of the neck. The angle of fusion is more acute in the male than in the female, accounting for the sexual dimorphism evidenced by this structure. Superiorly, this prominence ends in the **superior thyroid notch** and, inferiorly, in the inferior thyroid notch. The superior and inferior borders of each lamina end posteriorly in a **superior** and **inferior cornu**, respectively.

The posterolateral surface of the cartilage bears the **oblique line**, extending from the superior to the inferior thyroid tubercles. The medial surface of the thyroid lamina is smooth and unremarkable.

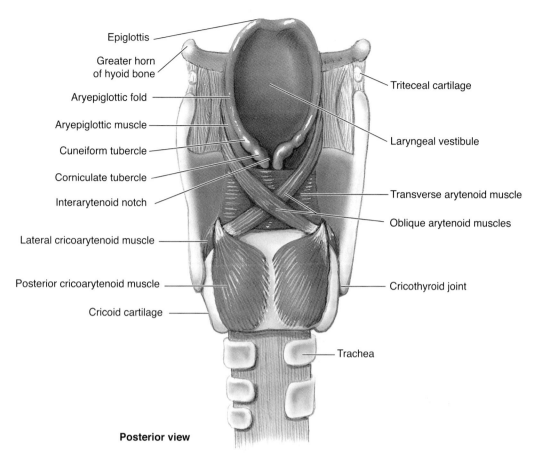

Epiglottis

Greater horn
of hyoid bone

Aryepiglottic fold

Aryepiglottic muscle

Cuneiform tubercle

Corniculate tubercle

Interarytenoid notch

Lateral cricoarytenoid muscle

Posterior cricoarytenoid muscle

Cricoid cartilage

Triteceal cartilage

Laryngeal vestibule

Transverse arytenoid muscle

Oblique arytenoid muscles

Cricothyroid joint

Trachea

Posterior view

Figure 16-8. Larynx (posterior view).

Cricoid Cartilage

The **cricoid cartilage** is a ring-shaped structure whose width is greater posteriorly than anteriorly. It comprises the anteroinferior and lateroinferior walls as well as most of the posterior wall of the larynx. It consists of a quadrilateral, dorsal lamina and a ventral, narrow arch. At each junction of the lamina and the arch are the facets for articulation of the cricoid with the inferior cornua of the thyroid cartilage.

The internal surface of the cricoid cartilage is smooth and unremarkable. The superior margin of the lamina on either side of the midline bears two elliptical depressions for articulation with the arytenoid cartilages.

Epiglottic Cartilage

The **epiglottic cartilage**, an unpaired, leaflike elastic cartilage, is attached by the thyroepiglottic ligament to the internal aspect of the laryngeal prominence, just inferior to the superior thyroid notch. This ligament attaches to the slender petiole, the narrow, inferior, stalklike extension of the epiglottic cartilage.

The broad, leaf-shaped, superior portion of the epiglottic cartilage extends craniad but in a posterior direction behind the tongue and hyoid bone, projecting above and anterior to the superior laryngeal aperture. Laterally, the aryepiglottic folds attach the epiglottis to the arytenoid cartilages.

The epiglottis is invested by a mucous membrane that is continuous with the mucosa of the root of the tongue and the lateral pharyngeal walls. The mucosa forms three folds between the tongue and the epiglottis: the single median glossoepiglottic fold and the two lateral glossoepiglottic folds. The depressions between these folds, on either side of the median glossoepiglottic fold, are known as the **epiglottic valleculae**.

Arytenoid Cartilage

The paired **arytenoid cartilages** are pyramidal structures located on the superior border of the lamina of the cricoid cartilage. The arytenoid cartilage has a concave base that articulates with the arytenoid articular surface of the cricoid lamina, a dorsomedially inclined apex to which the corniculate cartilage attaches, and three surfaces that provide attachments for muscles and ligaments.

The base has two free processes: the lateral angle, which is the **muscular process**, the point of insertion for the posterior and lateral cricoarytenoid muscles, and the anterior angle, or **vocal process**, to which the vocal cord attaches.

The posterior surface serves for the attachments of the transverse arytenoid muscles. The ventrolateral surface presents a superiorly positioned, triangular fovea containing mucous glands and providing attachment to the vestibular ligament. Positioned inferiorly is an oblong fovea that is the site of attachment for the vocalis and, frequently, the lateral cricoarytenoid muscles. The medial surface is smooth and is invested by a mucous membrane.

Corniculate and Cuneiform Cartilages

The **corniculate and cuneiform cartilages** are tiny pieces of elastic cartilage. The former articulates with the arytenoid apex, whereas the latter is attached to the aryepiglottic fold just anterior to the corniculate cartilage.

Membranes, Ligaments, and Muscles

> **Summary Bite** The larynx is composed of several membranes and ligaments, which are associated with the muscles that move the cartilages. Tensions and movements of the vocal ligaments and vocal cords modulate the air passage through the larynx producing audible sounds.

Deep to the laryngeal mucosa is a thick, intrinsic membrane of elastic lamina whose cranial portion is referred to as the **quadrangular membrane** and whose caudal portion is the **elastic cone**.

The inferior free edge of the quadrangular membrane assists in the formation of the ventricular vocal cords. The elastic cone has a well-defined anterior portion, known as the **median cricothyroid ligament**, and two thickened lateral portions, the **vocal ligaments**, whose free edges assist in formation of the vocal cords. Two extrinsic membranes of interest are the **thyrohyoid** and **cricothyroid membranes**. The former is a thick, fibroelastic membrane suspended between the body and greater cornua of the hyoid bone superiorly and the cranial aspect of the thyroid cartilage inferiorly. It becomes thicker in its median portion, thus its name, median thyrohyoid ligament, whereas the lateral portions are called lateral thyrohyoid ligaments. The median cricothyroid ligament is a narrow band of fibroelastic tissue connecting the superior rim of the cricoid cartilage with the inferior

rim of the thyroid cartilage. Issuing from the inferior rim of the cricoid cartilage and attaching to the superior rim of the first tracheal cartilage is the cricotracheal ligament.

Muscles of the Larynx

> **Summary Bite** The muscles of the larynx may be classed into extrinsic and intrinsic groups. The extrinsic muscles have been described previously. There are six bilateral pairs of intrinsic muscles.

The intrinsic muscles of the larynx are the cricothyroid, lateral cricoarytenoid, posterior cricoarytenoid, arytenoid, and thyroarytenoid, and the vocalis (see Fig. 16-8 and Table 16-2).

Cricothyroid Muscle

The **cricothyroid muscle** is situated on the ventrolateral aspect of the larynx, bridging the space between the cricoid and thyroid cartilages (Fig. 16-6). It originates on the arch of the cricoid cartilage and fans out to insert onto the inferior margin of the lamina and the inferior cornu of the thyroid cartilage.

The external branch of the superior laryngeal branch of the vagus nerve supplies the cricothyroid muscle. This muscle acts to elevate and tip the thyroid cartilage ventrally, thus placing tension on the vocal cords.

Lateral Cricoarytenoid Muscle

The **lateral cricoarytenoid muscle** is a small muscle originating on the arch of the cricoid cartilage to insert onto the muscular process of the arytenoid cartilage (Fig. 16-6). This muscle is frequently fused with the thyroarytenoid muscle.

Inferior laryngeal branches of the recurrent laryngeal nerve, a branch of the vagus nerve, supply motor innervation to this muscle. The lateral cricoarytenoid muscle acts to adduct the vocal cord by rotating the vocal process of the arytenoid cartilage in a medioinferior direction. This movement approximates the two vocal cords, narrowing the rima glottidis.

Posterior Cricoarytenoid Muscle

The **posterior cricoarytenoid muscle** arises from most of the inferomedial aspect of the cricoid lamina to insert on the muscular process of the arytenoid cartilage (Figs. 16-6 and 16-8).

It receives motor fibers from the inferior laryngeal branches of the recurrent laryngeal nerve, a branch of the vagus nerve, and acts to tense the vocal cords and draw them away from each other.

Table 16-2 Intrinsic Muscles of the Larynx

Name	Origin	Insertion	Innervation	Action
Cricothyroid	Arch of the cricoid cartilage	Lamina and inferior cornu of thyroid cartilage	External branch of superior laryngeal nerve	Tenses vocal cords
Lateral cricoarytenoid	Arch of the cricoid cartilage	Muscular process of arytenoid cartilage	Inferior laryngeal nerve	Adducts vocal cords
Posterior cricoarytenoid	Lamina of the cricoid cartilage	Muscular process of arytenoid cartilage	Inferior laryngeal nerve	Abducts vocal cords
Arytenoid Transverse	Posterior surfaces of the two arytenoid cartilages		Inferior laryngeal nerve	Adducts vocal cords
Oblique	Muscular process of one arytenoid cartilage	Apex of opposite arytenoid cartilage	Inferior laryngeal nerve	Adducts vocal cords
Thyroarytenoid	Thyroid lamina and cricothyroid ligament	Lateral margin and base of the arytenoid cartilage	Inferior laryngeal nerve	Adducts vocal cords
Vocalis	Thyroid lamina and cricothyroid ligament	Vocal ligament	Inferior laryngeal nerve	Modifies tension on vocal cord

Arytenoid Muscle

The **arytenoid muscle**, located on the dorsal aspect of the arytenoid cartilages, consists of transverse and oblique portions. The transverse portion **(transverse arytenoid)** is attached to the posterior surface of the lateral aspect of the two arytenoid cartilages. The oblique portion of the arytenoid muscle **(oblique arytenoid)** consists of two slender muscular filaments that cross over each other on the dorsal surface of the transverse arytenoid muscle. The oblique portion originates on the muscular process of one arytenoid cartilage to insert on the apex of the next (Figs. 16-6 and 16-8).

The muscle fibers frequently continue in the aryepiglottic region of the quadrangular membrane. This portion of the muscle is then called the **aryepiglotticus muscle**.

The arytenoid muscle is innervated by the inferior laryngeal branch of the recurrent laryngeal nerve, a branch of the vagus nerve. This muscle draws the arytenoid cartilages toward each other, thus closing the rima glottidis.

Thyroarytenoid Muscle

The **thyroarytenoid muscle** is located on the lateral aspect of the larynx deep to the thyroid lamina. It originates on the medial aspect of the thyroid lamina and from the cricothyroid ligament to insert into the lateral margin and base of the arytenoid cartilage (Figs. 16-6 and 16-8).

The thyroarytneoid muscle is innervated by the inferior laryngeal branch of the recurrent laryngeal nerve, a branch of the vagus nerve. This muscle adducts the vocal cords.

Vocalis Muscle

Although some authors do not recognize the **vocalis muscle** as a separate entity, it will be so recognized here.

The vocalis is described as arising from the thyroid lamina and cricothyroid ligament to insert into the lateral margin and base of the vocal ligament. It is often regarded as a slip of the thyroarytenoid muscle that inserts into the vocal process of the arytenoid cartilage and is attached to the vocal ligament.

The thyroarytenoid and the vocalis muscles are innervated by the inferior laryngeal branch of the recurrent laryngeal nerve. These muscles act on the arytenoid cartilages and vocal ligament to decrease the rima glottidis by approximating the vocal cords.

Movements of the Vocal Folds

Summary Bite Movements of the vocal folds toward each other (adduction) or away from each other (abduction) either open or restrict the air passage through the rima glottides, thus causing the tensed vocal folds to vibrate differentially, thereby producing sounds of various pitch.

The vocal folds may be adducted, that is, moved toward each other, so that the intervening space, the rima glottidis, is almost obliterated. They may also be abducted, that is, moved apart, so that the rima glottidis is opened. Air passing from the trachea through the rima vibrates the tensed vocal folds, producing sounds.

The rima glottidis may be thought of as having two regions, an intermembranous region, between the vocal folds, and an intercartilaginous region, between the arytenoid cartilages.

During normal breathing, the intermembranous portion is triangular and the intercartilaginous portion is rectangular in outline. During forced breathing, the arytenoid cartilages are rotated laterally so that the vocal folds are abducted greatly, describing a triangle whose apical angle is less acute than in normal respiration. The intercartilaginous portion of the rima also becomes triangular; thus the rima is shaped like a rhomboid.

During phonation, the rima is reduced to a thin slit in both its intermembraneous and intercartilaginous portions, and the vocal folds are tensed by the cranial tilting of the cricoid cartilage by the cricothyroid muscle. The pitch of the sound is directly dependent on the degree of tilting.

During soft speech, the intercartilaginous portion of the rima opens, whereas the intermembraneous portion is almost obliterated.

Vascular and Nerve Supply

Vascular Supply

Summary Bite. The vascular supply to the larynx is provided by branches from superior thyroid artery and a branch of the thyrocervical trunk. Venous drainage of the larynx is via the superior and inferior laryngeal veins.

The arterial supply of the larynx is derived mainly from the superior thyroid artery and the inferior thyroid branch of the thyrocervical trunk (Fig. 16-9). These vessels provide superior and inferior laryngeal branches, respectively, which vascularize the larynx. The cricothyroid branch of the superior thyroid artery also serves the larynx.

Venous drainage is accomplished by the superior and inferior laryngeal veins, tributaries of the superior and inferior thyroid veins, respectively.

Sensory and Motor Innervation

Summary Bite. Sensory and motor innervation to the larynx is provided by several branches originating from major branches of the vagus nerve in the neck and from recurrent branches of the vagus arising within the thorax.

Sensory innervation of the larynx, above the vocal cords, is via the internal laryngeal branch of the superior laryngeal nerve of the vagus (Fig. 16-9). The

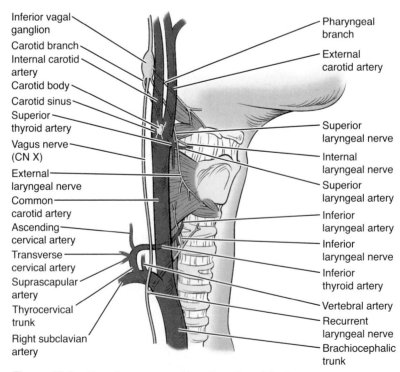

Figure 16-9. Vessels, nerves and lymph nodes of the larynx.

internal laryngeal nerve accompanies the superior laryngeal branch of the superior thyroid artery, pierces the thyrohyoid membrane, and distributes deep to the mucosa of the epiglottis, aryepiglottic fold, and larynx. Taste buds of this region are also supplied by the internal laryngeal nerve.

Sensory innervation below the vocal cords is via sensory fibers of the recurrent laryngeal branches of the vagus nerve.

Motor innervation of the larynx has been detailed earlier but, in summary, all intrinsic muscles of the larynx except the cricothyroid are innervated by the recurrent laryngeal branch of the vagus nerve. The cricothyroid muscle is served by the external la-ryngeal branch of the superior laryngeal nerve, a branch of the vagus nerve.

TRACHEA

Summary Bite. The trachea begins at the inferior border of the larynx and continues into the thorax, where it bifurcates into right and left bronchi. It is a membranous structure whose patency is maintained by incomplete cartilaginous rings.

Clinical Considerations

Heimlich Maneuver

Foreign objects, such as a piece of meat, can be aspirated into the inlet of the larynx and become lodged in the laryngeal vestibule above the vestibular folds, causing muscle spasms that tense the vocal folds, thus closing the rima glottidis. At this point, depending upon the degree of constriction, air movement into the trachea is restricted or may be completely obstructed from entering the trachea. The individual may start choking and perhaps will be unable to speak. The obstruction may result is complete asphyxiation and the person may die within approximately five minutes. Depending on the severity and condition of the patient, the Heimlich maneuver is performed to dislodge the obstruction by sudden compression of the abdomen to force a blast of air out of the lungs through the trachea and into the larynx, expelling the foreign object. When this procedure is unsuccessful, an emergency airway must be made into the trachea with a large-bore needle through the cricothyroid ligament.

Larynx

The intrinsic laryngeal musculature is served by two nerves, the inferior laryngeal branch of the recurrent laryngeal nerve and the external branch of the superior laryngeal nerve, both branches of the vagus nerve. Because these two nerves are prone to damage, it is essential that they be protected from injury during surgical procedures. The external laryngeal nerve, passing deep to the superior thyroid artery, supplies only a single muscle, the cricothyroid. Its section does not cause excessive damage to phonation. It will, however, affect the ability to tense the vocal cords and the ability of the patient to produce high-pitched sounds. In addition, damage to it causes some hoarseness and easy tiring of the voice.

Damage to the recurrent laryngeal or the inferior laryngeal nerves will result in serious complications, whose severity depends on the degree of damage and whether the injury is bilateral. Involvement may range from slight hoarseness to complete inability to vocalize and breathe, necessitating performance of a tracheotomy.

Tracheotomy

Tracheotomy is a surgical procedure performed to provide an airway passage to relieve dyspnea. This procedure is now generally used only for long-term maintenance of airway passage. Although the procedure may be performed any place along the trachea between the cricoid cartilage and the jugular notch, several complications may result because of the possibility of severing major venous channels and the isthmus of the thyroid gland overlying the trachea.

A much safer emergency procedure for opening the airway is **cricothyrotomy**, in which opening the passageway is accomplished by incising the cricothyroid membrane between the thyroid and cricoid cartilages. This procedure is easily performed, having few possible complications.

The trachea begins at the inferior border of the larynx, to which it is attached by the cricotracheal ligament (Figs. 16-3 and 16-6). The trachea enters the thoracic cavity, where it bifurcates, forming the right and left bronchi.

The cervical portion of the trachea is superficial, being only partially covered by the infrahyoid muscles. Its superior portion may be palpated between the sternal heads of the sternocleidomastoid muscles as well as in the jugular notch. It is a membranous structure, whose lumen is maintained by incomplete cartilaginous rings distributed more or less evenly along the length of the tube. The complete portion of the ring is placed anteriorly, and the posteriorly placed interval contains smooth muscle fibers that are able to regulate the size of the lumen to a limited extent.

DEGLUTITION

Summary Bite. Deglutition (swallowing) is a complex and incompletely understood process. Generally, there is agreement that the process, though continuous, is divided into three stages: voluntary, involuntary, and final stages.

Deglutition, or the act of swallowing, is a complex neuromuscular phenomenon that is only incompletely understood. For this reason, the anatomy of deglutition is an area rife with disagreement. The present discussion focuses on generally accepted aspects of deglutition.

Although the act of swallowing, once initiated, is a continuous process, it is divided into three phases here for the sake of convenience: voluntary, involuntary, and final stages.

- The **voluntary**, or first, stage involves formation of the bolus of food by the actions of the tongue against the hard palate and by the assistance of the soft palate as it approximates the back of the tongue. Once the bolus is ready, the suprahyoid muscles fix the hyoid bone and the tongue forces the bolus through the oropharyngeal isthmus.
- The **involuntary** or second, stage of deglutition is initiated when the bolus enters the oral pharynx. The levator veli palatini and tensor veli palatini muscles elevate and tense the soft palate, which comes into contact with the bar of Passavant, thus isolating the nasopharynx from the oral pharynx.
- The **final stage** of deglutition begins when the inferior constrictor muscle contracts, thereby forcing the bolus of food into the esophagus, whose cranial portion is completely relaxed. The esophagus, via its musculature, then performs peristaltic actions to transmit the bolus of food into the stomach.

The actions of the tensor veli palatini and salpingopharyngeus muscles also open the auditory tube.

The paired palatoglossus muscles also contract, bringing the palatoglossal folds in close proximity to the back of the tongue. Thus, the bolus cannot pass laterally, superiorly, or ventrally—only inferiorly.

Simultaneously, the stylopharyngeus, palatopharyngeus, salpingopharyngeus, and thyrohyoid muscles elevate the larynx and pharynx in a dorsal direction, approximating the laryngeal part of the pharynx to the descending bolus and pulling the laryngeal inlet out of the way.

To protect the larynx, the aryepiglottic, thyroarytenoid, and oblique arytenoid muscles contract to bring the aryepiglottic folds medially, creating a chute leading to the piriform recess. The bolus of food, sliding along the sides of the epiglottis, descends via this chute to the piriform recess.

Brain and Spinal Cord

17

Key Terms

The Brain develops from five primordia. Later, as certain divisions become greatly enlarged, they overgrow other regions of the developing brain so that the adult brain, on a cursory inspection, presents only three divisions: the cerebral hemispheres, the cerebellum, and the brainstem. The largest portion of the adult brain is the cerebral hemispheres, which are generally responsible for analyzing sensory input, memory, learning, motor function, etc. The cerebellum is generally responsible for coordination, balance, and influences on muscle. The brainstem, the third part, is responsible for many basic vital life functions such as heartbeat, breathing, blood pressure, etc. Additionally, all of the cranial nerves emanate from the brainstem.

Cerebrospinal Fluid (CSF) bathes the entire central nervous system (CNS). The CNS develops from a hollow tube that later expands to form ventricles within the brain and the central canal of the spinal cord. This lumen is filled with CSF, which is produced by the choroid plexus in the ventricles. The CSF enters the subarachnoid space via certain foramina, where it circulates and is eventually resorbed into the superior sagittal sinus by elements from both the pia and the arachnoid called the **arachnoid granulations**. The CSF may act as a hydrodynamic protective cushion to absorb sudden traumas, in addition to providing nutrient functions.

Meninges are the three layers of membrane that cover the central nervous system (CNS). The fibrous outer layer is called the dura mater. It is firmly attached the interior of the bony cranium, whereas it is unattached to the vertebral column as it houses the spinal cord. The arachnoid, middle layer, is separated from the dura only by a simple layer of epithelium. Weblike processes extend from it into cerebrospinal fluid-filled subarachnoid space housing blood vessels between the arachnoid and the innermost of the meninges, the pia mater. The pia is closely adhered to the surface of the brain.

The Spinal Cord is a continuation of the medulla, extending from the first cervical vertebra to the first or second lumbar vertebra where the spinal cord ends as the conus medullaris. However, lumbar and sacral spinal nerves continue as the cauda equinae to exit their respective intervertebral foramina. The subarachnoid space in the spinal cord houses CSF. In cross section, the periphery of the spinal cord is white matter, whereas the central gray matter is arranged in the shape of an H. The horizontal cross bar represents the dorsal and ventral gray commissures. The legs of the H represent dorsal horns and ventral horns. The ventral horns house motor neurons, whereas the dorsal horns receive sensory fibers. At thoracic levels (T1–L2), the **intermediolateral cell column** (gray matter) houses all presynaptic sympathetic cell bodies.

The brain and spinal cord together comprise the receiving, integrating, analyzing, and responding portion of the body, called the central nervous system (CNS). These are delicate, almost gelatinous structures that consist of cells with little intercellular connective tissue material. Because the CNS is so fragile and so important for the life and proper functioning of the individual, the brain and spinal cord are housed in bony compartments that protect them from injury. To provide further protection, the brain and spinal cord are surrounded by meningeal membranes and are bathed in cerebrospinal fluid (CSF).

This chapter does not provide a thorough account of the CNS; that is to be found in textbooks of neuroanatomy. Instead, a general account is included here to provide students with some terminology and a descriptive introduction to the morphology of the meninges, brain, and spinal cord.

MENINGES

Summary Bite. Three layers of mengines cover, support, and protect the brain: the innermost layer is the pia mater, the intermediate layer is the arachnoid, and the external fibrous layer is the dura mater.

The brain and spinal cord are invested by three layers of membranes that, in addition to providing support and protection, act as a covering for blood vessels that supply the CNS. These three layers include the external-most dura mater, the middle arachnoid, and the inner-most pia mater.

The **dura mater**, the outer, coarse, fibrous covering of the brain, also covers the spinal cord, and the two are continuous with each other through the foramen magnum. The dura of the brain is described in Chapter 9 (see Figs. 9-1 and 9-2); that of the spinal cord is similar in concept, but it forms no reflections as does the cranial dura. Instead, the spinal dura is a cylindrical sheath that surrounds the spinal cord as well as the spinal nerve roots that pass through the intervertebral foramina.

The external aspect of the spinal dura is not attached to bone; instead, a fatty connective tissue layer, the **epidural fat**, separates it from the periosteum and provides further cushioning of the spinal canal. The epidural fat contains the internal vertebral venous plexus, which empties into the venous sinuses of the cranial dura.

The internal aspect of the cranial and spinal dura mater is lined by a simple, squamous type of epithelium, which separates the dura from the arachnoid. A potential space, the **subdural space**, is interposed between the epithelial linings of the dura and the arachnoid.

The **arachnoid**, a thin, avascular layer, is covered by a simple, squamous epithelium and extends thin, weblike processes into the **subarachnoid space**, a CSF-filled region between the arachnoid and pia mater.

The arachnoid and dura, although separated from each other by the potential subdural space, follow each other's contours. These membranes display connections at the spinal and cranial nerves, at the infundibulum of the hypophysis, in regions where vessels penetrate the dura to and from the subarachnoid space, as well as at the points where the **denticulate ligaments** of the pia attach and fix the pia to the dura.

The subarachnoid space contains blood vessels and CSF. This fluid exits the subarachnoid space via the specialized **arachnoid granulations**, which, piercing the meningeal dura in the parietal region, deliver the CSF into the **lacunae lateralis**, located in the fovea granularis of the parietal bone. These lacunae are drained by vessels that empty into the superior sagittal sinus.

The subarachnoid space becomes dilated in certain regions, forming cisterns, which are detailed later in this chapter.

The **pia mater** is a delicate, cellular membrane that closely follows the contours of the brain and spinal cord, as well as the nerves emanating from them. Blood vessels passing through the subarachnoid space branch extensively on the superficial surface of the pia, which they pierce to enter the substance of the brain. Here, glial cells (supporting cells of the CNS) form a protective coating around the vessels, assisting in the establishment of an effective **blood–brain**

barrier, controlling the entry of materials into the extracellular spaces of the brain and spinal cord.

The CNS is a hollow structure lined by a special type of epithelium known as **ependyma**. This epithelium, which is modified in certain areas of the brain, surrounds vascular intrusions of pial elements to form the **choroid plexus**, which functions in the elaboration of CSF.

BRAIN

 Summary Bite. The brain is protected by its meninges as well as by its bony housing, the skull.

The brain is an immensely complex structure whose organizational hierarchy is not completely understood. This section of the chapter does not attempt to discuss the functional aspects of neuroanatomy; instead, only the gross morphology of the brain is described.

Divisions

 Summary Bite. During early embryogenesis, the brain is noted to be composed of five divisions. Some of these divisions greatly enlarge to overgrow other divisions, causing the brain to fold upon itself such that only three regions are immediately visible in the adult brain: the cerebral hemispheres, the cerebellum, and the brainstem.

The brain, during embryogenesis, is noted to be clearly divided into five continuous parts: the telencephalon, diencephalon, mesencephalon, metencephalon, and myelencephalon, arranged in an anteroposterior (rostrocaudal) direction.

Regions of the developing brain become greatly enlarged and some of these portions overgrow others such that the brain begins to fold on itself, so much so that parts of the brain become submerged and surrounded by more rapidly growing elements. Hence, only three regions are evident on cursory examination of the whole adult brain: the cerebral hemispheres, the cerebellum, and the brainstem.

Cerebral Hemispheres

The largest portion of the brain is composed of the two cerebral hemispheres. The two hemispheres, derived from the telencephalon, are partly separated from each other by the deep **longitudinal fissure**, a space occupied by the falx cerebri (Figs. 17-1 through 17-3).

The surface of the brain is intimately invested by the almost invisible pia mater, which follows the convoluted elevations and depressions of the surface. Each elevation, or **gyrus**, is bounded by the depressions, or **sulci**. The locations of these sulci and gyri are relatively constant.

The cerebral hemispheres completely fill the supratentorial space of the skull and may be subdivided into regions reflecting their anatomic position. Hence, there are frontal, parietal, temporal, occipital, and insular lobes.

The surface of each cerebral hemisphere is the cortex, consisting of **gray matter**. Deep to the cortex is **white matter**, consisting of fiber tracts passing to and from the cortex and other parts of the brain.

Deep within this fibrous region of the cerebrum reside **subcortical nuclei**, groups of cell bodies that constitute the **basal ganglia** associated with somatic motor functions.

The lateral convex surface of the cerebral hemisphere resembles a boxing glove, of which the thumb, pointing inferiorly, is the temporal lobe. A deep fissure, the **lateral sulcus**, separates the temporal from the frontal and parietal lobes (Fig. 17-1).

Deep to the temporal lobe, forming the floor of the lateral fissure, is the insula, a cortical lobe also covered by the frontal and parietal lobes.

The occipital lobe, a relatively small, triangular portion of the cerebrum, lies caudal to the parietal lobe, forming the posterior terminus of the cerebrum.

The **central sulcus**, running obliquely from just behind the center of the hemisphere to, but not into, the lateral fissure, separates the frontal and parietal lobes. The gyri, anterior and posterior to the central sulcus, are known as the **precentral gyrus** and the **postcentral gyrus**, respectively. The former is a motor area, whereas the latter is a sensory area of the cortex. The sulcus caudal to the postcentral gyrus is the **postcentral sulcus** and the one anterior to the precentral gyrus is the **precentral sulcus**.

The largest, or **frontal lobe**, of the cerebral hemisphere is bounded anteriorly by the anterior pole, posteriorly by the central sulcus, and inferiorly by the lateral sulcus. The precentral sulcus and precentral gyrus complete the frontal lobe. The region of the frontal lobe that covers the insula is known as the **frontal operculum**. The operculum and part of the inferior frontal gyrus function in speech.

The **parietal lobe** is incompletely defined morphologically. Its anterior boundary is the central sulcus, whereas posteriorly the lobe is separated from the occipital lobe by an imaginary line extending from the **parieto-occipital sulcus** to the **preoccipital notch**. The region of the parietal lobe covering the insula is the **parietal operculum**.

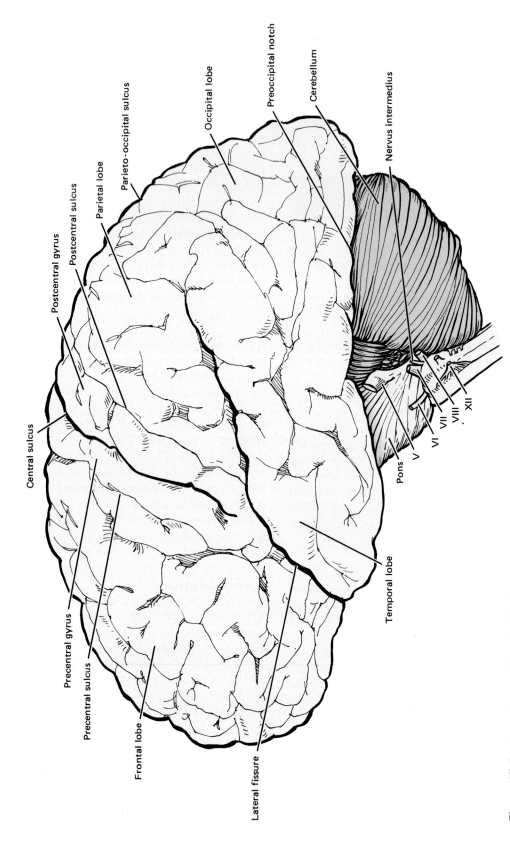

Central sulcus

Postcentral gyrus

Postcentral sulcus

Parietal lobe

Parieto-occipital sulcus

Occipital lobe

Preoccipital notch

Cerebellum

Nervus intermedius

Precentral gyrus

Precentral sulcus

Frontal lobe

Lateral fissure

Temporal lobe

Pons

V

VI

VII

VIII

XII

Figure 17-1. Lateral view of the whole brain.

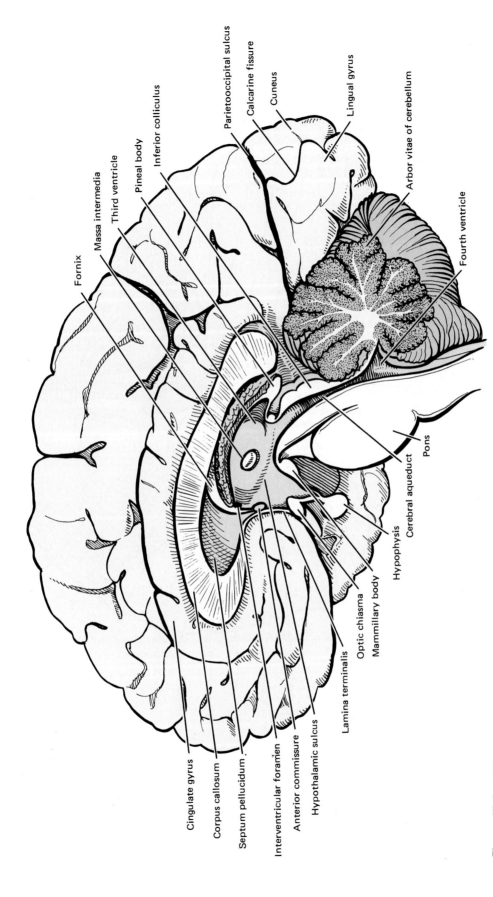

Figure 17-2. Midsagittal section of the whole brain.

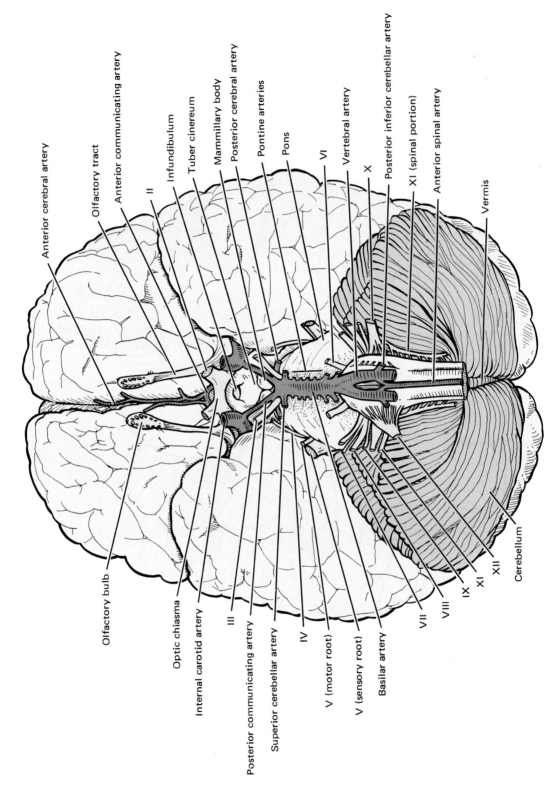

Figure 17-3. Ventral view of the whole brain and its major arterial supply.

Anterior cerebral artery

Olfactory tract

Anterior communicating artery

II

Infundibulum

Tuber cinereum

Mammillary body

Posterior cerebral artery

Pontine arteries

Pons

VI

Vertebral artery

X

Posterior inferior cerebellar artery

XI (spinal portion)

Anterior spinal artery

Vermis

Olfactory bulb

Optic chiasma

Internal carotid artery

III

Posterior communicating artery

Superior cerebellar artery

IV

V (motor root)

V (sensory root)

Basilar artery

VII

VIII

IX

XI

XII

Cerebellum

The **temporal lobe** has well-defined superior and inferior boundaries—the lateral sulcus and the inferior extent of the convexity of the cerebrum—and its posterior boundary is the imaginary line between the parieto-occipital sulcus and the preoccipital notch. Several short gyri may be observed on the inner aspect of the temporal lobe forming the inferior border of the lateral sulcus. These transverse gyri represent the primary auditory cortex.

The **occipital lobe** is the posterior-most aspect of the cerebral hemisphere and is separated from the parietal and temporal lobes by the imaginary line connecting the parieto-occipital sulcus and the preoccipital notch. The occipital lobe functions as the visual cortex.

The **insula** is the region of the cerebral hemispheres that is hidden from view by the parietal, the frontal, and especially the temporal opercula. It forms the floor of the lateral sulcus and is reported to function in taste.

The two cerebral hemispheres are structurally and functionally connected to each other by commissures, the larger of which is the **corpus callosum**, a midline structure forming the floor of the longitudinal fissure. The other commissure is the much smaller **anterior commissure**. The **fornix** also contains some commissural fibers, although these are not well developed in the human brain. The corpus callosum is best appreciated in the midsagittal view, where it is noted as a white, dense, salient feature of the brain (Fig. 17-2). Fortuitous hemisection of the brain displays the **septum pellucidum** (stretched between the inferior aspect of the corpus callosum and the fornix), which intervenes between the two **lateral ventricles** of the cerebral hemisphere. The two lateral ventricles communicate with each other and with the third ventricle via the **interventricular foramina (of Monro)**, which are located just inferior to the anterior portion of the fornix. The medial aspect of the hemisected brain displays the **cingulate gyrus**, located superior to the corpus callosum. The well-defined parieto-occipital sulcus, delineating the anterior border of the occipital lobe, is also evident. The occipital lobe is subdivided into a superior **cuneus** and an inferior **lingula** by the **calcarine fissure**.

When the cerebral hemisphere is viewed from the inferior perspective, the occipital and part of the temporal lobes are hidden by the cerebellum and the brainstem (Fig. 17-3). The anteroinferior aspect presents the midline longitudinal cerebral fissure, lateral to which is the thin **gyrus rectus** and the **olfactory sulcus** with the attendant **olfactory bulb** and **tract**. Olfactory nerves synapse in the inferior aspect of the bulb after passing through the cribriform plate of the ethmoid bone.

Cerebellum

The cerebellum is a large structure displaying thin, leaflike plates, the cerebellar folia, giving the cerebellum its distinctive appearance. The cerebellum lies deep to the tentorium cerebelli and is composed of two **cerebellar hemispheres** and the intervening **vermis** (Figs. 17-1 through 17-3). This portion of the brain is derived from the metencephalon. The cerebellum consists of a thin gray-matter mantle known as the **cerebellar cortex**, overlying the centrally located white matter containing several nuclei. Functionally, the cerebellum may be divided into three areas. The **neocerebellum** is responsible for precise coordination of muscle action, especially that related to movements of the hand. The **paleocerebellum** functions in maintaining proper posture in response to gravity. The **archicerebellum** is responsible for proprioception, especially that involved with spatial orientation.

Brainstem

The brainstem, the oldest part of the CNS, is obscured by the large cerebral and cerebellar hemispheres to such an extent that only its ventral and lateral aspects are visible in the whole brain. Removal of the cerebrum and cerebellum exposes the entire brainstem, which extends from the diencephalon rostrally to the myelencephalon (medulla oblongata) caudally. All cranial nerves arise from the ventral aspect of the brainstem, except for the trochlear nerve, which originates from its dorsal surface (Fig. 17-4).

Diencephalon

Summary Bite. The diencephalon is the rostral-most portion of the brainstem. It is composed of four regions: the epithalamus, thalamus, hypothalamus, and subthalamus.

The diencephalon surrounds an ependymal-lined space, the third ventricle, which communicates with the lateral ventricles of the cerebrum via the **interventricular foramen** and with the fourth ventricle through the **cerebral acqueduct** (Fig. 17-5).

The **epithalamus** is the dorsal surface of the diencephalon and is composed of the **pineal body** (an endocrine gland), the **stria medullaris**, and the **habenular trigone**, whose nuclei and interhabenular connections are associated with the olfactory system.

The **thalamus** is the largest portion of the diencephalon and is separated into right and left halves by the third ventricle. The two thalami are interconnected by a bridge of gray matter, the **massa intermedia** (or interthalamic adhesion) (Fig. 17-2).

All sensory stimuli, with the exception of olfaction, enter the thalamus and are redistributed to the sensory cortex for finer perception via the thalamocortical

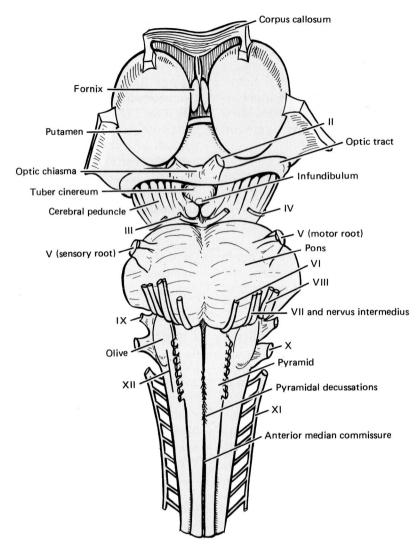

Figure 17-4. Ventral view of the brainstem.

radiations. The thalamus contains many nuclei, some of which create prominent bulges on the surface of the diencephalon. The **pulvinar** is one such large caudal region of the thalamus, located just above the midbrain. Two other nuclei, the **medial** and **lateral geniculate bodies**, associated with hearing and sight, respectively, are located in the vicinity of the pulvinar.

The **hypothalamus** is separated from the thalamus by a groove, the hypothalamic sulcus, located on either wall of the third ventricle. This small region of the diencephalon is associated with endocrine function, sleep, emotion, and regulation of temperature. Structures of the hypothalamus evident on the ventral surface of the brainstem are the **hypophysis** (pituitary gland); the small, elevated **tuber cinereum** with the attendant **infundibulum** of the hypophysis; and the two **mamillary bodies**, located caudal to the tuber cinereum (Figs. 17-2 and 17-4).

The **subthalamus** contains one major nucleus, the subthalamic nucleus, and a few small bundles of fiber tracts. This subdivision of the diencephalon is associated with somatic efferent functions.

Mesencephalon

Summary Bite. The mesencephalon (midbrain) is a short segment surrounding the cerebral aqueduct situated between the diencephalon and the pons.

The dorsal aspect, or **tectum**, contains four marked elevations: the **corpora quadrigemina**, consisting of the two rostrally placed **superior colliculi**, functionally related to the visual system, and the two caudally placed **inferior colliculi**, associated with hearing. The lateral geniculate body is connected to the superior colliculus via fiber bundles, the **brachium of the superior**

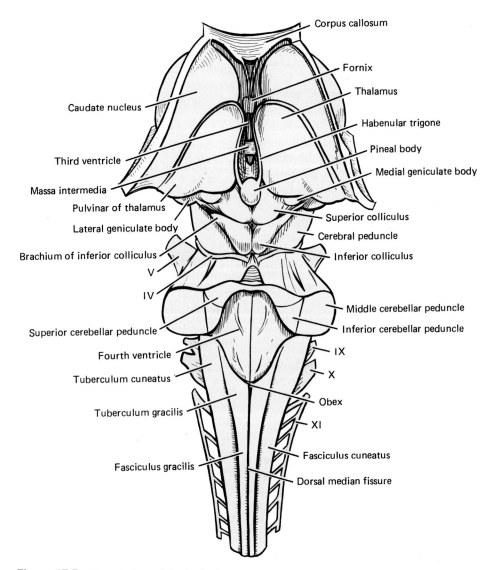

Figure 17-5. Dorsal view of the brainstem.

colliculus, whereas the **brachium of the inferior colliculus** connects the inferior colliculus to the medial geniculate body. Just inferior to this colliculus, the slender trochlear nerve (cranial nerve IV) emerges from the mesencephalon (Fig. 17-5). This is the only cranial nerve to leave the dorsal aspect of the brainstem. The two **cerebral peduncles**, fiber tracts connecting the cerebrum to the brainstem, are located ventrally, below the cerebral aqueduct in a region known as the tegmentum. The **interpeduncular fossa**, between the two peduncles, displays the oculomotor nerve (cranial nerve III) leaving the brainstem.

Metencephalon

Summary Bite. The metencephalon is hidden from view by the cerebellum, but its ventral surface is clearly visible as the bulging **pons**.

The metencephalon is separated from the mesencephalon by the superior pontine sulcus and from the myelencephalon by the inferior pontine sulcus. The dorsal aspect of the pons, which forms the floor of the fourth ventricle, is known as the **tegmentum**.

The tegmentum contains the nuclei of cranial nerves V, VI, VII, and VIII. As the facial nerve passes over the nucleus of cranial nerve VI, it forms a bulge on the floor of the fourth ventricle, the **facial colliculus**. The **superior** and **middle cerebellar peduncles** connect the cerebellum to the brainstem, and cranial nerve V pierces the rostal part of the middle cerebellar peduncle (Fig. 17-5). The other three cranial nerves associated with the metencephalon leave this structure at the inferior pontine sulcus.

Myelencephalon

 Summary Bite. The myelencephalon (**medulla oblongata**) is the caudal-most portion of the brainstem. It extends from the inferior pontine sulcus to the spinal cord, demarcated approximately by the foramen magnum.

The V-shaped lateral walls of the myelencephalon close over the fourth ventricle at the apex, the **obex**.

Bilateral, cylindrical structures, the **pyramids**, are evident on the ventral surface of the medulla. **Pyramidal decussations**, or crossings of fibers, appear across the anterior midline fissure from one pyramid to the other (Fig. 17-4). Lateral to each pyramid is an olive pit-shaped bulge, the **olive**.

Filaments of cranial nerve XII are lodged in the groove (**anterior lateral sulcus**) between the pyramid and the olive, whereas cranial nerves IX, X, and XI are located in the groove dorsal to the olive (Fig. 17-4).

Fiber connections between the medulla and the cerebellum are via the **inferior cerebellar peduncle**. Located in the midline of the dorsal surface of the medulla is the **posterior median fissure**, lateral to which is the **tuberculum gracilis**, a swelling demarcating the underlying **nucleus gracilis**, on which many lower sensory neurons synapse. Lateral to the tuberculum gracilis is a similar swelling, the **tuberculum cuneatus** with the underlying **nucleus cuneatus**, where many sensory neurons from the upper part of the body synapse. The most lateral swelling is the **tuberculum cinereum**, representing the descending tract of the trigeminal nerve.

Cerebrospinal Fluid and Ventricles

Cerebrospinal Fluid

The CNS develops from a hollow cylindrical tube and retains this space in the adult as the ventricles of the brain and the central canal of the spinal cord.

The ventricles and the central canal form a continuous channel filled with **CSF**, a clear, colorless, acellular liquid produced by specialized structures, the **choroid plexus**, located mostly in the ventricles.

CSF is elaborated continuously, bathing the CNS. Some of the fluid enters the subarachnoid space via specialized foramina of the myelencephalon, the paired lateral **foramina of Luschka** and the single, medial **foramen of Magendie**.

The CSF circulates in the subarachnoid space, eventually to be transported into the superior sagittal sinus by **arachnoid granulations**, structures composed of elements from both the pia and the arachnoid (Fig. 17-6).

The subarachnoid space closely follows the contours of the brain, except in certain regions where the arachnoid diverges, forming larger spaces known as **cisterns**. The three foramina of the myelencephalon empty into the **cisterna magna (cisterna cerebellomedullaris)**, the largest of the cisterns, located between the cerebellum and the medulla oblongata.

Two other large cisterns in the head are worthy of mention, the **cisterna superior**, between the cerebellum and the midbrain, and the **cisterna interpeduncularis**, located between the two cerebral peduncles. Hence, the CNS is completely surrounded by CSF, which may act as a hydrodynamic protective cushion, absorbing sudden traumas in addition to providing possible nutrient functions.

Ventricles

 Summary Bite. The four ventricles of the brain are ependymal-lined spaces containing CSF.

The four ventricles of the brain containing CSF are the paired **lateral ventricles** of the cerebral hemispheres and the **third** and **fourth ventricles**. The paired lateral ventricles, the largest of the four, hollow out the cerebral hemispheres. These two ventricles

Clinical Considerations

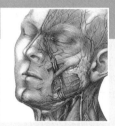

Myelencephalon

Disease of or trauma to the myelencephalon is often fatal because this region of the brain is responsible for the vital functions of the body such as respiration and control of circulation.

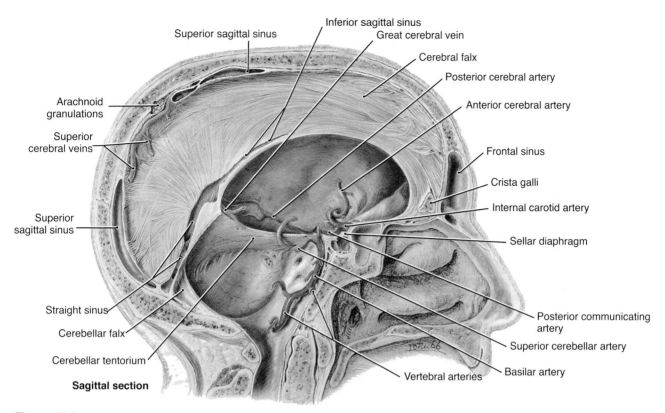

Superior sagittal sinus
Inferior sagittal sinus
Great cerebral vein
Cerebral falx
Posterior cerebral artery
Anterior cerebral artery
Arachnoid granulations
Superior cerebral veins
Frontal sinus
Crista galli
Internal carotid artery
Superior sagittal sinus
Sellar diaphragm
Straight sinus
Cerebellar falx
Cerebellar tentorium
Posterior communicating artery
Superior cerebellar artery
Basilar artery
Vertebral arteries
Sagittal section

Figure 17-6. Dural reflections (midsagittal view).

are separated from each other by the intervening **septum pellucidum**, although a connection, the **interventricular foramen**, permits communication between the lateral ventricles and the third ventricle (Fig. 17-2). Each lateral ventricle has a body and anterior, posterior, and inferior horns.

The third ventricle is surrounded by the right and left halves of the thalamus and is interrupted by a mass of gray matter, the massa intermedia, which crosses this ventricle. The third ventricle communicates with the fourth ventricle by the **cerebral aqueduct**.

The fourth ventricle is located in the hindbrain and also communicates with the central canal of the medulla. CSF, as indicated previously, leaves the fourth ventricle to enter the subarachnoid space by way of the paired lateral foramina of Luschka and the median foramen of Magendie.

Blood Supply

Arterial Supply

Summary Bite. Branches of the two vertebral arteries and the two internal carotid arteries provide the arterial supply to the brain.

Arterial supply to the brain is derived from the two vertebral and two internal carotid arteries (Fig. 17-3 and 17-7). The vertebral arteries enter the cranial cavity through the foramen magnum and, just before reaching the pons, fuse to form the single basilar artery.

The two internal carotid arteries gain access to the cranial cavity via the carotid canals, pass through the cavernous sinus, and give branches to the brain.

The vertebral artery, a branch of the first part of the subclavian artery, supplies three named branches to the CNS: the single anterior spinal artery and the posterior spinal artery, serving the medulla and the spinal cord; and the **posteroinferior cerebellar artery**, vascularizing the inferior aspect of the caudal portion of the cerebellum. The vertebral arteries of the two sides join to form the single **basilar artery**, which travels along the ventral aspect of the pons in the basilar groove. Branches of the basilar artery are the anteroinferior cerebellar, labyrinthine, pontine, superior cerebellar, and posterior cerebral arteries.

The **anteroinferior cerebellar artery**, the caudalmost branch of the basilar artery, supplies the inferior aspect of the anterior portion of the cerebellum. The small **labyrinthine artery** serves the cochlea and

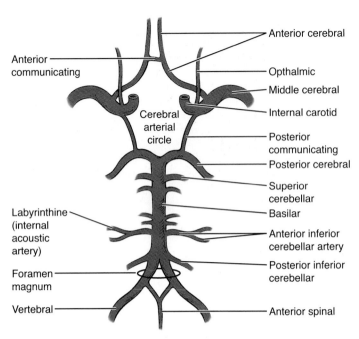

Figure 17-7. Cerebral arterial circle (circle of Willis).

vestibular apparatus. Several small **pontine arteries** vascularize the pons, whereas the **superior cerebellar artery** passes between the cerebral hemispheres and the cerebellum to serve the superior aspect of the latter structure.

The basilar artery bifurcates to give rise to the two **posterior cerebral arteries**, which serve the inferomedial aspect of the temporal and occipital lobes of the cerebrum. The posterior cerebral artery possesses an arterial connection to the internal carotid artery, the **posterior communicating artery**, thus forming the posterior arch of the **cerebral arterial circle of Willis** (Fig. 17-7).

Branches of the internal carotid artery are the anterior choroidal, middle cerebral, anterior cerebral, and ophthalmic arteries.

■ The **anterior choroidal artery** supplies the choroid plexus and portions of the cerebral hemispheres.

■ The **middle cerebral artery** courses laterally to pass between the temporal and parietal lobes. It supplies the lateral surfaces of most of the frontal, parietal, and temporal lobes.

■ The **anterior cerebral artery** passes anteriorly, on the inferomedial aspect of the gyrus rectus, to vascularize the medial and superior aspects of the frontal and parietal lobes. The two anterior cerebral arteries are interconnected by the short.

■ **Anterior communicating artery**, thus completing the cerebral arterial circle.

This arterial circle, circumscribing the mamillary bodies, the hypophysis, and the optic tracts, is composed

Clinical Considerations

Arterial Occlusion or Rupture

The deeper regions of the brain, unlike most areas of the body, do not possess arterial anastomoses. Therefore, when an artery (e.g., one of the named branches of the circle of Willis) is occluded or ruptures, the area of the brain that is affected is often widespread and, because nerve tissue does not repair itself, the damage produced is permanent.

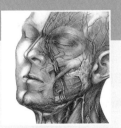

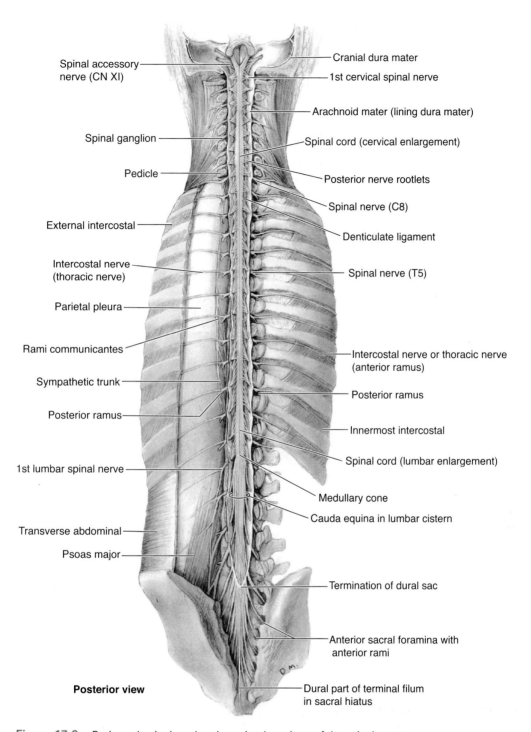

Spinal accessory nerve (CN XI)

Cranial dura mater

1st cervical spinal nerve

Arachnoid mater (lining dura mater)

Spinal ganglion

Spinal cord (cervical enlargement)

Pedicle

Posterior nerve rootlets

Spinal nerve (C8)

External intercostal

Denticulate ligament

Intercostal nerve (thoracic nerve)

Spinal nerve (T5)

Parietal pleura

Rami communicantes

Sympathetic trunk

Intercostal nerve or thoracic nerve (anterior ramus)

Posterior ramus

Posterior ramus

Innermost intercostal

1st lumbar spinal nerve

Spinal cord (lumbar enlargement)

Medullary cone

Cauda equina in lumbar cistern

Transverse abdominal

Psoas major

Termination of dural sac

Posterior view

Anterior sacral foramina with anterior rami

Dural part of terminal filum in sacral hiatus

Figure 17-8. Brain and spinal cord and proximal portions of the spinal nerves.

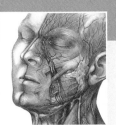

Clinical Considerations

Stroke

Stroke results from ischemic blood flow usually caused by occlusion of a cerebral artery in the brain, causing the patient to develop sudden neurological deficits. Although the first attack is not usually fatal, the patient is left neurologically impaired. Vessels of the circle of Willis provide collateral circulation to the damaged area, thus permitting some degree of rehabilitation for the patient.

---

of the two posterior cerebral, two posterior communicating, two internal carotid, two anterior cerebral, and the single anterior communicating arteries.

The **ophthalmic artery** is not associated with vascularization of the brain. It passes through the optic foramen to enter and supply the orbit and its contents.

Venous Drainage

Venous drainage of the brain arises from the pial venous plexus derived from the confluence of minute venous vessels. The cerebral veins are divisible into external and internal groups.

▨ The external veins drain into the regional venous sinuses. Venous drainage of the deeper regions of the brain eventually empty into the straight sinus via the **great cerebral vein**. Cerebellar veins also are of two groups, **superior** and **inferior cerebellar veins**. These drain into the straight sinus or other regional sinuses.

SPINAL CORD

The spinal cord is an anteroposteriorly flattened cylindrical continuation of the medulla, extending from the cranial border of the first cervical vertebra to the first or second lumbar vertebra. Thus, the spinal cord of the adult does not fill the whole vertebral canal, but ends in a conical structure, the **conus medullaris**. The pial covering continues as a threadlike filament, the **filum terminale**, anchoring the conus medullaris to the coccyx (Fig. 17-8).

The spinal cord is fixed also to the lateral wall of the dural covering by toothlike extensions of pia, the **denticulate ligaments**, located equidistant between the ventral and dorsal roots of each spinal nerve.

Although the spinal cord extends only to L1 or L2 vertebral levels, the dural covering continues to line the entire extent of the vertebral canal, creating a large, fluid-filled subarachnoid space, the **lumbar**

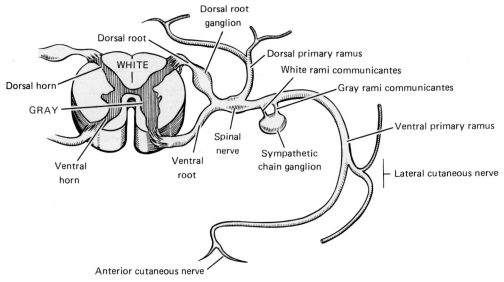

Figure 17-9. Typical thoracic spinal cord segment and spinal nerve.

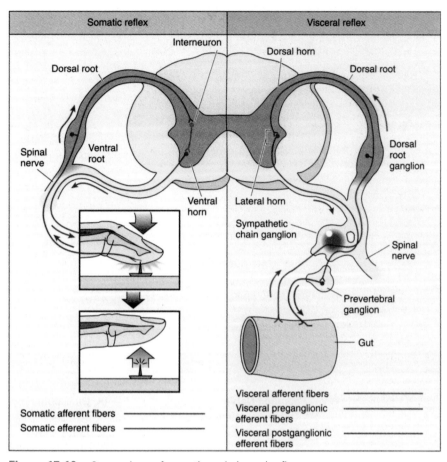

Somatic reflex	Visceral reflex

Interneuron

Dorsal horn

Dorsal root

Dorsal horn

Dorsal root

Spinal nerve

Ventral root

Ventral horn

Lateral horn

Sympathetic chain ganglion

Dorsal root ganglion

Spinal nerve

Prevertebral ganglion

Gut

Somatic afferent fibers ———————
Somatic efferent fibers ———————

Visceral afferent fibers ———————
Visceral preganglionic efferent fibers ———————
Visceral postganglionic efferent fibers ———————

Figure 17-10. Comparison of somatic and visceral reflexes.

cistern, used for spinal fluid taps and lumbar punctures. The lumbar cistern contains, in addition to the filum terminale and CSF, the **cauda equinae**, root filaments of lumbar, and sacral spinal nerves, which must pass from the spinal cord to the intervertebral foramina of their destination.

The spinal cord, in cross section, displays the peripheral white matter, with the central gray matter arranged in a characteristic H-shaped configuration (Fig. 17-9). The horizontal crossbar of the H is represented by the **dorsal** and **ventral gray commissures**, posterior and anterior to the ependyma-lined central canal, respectively.

The legs of the H are represented by the ventral and dorsal horns. The **ventral horns** house the motor

neurons, whose axons leave the spinal cord as ventral rootlets (Fig. 17-10). Sensory fibers enter the spinal cord as dorsal rootlets via the **dorsal horns.** Internuncial cell bodies occupy the **dorsal gray column**, whereas, at thoracic levels (T1–L2), the **intermediolateral cell column** houses all presynaptic sympathetic cell bodies.

The right and left sides of the spinal cord are partly separated from each other by the **dorsal median septum** and the somewhat wider **ventral median fissure**, neither of which penetrates the gray matter. Each half of the spinal cord is an apparent mirror image of the other, and the white matter of each half contains groups of nerve fiber tracts (or fasciculi) ascending or descending in the cord.

Cranial Nerves

18

Key Terms

Cranial Nerve Modalities represent the seven specific functional components transmitted within the cranial nerves, including afferent (sensory) as well as efferent (motor) modalites. Although each cranial nerve may transmit one to several modalities, none carry all of them; thus, each cranial nerve possesses specific modalities that are responsible for receiving sensory input from receptors or delivering output from its motor component. An additional component, general proprio-

ception (GP), is generally understood, if not specified, as sensory input from within the muscles innervated by those cranial nerves.

Motor Modalities:
General somatic efferent (GSE) represents motor innervation to skeletal muscles developed from somites.

General visceral efferent (GVE) represents motor fibers that innervate

smooth muscles, cardiac muscles, and glands.

Special visceral efferent (SVE) represents motor fibers to skeletal muscles of branchiomeric origin (pharyngeal arch origin).

Sensory Modalities:
General somatic afferent (GSA) represents general sensation (touch, pressure, temperature, pain) from the skin about the anterior face and lateral head.

General visceral afferent (GVA) represents general sensation from the viscera, generally perceived as pressure and/or pain.

Special somatic afferent (SSA) represents special sensation from the eye (vision) and the ear (auditory and equilibrium).

Special visceral afferent (SVA) represents visceral sensations of smell (olfaction) and taste (gustatory).

CRANIAL NERVES

Twelve pairs of cranial nerves originate in the brain, leave its surface, and pass through certain foramina of the skull to be distributed in and about the head and neck. One cranial nerve, the vagus, continues into the thorax and abdomen to innervate some of the viscera. The cranial nerves are named and numbered sequentially with roman numerals, progressing rostrally to caudally:

I.   Olfactory
II.   Optic
III. Oculomotor
IV.   Trochlear
V.   Trigeminal
VI.   Abducens
VII. Facial
VIII. Vestibulocochlear
IX.   Glossopharyngeal
X.   Vagus
XI.   Accessory
XII. Hypoglossal

Three figures appearing earlier in the book can be reviewed to observe the relative positions of the cranial nerves emerging from the brain (Figs. 17-3 and 17-4) and their relative positions in the floor of the cranial vault (Fig. 9-2).

As explained earlier, peripheral nerves consist of several nerve fiber types specific for their function. Typically, each peripheral nerve contains somatic and visceral components, each with afferent and efferent fibers.

Peripheral nerves emanating from the brain (known as cranial nerves) are more complex than those arising from the spinal cord, since these nerves serve special sensory functions—such as hearing, seeing, smelling, and tasting—in addition to supplying special skeletal muscles of branchiomeric origin.

The cranial nerves, then, carry certain components in addition to the general somatic and general visceral components carried by spinal nerves, designated as special somatic afferent, special visceral afferent, and special visceral efferent.

CRANIAL NERVE MODALITIES

General somatic afferent (GSA)—General sensation in function. For example, the trigeminal nerve serves much of the skin and the mucous membranes of the face, whereas the facial, glossopharyngeal, and vagus nerves serve the area of the ear with general sensation.

General somatic efferent (GSE)—General motor in function to skeletal muscles. This grouping is carried by the oculomotor, trochlear, abducent, and hypoglossal nerves innervating musculature derived from somites.

General visceral afferent (GVA)—General sensation from the viscera included in the facial, glossopharyngeal, and vagus nerves.

General visceral efferent (GVE)—Visceral motor (parasympathetic) to the viscera. Only four cranial nerves transmit parasympathetic fibers: the oculomotor, facial, glossopharyngeal, and vagus nerves.

Special somatic afferent (SSA)—Special sensory in function from the eye and ear. The cranial nerves carrying this component are the optic and vestibulocochlear nerves.

Special visceral afferent (SVA)—Special sensory in function from the viscera. These fibers are associated with the special senses of smell, carried in the olfactory nerve; and taste, transmitted in the facial, glossopharyngeal, and vagus nerves. An easy way to remember the difference between SSA and SVA fibers is that for SVA fibers to be activated, the material has to be dissolved in a fluid (saliva or mucus).

Special visceral efferent (SVE)—Special motor to the branchiomeric musculatures. This component is carried to the muscles derived from the pharyngeal arches and is transmitted by the nerves of those arches: the trigeminal, facial, glossopharyngeal, accessory (contributions to the pharyngeal plexus), and vagus nerves.

As with the typical spinal nerve, cell bodies of afferent nerve fibers of cranial nerves are located in sensory ganglia outside the central nervous system, that is, outside the brain. Central processes of these fibers pass via the cranial nerves into the brain to terminate on neurons that relay impulses for processing, sorting out, and coordinating the information before initiation of a motor response that may or may not be at a conscious level.

All of the interconnections and workings of the brain are extremely complicated and beyond the scope of this text. Readers who want more information about this subject are referred to standard textbooks of neuroanatomy.

Each of the 12 cranial nerves is described in the following sections, including information on the location of the cell bodies, the components carried, connections with other nerves, and finally the distribution and function. A summary of this information is presented in tabular form in Table 18-1.

Table 18-1 Cranial Nerves

Nerve	Components	Cell Bodies	Peripheral Distribution	Function
I Olfactory	SVA	Olfactory epithelial cells	Olfactory nerves	Smell
II Optic	SSA	Ganglion cells of retina	Rods and cones	Vision
III Oculomotor	GSE	Nucleus III	Levator palpebrae; recti: superior, medial, inferior; and inferior oblique	Eye movement
	GVE	Edinger-Westphal nucleus	Ciliary ganglion—Ciliary body—Sphincter pupillae	Contraction of pupil and accomodation
	GP	Mesencephalic nucleus V	Ocular muscles	Kinesthetic sense
IV Trochlear	GSE	Nucleus IV	Superior oblique	Ocular movement
	GP	Mesencephalic nucleus V	Superior oblique	Kinesthetic sense
V Trigeminal	GSA	Trigeminal ganglion	Ophthalmic, maxillary, and mandibular divisions to mucous membranes and skin of face and head	General sensation
	SVE	Motor nucleus V	Temporalis, masseter, pterygoids, anterior belly of digastric, mylohyoid, tensors palatini and tympani	Mastication
	GP	Mesencephalic nucleus V	Muscles of mastication	Kinesthetic sense
VI Abducens	GSE	Nucleus VI	Lateral rectus	Eye movement
	GP	Mesencephalic nucleus V	Lateral rectus	Kinesthetic sense
VII Facial	SVE	Motor nucleus VII	Muscles of facial expression, stapedius, stylohyoid, post, belly of digastric	Facial expression
	GVE	Salivatory nucleus	Greater petrosal— pterygopalatine ganglion—nasal mucosa, lacrimal gland; chorda tympani—lingual nerve, submandibular ganglion—submandibular, sublingual glands	Secretomotor
	SVA	Geniculate ganglion	Chorda tympani—lingual nerve-taste buds anterior two-thirds tongue	Taste
	GVA	Geniculate ganglion	Greater petrosal, chorda tympani	Visceral sensation
	GSA	Geniculate ganglion	Auricular branch—ear and mastoid	Cutaneous sensation

(continued)

Table 18-1 Cranial Nerves

Nerve	Components	Cell Bodies	Peripheral Distribution	Function
VIII Vestibulocochlear	SSA SP	Spiral ganglion Vestibular ganglion	Organ of Corti Vestibular mechanism	Hearing Balance
IX Glosso-pharyngeal	SVA	Inferior ganglion IX	Lingual br.—taste buds posterior one-third tongue, circumvallate papillae	Taste
	GVA	Inferior ganglion IX	Tympanic nerve—middle ear, pharynx, tongue, carotid sinus	Visceral sensation
	GVE	Salivatory nucleus	Tympanic—lesser petrosal—otic ganglion auriculotemporal to parotid gland	Secretomotor
	GSA	Inferior ganglion IX	External ear	Cutaneous sensation
	SVE	Nucleus ambiguns	Stylopharyngeus	Swallowing
X Vagus	GVE	Dorsal motor nucleus X	Cardiac nerves and plexus, ganglia on heart; pulmonary plexus, ganglia respiratory tract; esophageal, gastric, celiac plexus; myenteric and submucous plexus—to transverse colon	Smooth muscle and glands
	SVE	Nucleus ambiguus	Pharyngeal br., superior, inferior laryngeal nerves	Swallowing, speaking
	GVA	Inferior ganglion X	All fibers in all branches	Visceral sensation
	SVA	Inferior ganglion X	Br. to epiglottis, base of tongue, taste buds	Taste
	GSA	Superior ganglion X	Auricular br.—ear, meatus	Cutaneous sensation
XI Accessory	SVE	Nucleus ambiguus	Communication to vagus—muscles of pharynx and larynx	Swallowing, speaking
	SVE (Assuming branchiomeric origin)	Upper spinal cord—lat. column	Spinal portion—sternocleidomastoid, trapezius	Movement, head and shoulder
XII Hypoglossal	GSE	Nucleus XII	Brs. intrinsic, extrinsic muscles of tongue	Tongue movement

GP, general proprioception; GSA indicates general somatic afferent; GSE, general somatic efferent; GVA, general visceral afferent; GVE, general visceral efferent; SP, special proprioception; SSA, special somatic afferent; SVA, special visceral afferent; SVE, special visceral efferent.

I. OLFACTORY NERVE

 Summary Bite. SVA is the only modality carried by the olfactory nerve.

Cell bodies of the olfactory nerve, the nerve of smell, are found in the olfactory mucosa situated over the superior nasal concha. Axons of the olfactory nerve pass through the cribriform plate of the ethmoid bone to terminate in the **olfactory bulb**, which is connected to the brain by the **olfactory tract**, technically a part of the brain (Fig. 18-1 and Tables 18-1 and 18-5).

II. OPTIC NERVE

 Summary Bite. SSA is the only modality carried by the optic nerve.

Cell bodies of the optic nerve, the nerve of sight, are located in the ganglionic layer of cells composing the retina. Axons of these cells are gathered into bundles that leave the bulb of the eye as the optic nerve, passing posteriorly through the orbit to exit through the optic foramen. Here the axons join the optic nerve of the opposite side, forming the **optic chiasma**. Optic tracts continue from the chiasma to enter the base of

Clinical Considerations

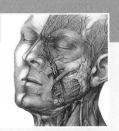

Anosmia

Anosmia results following a unilateral lesion either within the olfactory epithelium or within the olfactory nerve, causing the patient to experience complete loss of the sense of smell on the side of the lesion.

the brain near the cerebral peduncle (Fig. 18-2 and Tables 18-1 and 18-5).

III. OCULOMOTOR NERVE

Summary Bite. GSE, GVE, and GP (general proprioception to the extraocular muscles for kinesthetic sense) are the modalities carried by the oculomotor nerve.

The oculomotor nerve serves all of the extrinsic muscles of the eye, excluding the superior oblique and the lateral rectus muscles, with general somatic efferent innervation. A specialized group of autonomic motor cells in the oculomotor nucleus within the brain is termed the **Edinger–Westphal nucleus.** These are preganglionic parasympathetic neurons whose fibers are destined for the ciliary ganglion within the orbit. Postganglionic fibers from the ciliary ganglion pass to the orb via short ciliary nerves and on to the ciliary body and sphincter pupillae muscles of the eye (see Table 18-2).

The oculomotor nerve exits the brain near the medial side of the cerebral peduncle, passes through the free and attached borders of the tentorium cerebelli, and then passes through the lateral wall of the cavernous sinus to enter the superior orbital fissure for distribution. While in the cavernous sinus, contributions from the carotid plexus are communicated to the oculomotor nerve. These communications are the postganglionic **sympathetic** fibers from the superior cervical ganglion destined for the dilatator pupillae muscle of the eye.

Once in the orbit, the oculomotor nerve divides into superior and inferior divisions, facilitating innervation of the extraocular muscles. The ciliary ganglion

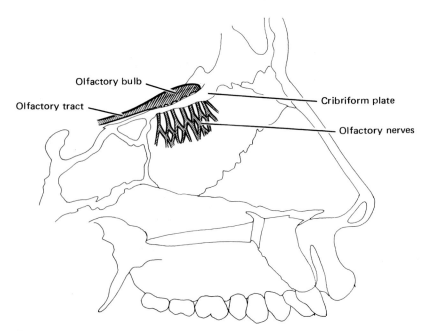

Olfactory bulb

Olfactory tract

Cribriform plate

Olfactory nerves

Figure 18-1. I. Olfactory nerve.

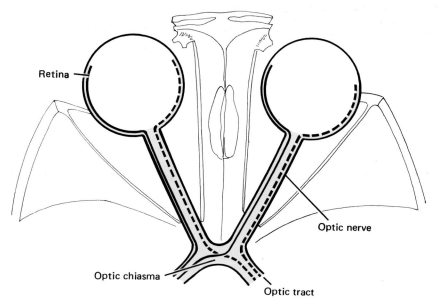

Figure 18-2. II. Optic nerve. Observe the crossing over of fibers at the optic chiasma.

Clinical Considerations

Myopia and Hyperopia

Changes in the longitudinal dimension of the optical axis will cause images to be focused either anterior (myopia) or posterior (hyperopia) to the retina. This is usually the result of changes in the refractive elements of the eye, notably the cornea, which experiences a slight change in shape. There may also occur an alteration in the dimension of the orb. Often, both processes occur as a function of aging. These conditions can be diagnosed and treated with prescription-ground glasses that can optically correct for the alteration in the longitudinal dimension of the optical axis.

Multiple Sclerosis (MS)

Multiple sclerosis is one of the demyelinating diseases that affects the optic nerve but not the other cranial nerves. This is because the myelin surrounding the optic nerves is produced by glial cells rather than by Schwann cells, as in other cranial nerves.

Detached Retina

The 10-layered retina is loosely attached to the choroid layer of the orb and is retained in that position by the vitreous body. Sudden jolts absorbed in the orbit may detach the retina, causing a medical emergency. The detached retina is sightless but sight can usually be restored by surgical reattachment of the retina.

Cataract

Cataract is an age-related condition where the lens loses its transparency and becomes clouded, causing blurred vision. It is the major cause of poor vision and blindness throughout the world. Modern techniques now permit surgical placement of plastic lenses, resulting in restored vision.

Presbyopia

Presbyopia is associated with aging. It results from the inability of the eye to focus on close objects (accommodation), which is related to the lens becoming less elastic, thus light cannot be focused properly on the retina.

Table 18-2 Parasympathetic Ganglia of the Head

Preganglionic Parasympathetic				Postganglionic Parasympathetic		
Nucleus of Origin	Cranial Nerve of Origin	Preganglionic Nerve	Parasympathetic Ganglion	Trigeminal Nerve Association	Delivery Nerve	Target: Smooth Muscle, Gland
Edinger-Westphal	Oculomotor III	Unnamed	**Ciliary** (GVE)	Ophthalmic (V₁)	Short ciliary from ganglion	Sphincter pupillae, ciliary body
Super salivatory	Facial VII	Greater petrosal	**Pterygopalatine** (GVE)	Maxillary (V₂)	Zygomatico-temporal to lacrimal of (V₁)	Lacrimal gland
Superior salivatory	Facial VII	Greater petrosal	**Pterygopalatine** (GVE)	Maxillary (V₂)	Greater; lesser palatine; post. sup. nasal, nasopalatine; post., middle, ant. sup. alveolars	Mucous glands of nasal cavity, max, sinus, and palate
Superior salivatory	Facial VII	Chorda tympani	**Submandibular** (GVE)	Mandibular (V₃)	Lingual	Submandibular and sublingual glands, minor glands in floor of mouth
Inferior salivatory	Glosso-pharyngeal IX	Lesser petrosal	**Otic** (GVE)	Mandibular (V₃)	Auriculotemporal	Parotid gland

GVE indicates general visceral efferent.

is suspended from the inferior division by the parasympathetic motor root of the ganglion. Additional communications to the ganglion are from the nasociliary nerve, a branch of the ophthalmic division of the trigeminal nerve. These communications are purely sensory, passing through the ganglion without synapsing there. Thus, these somatic sensory nerves reach their destination in the orb by way of the short ciliary nerves. Postganglionic sympathetic fibers may also communicate with the ganglion in a fashion similar to that of the nasociliary nerve; however,

these sympathetic fibers are destined for the dilatator pupillae muscle. The functions of these intrinsic muscles of the eye are detailed in Chapter 10.

Proprioceptive fibers of the extraocular muscles are carried in the oculomotor nerve, then transmitted to the ophthalmic division of the trigeminal nerve to join it in the orbit, or via communications while it passes through the walls of the cavernous sinus. Terminations of these fibers are described in the section on the trigeminal nerve (Fig. 18-3 and Tables 18-1, 18-2, and 18-5).

Clinical Considerations

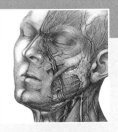

Oculomotor Nerve Injury

Injury to the oculomotor nerve will result in palsy on the ipsilateral side with dilated pupil and ptosis. Additionally, the bulb of the eye will turn down and out with a con-comitant inability to move the eye either up or down; moreover, the pupillary reflex will be lost.

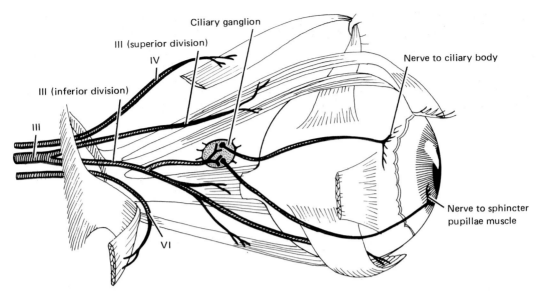

Figure 18-3. III. Oculomotor nerve. IV. Trochlear nerve. VI. Abducens nerve. Observe that the trochlear and abducens nerves innervate only one muscle each. Note the ciliary ganglion and the distribution of the postganglionic parasympathetic fibers from it.

IV. TROCHLEAR NERVE

Summary Bite. GSE and GP (general proprioception fibers to the extraocular muscle for kinesthetic sense) are the modalities carried by the trochlear nerve.

The trochlear nerve, the smallest of the cranial nerves, supplies the superior oblique muscle of the eye with motor innervation. This is the only cranial nerve originating on the dorsal surface of the brainstem. From there, it passes around the midbrain to pierce the tentorial dura, thus entering the cavernous sinus. While coursing through the wall of the cavernous sinus, the trochlear nerve communicates with the carotid plexus and the ophthalmic division of the trigeminal nerve. Proprioceptive fibers from the superior oblique muscle are thought to communicate with the ophthalmic nerve at that point. On entering the orbit through the superior orbital fissure, the nerve terminates in the superior oblique muscle, which it provides with motor innervation (Fig. 18-3 and Tables 18-1 and 18-5).

V. TRIGEMINAL NERVE

Summary Bite. GSA, SVE, and GP (general proprioception fibers to the muscles of mastication for kinesthetic sense) are the modalities carried by the trigeminal nerve.

The largest of the cranial nerves, the trigeminal nerve serves much of the face, the teeth and supporting structures, most of the anterior portion of the oral cavity, and the mucous membranes of the head with cutaneous sensation. Also, it provides motor innerva-

Clinical Considerations

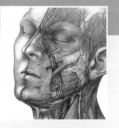

Trochlear Nerve Injury

The trochlear nerve provides motor innervation only to the superior oblique muscle. When this cranial nerve is injured, the superior oblique muscle on the ipsilateral side will be paralyzed, causing the eyeball to rotate outward, resulting in double vision.

tion to the muscles of mastication. The nerve has two roots emanating from the pons. The larger, sensory root, which lies lateral to the motor root, contains the central processes of the neurons whose cell bodies are found in the **trigeminal (semilunar) ganglion**, the sensory ganglion of the trigeminal nerve. This ganglion is located under the cover of the dura in a pocket (the Meckel cave) on the trigeminal impression located near the apex of the petrous portion of the temporal bone. Peripheral processes of the sensory neurons located in the flat, semilunar-shaped ganglion are gathered in three separate bundles. These bundles leave the ganglion as the ophthalmic, maxillary, and mandibular divisions of the trigeminal nerve. The motor root courses beneath the trigeminal ganglion, proceeds medial to the sensory root, and the two leave the skull via the foramen ovale and then join each other to form the mandibular division of the trigeminal nerve. Thus, the mandibular division is mixed in function. The ophthalmic and maxillary divisions are purely sensory, and they leave the cranial vault via the superior orbital fissure and foramen rotundum, respectively.

The four parasympathetic ganglia of the head are in close association with the trigeminal nerve, although, functionally, these ganglia are not part of the trigeminal nerve. Postganglionic parasympathetic fibers arising in these ganglia are transmitted to the structures they serve by joining branches of the trigeminal nerve for distribution. The parasympathetic ganglia, the preganglionic motor root, and the associated divisions of the trigeminal nerve are listed in Table 18-2 (Figs. 18-4 through 18-7 and Tables 18-1 and 18-3 through 18-5).

OPHTHALMIC NERVE V₁

Summary Bite. GSA is the only modality carried by the ophthalmic division of the trigeminal nerve.

The ophthalmic nerve supplies the bulb and conjunctiva of the eye, the lacrimal gland, the skin of the forehead and nose, and the mucous membranes of the paranasal sinuses with sensory innervation. The ophthalmic nerve leaves the superior aspect of the trigeminal ganglion, then lies in the lateral wall of the cavernous sinus as it courses to the orbit (Fig. 18-4 and Tables 18-3 and 18-5). Along the way, tentorial branches are supplied to the tentorium. Just before

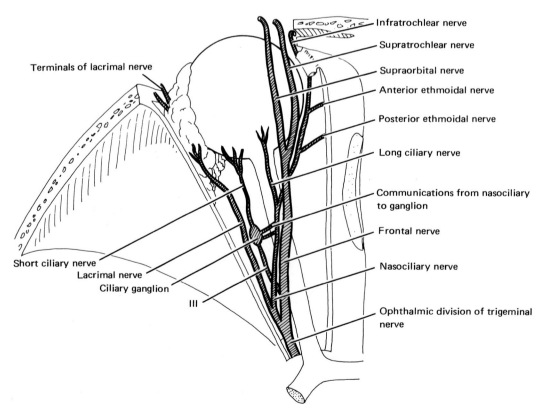

Figure 18-4. V. Trigeminal nerve, ophthalmic division. Note the communications to the ciliary ganglion from the nasociliary nerve.

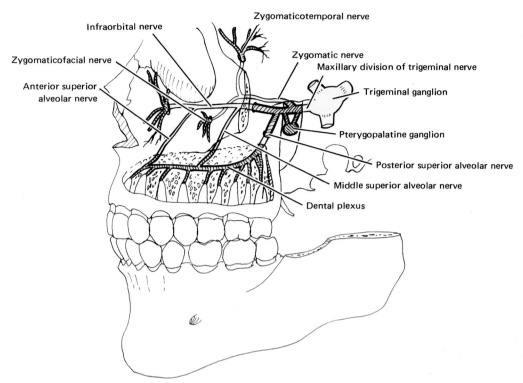

Figure 18-5. V. Trigeminal nerve, maxillary division.

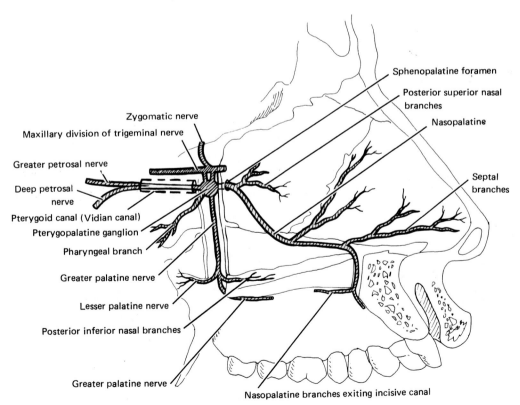

Figure 18-6. Pterygopalatine ganglion and connections.

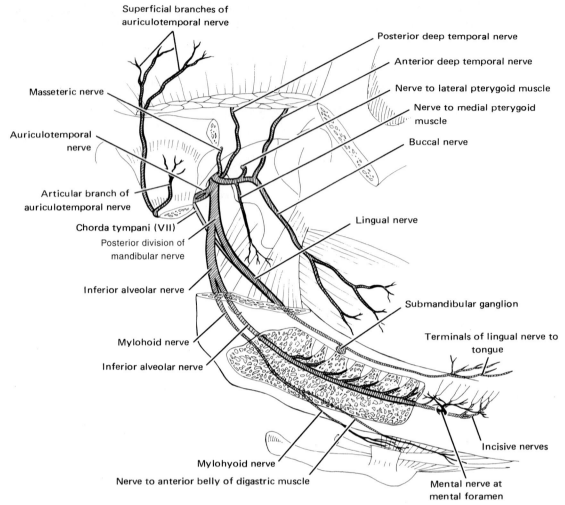

Superficial branches of auriculotemporal nerve

Posterior deep temporal nerve

Anterior deep temporal nerve

Nerve to lateral pterygoid muscle

Nerve to medial pterygoid muscle

Masseteric nerve

Buccal nerve

Auriculotemporal nerve

Articular branch of auriculotemporal nerve

Lingual nerve

Chorda tympani (VII)

Posterior division of mandibular nerve

Inferior alveolar nerve

Submandibular ganglion

Terminals of lingual nerve to tongue

Mylohoid nerve

Inferior alveolar nerve

Incisive nerves

Mylohyoid nerve

Nerve to anterior belly of digastric muscle

Mental nerve at mental foramen

Figure 18-7. V. Trigeminal nerve, mandibular division. Observe the chorda tympani from the facial nerve joining the lingual nerve.

entering the orbit through the superior orbital fissure, the nerve divides into three separate nerves: the lacrimal, frontal, and nasociliary nerves. In its course, the ophthalmic nerve communicates with the carotid plexus in the cavernous sinus and with other cranial nerves represented in the orbit. However, discussion of these communications is not warranted here.

Lacrimal Nerve

The lacrimal nerve, the smallest branch of the ophthalmic division, runs along the lateral rectus muscle distributing to the lacrimal gland and adjacent conjunctiva. It then exits the orbit to be distributed to the skin of the lateral aspect of the upper eyelid (Fig. 18-4). While in the orbit, it communicates with the zygomaticotemporal branch of the zygomatic nerve of the maxillary division of the trigeminal nerve, which is carrying postganglionic parasympathetic fibers communicated to it from the pterygopalatine ganglion.

These parasympathetic fibers are then transmitted to the lacrimal gland via the lacrimal nerve, thus providing it with secretomotor innervation (see Table 18-2).

Frontal Nerve

The frontal nerve, the largest branch of the ophthalmic nerve, divides shortly after entering the superior aspect of the orbit into a smaller supratrochlear and a larger supraorbital nerve. The former passes medial to the latter as the nerves course anteriorly above the levator palpebrae superioris muscle (Fig. 18-4). The **supratrochlear nerve** bends to pass superior to the pulley of the superior oblique muscle. Here it provides sensory innervation to the conjunctiva and skin of the medial aspect of the upper eyelid before leaving the orbit to turn upward to supply the skin over the forehead. The **supraorbital nerve** continues forward to exit the orbit at the supraorbital notch. While passing the notch, it sends a filament

Table 18-3 Trigeminal Nerve—Sensory Components

Division of Trigeminal Nerve	Modality	Nerve Branch(es)	Foramen of Passage	Associated Parasympathetic Ganglion/Nerve	Sensory Region Served
Ophthalmic (V₁)	GSA	**Lacrimal**	*Exits* Superior orbital fissure	Zygomaticotemporal of V₂, delivers post. para. from pterygopalatine ganglion (VII) for lacrimal gland (GVE)	Lacrimal gland, adjacent conjunctiva, lateralaspect of skin of upper eyelid
		Frontal	*Exits* Superior orbital fissure		
		Supratrochlear			Conjunctiva and skin of the medial portion of the eye and skin over the forehead
		Supraorbital			Filament to frontal sinus, upper eyelid, forehead, and scalp
		Nasociliary	*Exits* Superior orbital fissure	Ciliary ganglion (III) & possibly post. sym. from carotid plexus (GVE) (Postganglionic sympathetic to dilatator pupillae)	
		Long ciliary			Orb, cornea
		Posterior ethmoidal			P.E. foramen—ethmoidal, sphenoidal, frontal sinuses
		Anterior ethmoidal			A.E. foramen—ethmoidal, sphenoidal, frontal sinuses
		Internal nasal			Mucous membranes
		External nasal			Ala and globus of nose
		Infratrochlear			Conjunctiva, eyelid, caruncula, lacrimal sac, side of nose
Maxillary (V₂)	GSA	**Zygomatic**	*Exits* Rotundum	Pterygopalatine ganglion (VII) delivers post. para. secretomotor fibers to zyygomaticotemporal nerve for distribution to lacrimal nerve to lacrimal gland (GVE)	
		Zygomaticofacial			Skin of the cheek
		Zygomaticotemporal		Delivers secretomotor fibers to lacrimal nerve for lacrimal gland	Skin of temporal region
Maxillary (V₂)	GSA	Pterygopalatine	These nerves serve as a functional connection to the pterygopalatine ganglion permitting passage of post. para. to zygomatic nerve and sensory fibers from maxillary through ganglion to become other named branches of the maxillary nerve		
		Orbital	*Enters* Inferior orbital fissure		Periorbita, ethmoid, and sphenoid sinuses

(continued)

Table 18-3   Trigeminal Nerve—Sensory Components *(continued)*

Division of Trigeminal Nerve	Modality	Nerve Branch(es)	Foramen of Passage	Associated Parasympathetic Ganglion/Nerve	Sensory Region Served
		Greater palatine	*Exits* Greater palatine	Pterygopalatine ganglion (VII) delivers post. para. secretomotor fibers to small glands of the nasal cavity, pharynx, and palate (GVE)	Adjacent soft palate, hard palate, gingiva, mucous membranes anteriorly to incisor teeth (communicates with nasopalatine)
		Lesser palatine	*Exits* Lesser palatine	Delivers secretomotor fibers to glands of soft palate	Soft palate, tonsil, and uvula. (Many of the afferents were communicated from facial nerve)
		Posterior superior nasal branches	*Exits* Sphenopalatine	Delivers secretomotor fibers to glands of nasal cavity	Nasal cavity supplying mucous memb. of sup. and middle conchae, median nasal septum and ethmoid sinus. Major trunk is nasopalatine
		Nasopalatine	*Exits* Incisive canal	Delivers secretomotor fibers to glands of nasal cavity	Between septum and mucous memb. to incisive canal. Serves anterior palate as far laterally as cuspid. (Communicates with greater palatine nerve)
		Pharyngeal br.	*Enters* Pharyngeal canal	Delivers secretomotor fibers to glands of nasopharynx and spheniod sinus	Enters pharyngeal canal. Serves m. memb. and nasopharynx to auditory tube
		Posterior superior alveolar[a]	*Enters* Poster or superior alveolar		Sometimes branched. Passes over max. tuberosity to serve m. memb. of cheek and adjacent gingiva. Enters P.S.A.F to distribute to max. sinus and to roots of 3 max. molars (except mesial buccal root of 1st molar)
Maxillary (V$_2$)	GSA	**Infraorbital**	This nerve is a continuation of the maxillary nerve into the floor of the orbit via the inferior orbital fissure and exiting the skull at the infraorbital foramen		
		Middle superior alveolar[a]			Lateral wall of max.sinus, enters mesial buccal root of 1st molar and all roots of premolars
		Anterior superior alveolar[a]			Anterior max. sinus, and roots of anterior teeth, and twigs to floor of nasal cavity serving inferior meatus, and adjacent m. membrane
		Inferior palpebral brs.	*Exits* Infraorbital		Skin and conjunctiva of the lower eyelid
		External nasal brs.	*Exits* Infraorbital		Skin about the lateral aspect of the nose

(continued)

Table 18-3 Trigeminal Nerve—Sensory Components

Division of Trigeminal Nerve	Modality	Nerve Branch(es)	Foramen of Passage	Associated Parasympathetic Ganglion/Nerve	Sensory Region Served
		Superior labial brs.	*Exits* Infraorbital		Skin and mucous memb. of the upper lip
Mandibular (V₃)	GSA	Sensory root	*Exits* Ovale	Sensory and motor roots join outside the skull (F. ovale) to form a mixed nerve. Some branches are sensory, some motor, whereas some are mixed	
		From trunk **Recurrent meningeal**	*Enters* Spinosum		Dura and mastoid air cells
		From anterior division **Buccal**			Skin of cheek over buccinator muscle passes through buccinator muscle to serve buccal mucosa and adjacent gingiva. (May communicate with facial nerve for distribution purposes)
		Articular br. to TMJ *From:* masseteric nerve[b]			TMJ
		From posterior division **Lingual**		Joined by chorda tympani (VII) delivering taste fibers (SVA) to ant. 2/3 of tongue, and pre. para to submandibular ganglion (VII) delivers post.para from ganglion to sublingual and minor salivary glands of the floor of the mouth (GVE)	Anterior 2/3 of tongue with GSA and delivers SVA (taste) from facial nerve to taste buds in anterior 2/3 of tongue. Post.para from submandibular ganglion pass directly to submandibular gland. Those destined for sublingual gland and other minor glands reenter the lingual and get distributed to the glands.
		Inferior alveolar	*Enters* Mandibular		Mandibular teeth and supporting tissues via a dental plexus, two terminals—main trunk continues to incisor teeth, other terminal is mental nerve
		Mental	*Exits* Mental		Skin of chin, lower lip including mucous membrane
		Auriculo-temporal		Otic ganglion (IX) communicates post. para fibers for distribution to the parotid gland (GVE)	Distribute superficial temporal nerves over skin of temple. Articular brs. toTMJ secretomotor fibers from otic ganglion to parotid gland

GSA indicates general somatic afferent; GVE, general visceral efferent; TMJ, temporomandibular joint.
[a]Posterior, middle, and anterior superior alveolar nerves communicate, forming a dental plexus before innervating the teeth.
[b]The masseteric nerve from the anterior division is a mixed nerve. Its sensory fibers are the articular branches to the TMJ.

Table 18-4 Trigeminal Nerve—Motor Components

Division of Trigeminal Nerve	Modality	Nerve Branch	Motor to Muscles
Mandibular (V₃)	SVE	Sensory and motor roots of the trigeminal nerve exit the foramen ovale and then join to form the trunk of the nerve, which then divides into anterior and posterior divisions. Some nerves are sensory, some motor, and some mixed. Only motor components are presented.	
		From Trunk	
		Nerve to medial pterygoid	Medial pterygoid
		Nerve to tensor tympani	Tensor tympani
		Nerve to tensor veli palatini	Tensor veli palatini
		From Anterior Division	
		Deep temporal nerves (anterior and posterior)	Temporalis
		Lateral pterygoid nerve	Lateral pterygoid
		Masseteric nerve	Masseter
		From Posterior Division	
		Mylohyoid nerve	Mylohyoid
		Nerve to anterior digastric	Anterior diagastric

SVE indicates special visceral efferent.

into the frontal sinus. The nerve supplies sensory innervation to the upper lid, forehead, and scalp as far posteriorly as the lambdoidal suture.

Nasociliary Nerve

The nasociliary nerve enters the orbit between the lateral rectus muscle and the oculomotor nerve. It then passes obliquely over the optic nerve to the medial wall of the orbit, where its terminal branch enters the anterior ethmoidal foramen (Fig. 18-4). Just before entering the foramen, the nasociliary nerve gives off an **infratrochlear branch**, which courses anteriorly along the medial wall of the orbit and exits at its medial margin. Along the way, the branch provides sensory innervation to the conjunctiva, eyelid, lacrimal sac, caruncula, and side of the nose. **Anterior** and **posterior ethmoidal branches** enter the same-named foramina to supply the ethmoidal, sphenoidal, and frontal sinuses. The **anterior ethmoidal nerve** continues through the ethmoid bone to enter the nasal cavity. **Internal nasal branches** arising from it innervate the mucous membranes of the nasal cavity. The anterior ethmoidal nerve continues anteriorly to exit the nasal cavity at the inferior border of the nasal bone as the **external nasal branch**, providing general sensation to the ala and globe of the nose.

While in the orbit, the nasociliary nerve sends **long ciliary nerves** to the eyeball as the nerve crosses the optic nerve. Other short filaments pass to the ciliary ganglion, establishing a close association with

this parasympathetic ganglion. The long ciliary nerves and those filaments that pass to the ganglion and on to the eyeball, as part of the short ciliary nerves are purely sensory and are destined for the iris and cornea. Postganglionic sympathetic fibers communicate to the ophthalmic nerve from the carotid plexus while passing through the cavernous sinus, or they may accompany the long ciliary nerves or the short filaments to the ganglion and on to the eyeball via the short ciliary nerves. These postganglionic sympathetic fibers are destined for the dilatator pupillae muscle within the iris.

Maxillary Nerve V₂

 Summary Bite. GSA is the only modality carried by the maxillary division of the trigeminal nerve.

The maxillary nerve, the second division of the trigeminal nerve, is purely sensory and serves the skin of the side of the nose; cheek; eyelids; mid-face; nasopharynx; tonsil; palate; maxillary sinus; and gingiva, teeth, and associated structures of the upper jaw. The nerve exits the cranial vault via the foramen rotundum after passing through the posterior portion of the cavernous sinus. From the foramen rotundum, the nerve courses through the pterygopalatine fossa to enter the floor of the orbit at the inferior orbital fissure. Here, the nerve becomes known as the infraorbital nerve, enters the infraorbital canal, and then

Table 18-5 Cranial Nerves—Clinical Testing

Cranial Nerve	Modality	Assessment Technique	Perceived Dysfunction
I Olfactory	SVA	Patient is asked to differentiate distinct odors (coffee, vanilla) with eyes covered. Test each side independently.	Damage such as an ethmoid fracture may result in anosmia (loss of sense of smell).
II Optic	SSA	Eye charts are used to assess visual acuity. Visual fields are determined by examining when patient observes an object moving from lateral to medial. Ophthalmoscope used for observing retina, optic disc, and blood vessels.	Damage to the retina usually results in blindness to the affected eye. Damage beyond the optic chiasma will present partial visual losses.
III Oculomotor	GSE	Patient is asked to follow with his or her eyes the examiner's finger as it moves up and down vertically and medially and laterally. Watch for crossing of eyes during convergence.	Damage to this modality may cause paralysis of all extraocular muscles except the superior oblique and lateral rectus. This produces lateral strabismus and inability to look vertically. Also ptosis (eyelid drooping). Damage to this modality will produce lack of pupillary reflex, dilated pupils, and lack of changes in pupil at close focus.
	GVE	Examine patient for pupillary reflex with light shining on and off in each eye. Observe and compare contractions and dilations in affected and unaffected eyes.	
IV Trochlear	GSE	Analysis of function is performed during testing of the oculomotor nerve.	Damage to this nerve causes double vision and inability to rotate the eye inferolaterally.
V Trigeminal Ophthalmic division (V_1)	GSA	Test for corneal reflex with whisp of cotton. Prick forehead with pin (pain), apply warm and cold objects (temperature).	Damage to this division will inhibit the corneal reflex and will reduce or inhibit sensation over the (V_1) zone.
Maxillary division (V_2)	GSA	Stroke sensory zone of (V_2) with eyes closed (light touch), prick with pin (pain), apply warm and cold objects (temperature).	Damage to this division will reduce or inhibit sensation over the (V_2) zone.
Mandibular division (V_3)	GSA	Stroke sensory zone of (V_3) with eyes closed (light touch), prick with pin (pain), apply warm and cold objects (temperature).	Damage to this division will reduce or inhibit sensation over the (V_3) zone.
Mandibular division (V_3)	SVE	Ask patient to clench jaws, open, then move jaw side to side with resistance. Muscle strength in the temporalis and masseter should be compared from side to side by palpation.	Damage in this modality may cause paralysis of the muscles of mastication, thus causing the jaw to deviate same side as the lesion.
VI Abducens	GSE	Analysis of function is performed during testing of the oculomotor nerve.	Damage to this nerve causes double vision and paralysis of the lateral rectus muscle, thus the eye remains rotated medially on the affected side.
VII Facial	SVA	Test for taste for sweet and salty on anterior 2/3 of tongue.	Damage to this modality will reduce or inhibit the sensation of taste on the anterior 2/3 of the tongue.
	GVE	Observe tearing with pungent fumes (ammonia).	Damage to this modality will reduce or inhibit the ability to secrete tears from the affected side. Mucus production in the nasal cavity and salivary gland secretions from the submandibular and sublingual glands is more difficult to evaluate.

(continued)

Table 18-5   Cranial Nerves—Clinical Testing *(continued)*

Cranial Nerve	Modality	Assessment Technique	Perceived Dysfunction
	SVE	Observe symmetry of face when asked to close eyes, frown, smile, whistle, raise eyebrows. Look for flacid sagging of face.	Damage to this modality, such as in stroke, causes a paralysis of the muscles of facial expression, which causes the face to sag and an inability to make facial expressions on the affected side.
VIII Vestibulocochlear Cochlear division	SSA	Test with a tuning fork by air and bone conduction.	Loss of hearing by air conduction indicates a lesion or damage to the middle ear. Loss by bone conduction indicates nerve deafness.
Vestibular division	GSA (SP)	Test walking a straight line, dizziness. Watch for rapid eye movements.	Damage to the vestibular division elicits dizziness, nausea, vomiting, and uncontrolled rapid eye movement.
IX Glossopharyngeal	GVA	Test for gag reflex and swallowing and position of the uvula during this procedure. Test touch reception on the posterior 1/3 of the tongue.[b]	Damage to this modality would reduce or inhibit the gag reflex and produce difficulty in swallowing. It would also reduce or inhibit general sensation on the posterior 1/3 of the tongue. Sensation to the carotid body and sinus would also be lost, thereby altering blood pressure and oxygen tension in the bloodstream.
	SVA	Test for bitter and sour taste on the posterior 1/3 of the tongue and on circumvallate papillae.	Damage to this modality would reduce or inhibit the sense of taste over the posterior 1/3 of the tongue and on the circumvallate papillae.
	GVE	Observe saliva flow from the parotid duct.	Damage to this modality would reduce or inhibit saliva secretion from the parotid gland.
X Vagus[c]	SVE	Have patient elevate the palate by saying "aahhhh," swallow, and speak.	Damage to this component will prevent the palate from being elevated and will make swallowing and speech difficult.
XI Accessory[d]	SVE	Have patient shrug shoulders and rotate head against resistance.	Damage to this modality would reduce or inhibit the movement of the head and shoulders.
XII Hypoglossal	GSE	Have patient protrude and retract tongue.	Damage to this nerve will cause the tongue to deviate toward the affected side on protrusion, and that side will appear shrunken and wrinkled.

GSA, general somatic afferent; GSE, general somatic afferent; GVE, general visceral efferent; SP, special proprioception; SSA, special somatic afferent; SVA indicates special visceral afferent; SVE, special visceral efferent.

[a]Note that some modalities associated with certain cranial nerves are not represented in this table because some areas of the head and neck receive overlapping innervation from more than one cranial nerve, thus complicating definitive testing. For example the area about the ear/auditory meatus receives sensory innervation from several cranial nerves in addition to contributions from the cervical plexus, thereby making assessment extremely difficult.

[b]Because there is close association and intermingling of nerve fibers of the glossopharyngeal, vagus, and accessory nerves, it is difficult to distinguish the affected nerve in clinical testing procedures. However, the gag reflex is generally considered the definitive test for glossopharyngeal nerve damage.

[c]Although the vagus nerve serves visceral structures in the thorax and abdomen, the contents of the table are restricted to its functions in the head and neck.

[d]This assumes that the SVE component of the accessory nerve that serves the sternocleidomastoid and trapezius muscles is from the cranial root of the accessory nerve. Remember that the SVE component of the vagus is also part of the cranial root of the accessory nerve. Therefore, damage to this root would affect both areas served by the vagus and the accessory nerves.

exits on the face through the infraorbital foramen (Figs. 18-5 and 18-6 and Tables 18-3 and 18-5).

Along its route, the maxillary nerve provides several branches in the cranial vault, pterygopalatine fossa, and orbit, as well as on the face. While in the cranial vault, its **middle meningeal nerve** supplies the dura. Several branches also arise from the nerve as it traverses the pterygopalatine fossa.

Zygomatic Nerve

The zygomatic nerve, the first branch to arise from the maxillary nerve while it traverses the pteryogpalatine fossa, passes into the orbit and divides into the **zygomaticofacial** and **zygomaticotemporal nerves**. Both of these nerves enter the zygomatic bone and exit it through the like-named foramina on its external surface (Fig. 18-5). The zygomaticofacial nerve exits on the face, providing sensation for the cheek. The zygomaticotemporal nerve exits in the temporal fossa to distribute to the skin of the side of the forehead. Before leaving the orbit, the zygomaticotemporal nerve supplies a branch to the lacrimal nerve. This communication is a postganglionic parasympathetic fiber derived from cranial nerve VII, passed to the zygomatic nerve from the pterygopalatine ganglion (see Table 18-2). The pterygopalatine ganglion lies in close association with the maxillary nerve within the pterygopalatine fossa and is connected to it via two **pterygopalatine nerves** (Fig. 18-6).

Pterygopalatine Nerves

The pterygopalatine nerves are part of the maxillary nerve rather than part of the pterygopalatine ganglion, although they serve as functional communications to the ganglion by permitting the passage of postganglionic parasympathetic fibers from the ganglion to the nerve trunk for distribution to the lacrimal gland (Fig. 18-6 and Table 18-2).

Additional postganglionic parasympathetic fibers are communicated from the pterygopalatine ganglion to branches of the maxillary nerve destined for glands in the palate and nasal cavity, where these parasympathetic fibers serve secretomotor function.

There are several branches of the maxillary nerve that appear to originate from the ganglion but actually are branches of the two pterygopalatine nerves. These branches emerge after the pterygopalatine nerves have passed through the ganglion. They are the orbital, palatine, posterior superior nasal, and pharyngeal branches.

Orbital Branches

The orbital branches enter the orbit to supply the periorbita and the posterior ethmoidal and sphenoidal sinuses.

Greater Palatine Nerve

The greater palatine nerve leaves the ganglion to enter and descend in the pterygopalatine canal, finally to emerge on the palate through the greater palatine foramen (Fig. 18-6).

The greater palatine nerve serves the anterior border of the soft palate, hard palate, gingiva, and mucous membranes of this region as far anteriorly as the incisive teeth, where it communicates with the nasopalatine nerve.

In its descent in the pterygopalatine canal, **posteroinferior nasal branches** are given off, innervating the inferior concha and the middle and inferior meatuses.

The greater palatine nerve splits while in the canal to form a **lesser palatine nerve**, which exits on the palate through two or three like-named foramina serving the soft palate, tonsil, and uvula (Fig. 18-6).

Many of the afferents to this region are from the facial nerve communicated to the lesser palatine nerve through the pterygopalatine ganglion by way of the greater petrosal nerve and the nerve of the pterygoid canal. These nerves are described with the facial nerve.

Posterior Superior Nasal Branches

Posterior superior nasal branches enter the nasal cavity from the sphenopalatine foramen to supply the mucous membrane over the middle and superior conchae, the median nasal septum, and the ethmoidal sinus (Fig. 18-6).

One of these branches, the **nasopalatine nerve**, is larger than the others and continues anteriorly between the median nasal septum and the mucous membrane to reach the incisive canal, through which it passes to communicate with its counterpart from the opposite side (Fig. 18-6). It serves the anterior palate as far posteriorly as the cuspid teeth, where it overlaps the distribution of the greater palatine nerve.

Pharyngeal Branch

A pharyngeal branch leaves the posterior aspect of the ganglion to enter the pharyngeal canal. It serves the mucous membrane and the nasopharynx as far as the auditory tube (Fig. 18-6).

Posterior Superior Alveolar Nerve(s)

Arising from the main trunk of the maxillary nerve, while still in the pterygopalatine fossa, is (are) the posterior superior alveolar nerve(s) (Fig. 18-5).

This nerve, which may display more than one terminal, passes down over the tuberosity of the maxilla providing branches to the mucous membrane of the cheek and the adjacent gingiva.

The posterior superior alveolar nerve then enters the same-named foramen to supply the maxillary sinus and the molar teeth, with the exception of the mesial buccal root of the first molar. Sensory innervation to this root is provided by the middle superior alveolar nerve, which is described in the next section.

Infraorbital Nerve

After traversing the pterygopalatine fossa, the maxillary nerve enters the floor of the orbit, thus becoming the infraorbital nerve (Fig. 18-5).

On entering the floor of the orbit, the infraorbital nerve sends a **middle superior alveolar nerve** over the lateral wall of the maxillary sinus, which it innervates. Branches of this nerve then enter the mesial buccal root of the first molar and all of the roots of the premolar teeth.

Continuing anteriorly, the infraorbital nerve provides an anterior superior alveolar nerve just before its exit from the infraorbital foramen. The **anterior superior alveolar nerve** supplies the anterior maxillary sinus and the roots of the anterior teeth. Also, small twigs of this nerve enter the nasal cavity to supply its floor, the inferior meatus, and adjacent mucous membrane.

The posterior, middle, and anterior superior alveolar nerves intermingle, forming a dental plexus before innervating the upper teeth.

As the infraorbital nerve exits the skull via the same-named foramen, it provides the following three major groups:

- **Inferior palpebral branches**, ascending to the lower eyelid.
- **External nasal braches**, serving the side of the nose.
- **Superior labial branches**, serving the upper lip.

Mandibular Nerve V₃

Summary Bite. GSA, SVE, and GP (general proprioception fibers to the muscles of mastication kinesthetic sense) are the modalities carried by the mandibular division of the trigeminal nerve.

The mandibular nerve, the largest division of the trigeminal nerve, is the only division containing both motor and sensory components. The sensory fibers serve the skin about the lower face, cheek and lower lip, ear, external acoustic meatus, temporomandibular joint, and skin about the temporal region. This sensory component also supplies the mucous membranes of the cheek, the mucosa of the anterior two thirds of the tongue, the mandibular teeth, and sup-

porting tissues and gingiva, mastoid air cells, the mandible, and portions of the dura.

The motor component supplies all of the musculature developed within the first pharyngeal arch: the muscles of mastication, including the temporalis, masseter, medial and lateral pterygoid muscles, as well as the tensors tympani and veli palatini, and the anterior belly of the digastric and the mylohyoid muscles (Fig. 18-7 and Tables 18-3 through 18-5).

As described earlier, the motor and sensory roots do not unite before exiting the skull. Rather, both roots pass through the foramen ovale and unite just outside the skull, forming the mandibular trunk. The latter is a mixed nerve that soon divides into a smaller, anterior division that is primarily motor and a larger posterior division that is mostly sensory in function.

Lying just outside the foramen ovale, immediately deep to the mandibular nerve trunk, is the otic ganglion. Although this parasympathetic ganglion (see Table 18-2) is in close association with the mandibular nerve via the nerve to the medial pterygoid muscle that passes through it, the preganglionic parasympathetic fibers synapsing within the ganglion are from the lesser petrosal nerve, a branch of the glossopharyngeal nerve.

Postganglionic fibers from the ganglion are secretomotor to the parotid gland and use the auriculotemporal nerve for distribution. The mandibular nerve possesses several branches: some from the nerve trunk, others from the anterior division, and still others from the posterior division; they are described in that order in the following sections.

Branches from the Mandibular Trunk

Two nerves branch from the trunk of the nerve: the recurrent meningeal nerve and the nerve to the medial pterygoid muscle.

The **recurrent meningeal nerve** leaves the mandibular trunk and ascends back into the skull through the foramen spinosum in company with the middle meningeal artery. This nerve supplies the dura, while some fibers supply the mastoid air cells.

The **medial pterygoid nerve** arises from the posterior aspect of the mandibular trunk, passes through the otic ganglion, and then enters the deep surface of the medial pterygoid muscle, supplying it with motor innervation (Fig. 18-7).

Two small branches arise from the medial pterygoid nerve: the **nerve to the tensor tympani muscle**, which penetrates the auditory tube cartilage to supply this muscle with motor innervation, and the **nerve to the tensor veli palatini muscle**, which enters that muscle near its origin, supplying it with motor innervation.

Branches from the Anterior Mandibular Division

The smaller anterior division, through its branches, supplies all of the remaining muscles of mastication with motor innervation (Fig. 18-7).

The **buccal nerve** is the only branch of the anterior division that is sensory in function. Arising from this division are the deep temporal, lateral pterygoid, masseteric, and buccal nerves.

The **deep temporal nerves** arise from the anterior division and ascend, usually as anterior and posterior branches, between the two heads of the lateral pterygoid muscle to enter the deep surface of the temporalis muscle, which they supply. Frequently, the anterior branch arises from the buccal nerve, whereas the posterior branch may arise in common with the masseteric nerve.

The **lateral pterygoid nerve** is very short and almost immediately enters the deep surface of the lateral pterygoid muscle, which it serves. This nerve may originate from the buccal nerve as that nerve passes between the two heads of the lateral pterygoid muscle.

The **masseteric nerve** passes above the lateral pterygoid muscle on its way to the mandibular notch, which it crosses to enter the masseter muscle in company with the same-named artery; it gives off a sensory twig to the temporomandibular joint before entering the muscle.

The origin of the **buccal nerve** (clinically sometimes referred to as the *long buccal nerve*) is not constant. Occasionally, it may arise from the trigeminal ganglion individually, reaching its destination via a separate foramen. Alternatively, it may arise from the inferior alveolar nerve of the posterior division. The description that follows assumes origin from the anterior division. The buccal nerve ascends, passing between the two heads of the lateral pterygoid muscle. Here it may give off branches to the temporalis and/or the lateral pterygoid muscles. It then descends to ramify over the buccinator muscle, supplying sensory innervation to the skin of the cheek in the area. Other branches pierce the muscle to provide sensory fibers to the buccal mucosa and adjacent gingiva. The buccal nerve communicates with the facial nerve, forming a complex over the buccinator muscle, presumably facilitating distribution of both nerves. It should be remembered that the buccal nerve is purely sensory and does not innervate the buccinator muscle (see the VII. Facial Nerve section).

Branches from the Posterior Mandibular Division

The larger posterior division of the mandibular nerve is mainly sensory in function, with the mylohyoid nerve being the only motor nerve of the division. Nerves arising from this division of the mandibular nerve are the lingual, inferior alveolar, and auriculotemporal nerves (Fig. 18-7).

The **lingual nerve** descends deep to the lateral pterygoid muscle, then courses forward between the medial pterygoid muscle and the mandible, where it is joined by the chorda tympani nerve, a branch of the facial nerve. The lingual nerve then descends over the superior pharyngeal constrictor and styloglossus muscles to reach the lateral aspect of the tongue adjacent to the hyoglossus muscle. Here it lies between that muscle and the submandibular gland.

The nerve proceeds anteriorly to the tip of the tongue, lying alongside the submandibular duct just beneath the mucosa.

Fibers of the lingual nerve, derived from the trigeminal nerve, provide sensory innervation to the mucous membranes of the anterior two thirds of the tongue, the lingual gingiva, and other structures adjacent to the tongue.

Fibers communicated to the lingual nerve from the facial nerve, via the chorda tympani, serve two functions:

- One group provides special sensory fibers for taste to the taste buds of the anterior two thirds of the tongue; these fibers are distributed by the lingual nerve.
- The other group supplies preganglionic parasympathetic fibers destined for the submandibular ganglion (see Table 18-2). The ganglion is suspended from the lingual nerve as that nerve lies between the hyoglossus muscle and the submandibular gland. Preganglionic fibers (contributed by the chorda tympani nerve) leave the lingual nerve to synapse on postganglionic cell bodies within the ganglion.

Postganglionic fibers pass directly to the submandibular gland or reenter the lingual nerve for distribution (as secretomotor fibers) to the sublingual gland and other minor salivary glands in the floor of the mouth.

The **inferior alveolar nerve** descends along with, but lateral to, the lingual nerve in company with the inferior alveolar artery on its way to the mandibular foramen.

The **mylohyoid nerve** arises from the inferior alveolar nerve just before the latter enters the mandibular foramen. The mylohyoid nerve descends in the mylohyoid groove on the mandible, then enters the mylohyoid muscle, which it provides with motor innervation. A portion of this nerve continues on the superficial surface of the muscle to the anterior belly of the digastric muscle, supplying it with motor innervation.

Upon entering the mandibular foramen, the inferior alveolar nerve proceeds in the bony mandibular canal, forming a dental plexus that provides sensory innervation to the mandibular teeth and supporting structures.

The nerve divides into two terminals: one, the **mental nerve**, exits the mental foramen to provide sensation to the skin of the lower lip and chin as well as to the mucous membrane of the lower lip; the other, the **incisive nerve**, continues to supply the anterior teeth and supporting tissues with sensory innervation.

The **auriculotemporal nerve** originates usually via two rootlets that arise from the trunk of the posterior division. One rootlet passes deep, whereas the other passes superficial to the middle meningeal artery, forming a loop around it, just prior to the artery entering the foramen spinosum. The two rootlets then unite, forming the auriculotemporal nerve, which courses deep to the lateral pterygoid muscle.

After emerging at the neck of the mandible, the nerve turns superiorly with the superficial temporal artery within the substance of the parotid gland. It continues to ascend between the auricula and temporomandibular joint, exiting the gland to pass over the zygomatic arch to distribute sensory fibers as **superficial temporal nerves** over the skin of the temporal region.

In its course, the auriculotemporal nerve sends **articular branches** to the temporomandibular joint, **anterior auricular branches** to the anterior portion of the external ear, **branches to the external acoustic meatus**, and **branches to the parotid gland**. Those branches to the parotid gland are postganglionic parasympathetic fibers whose cell bodies are located in the otic ganglion. These fibers, which supply secretomotor innervation to the gland, are communicated to the rootlets of the auriculotemporal nerve from the otic ganglion for distribution to the parotid gland (see Table 18-2).

Preganglionic parasympathetic fibers to the ganglion are supplied by the lesser petrosal branch of the glossopharyngeal nerve.

Although the auriculotemporal nerve is strictly sensory, it and the facial nerve communicate freely about the parotid gland, each facilitating distribution.

VI. ABDUCENS NERVE

Summary Bite. GSE and GP (general proprioception fibers to an extraocular muscle for kinesthetic sense) are the modalities carried by the abducens nerve.

The abducens nerve arises from the brain between the pons and the medulla. On its course to the orbit, the nerve pierces the dura covering the dorsum sel-

Clinical Considerations

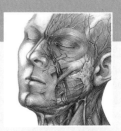

Unilateral Lesion of the Motor Root of the Trigeminal Nerve

Lesion of the motor root of the trigeminal nerve of one side results in ipsilateral flaccid paralysis and muscular atrophy of the muscles of mastication and all other muscles receiving motor supply from the mandibular division of the trigeminal nerve. Additionally, hyperacusis in one ear results from inactivity of the ipsilateral tensor tympani muscle.

The ipsilateral general somatic afferent modality will result in diminished sensation in the orofacial and nasal structures.

Trigeminal Neuralgia

Trigeminal neuralgia (tic douloureux), an extremely painful, debilitating condition involving pain fibers of the

trigeminal nerve, is caused by an unknown etiology but occasionally it may be associated with dental carious lesions. The pain is often excruciating and is experienced over the face, teeth, gingivae, nasal, and paranasal cavities, as well as the external ear canal. These are the areas served by the maxillary and mandibular divisions, although infrequently the area served by the ophthalmic division of the trigeminal nerve may be affected. Treatment varies from alcohol injection into the trigeminal division affected to sectioning of the trigeminal nerve between the pons and the ganglion.

Clinical Considerations

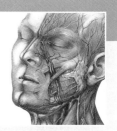

Abducens Nerve Injury

The abducens nerve provides motor innervation to the lateral rectus muscle. When affected, the muscle on the ipsilateral side will be paralyzed, causing the eyeball to deviate medially, resulting in double vision.

lae of the sphenoid bone and enters the cavernous sinus, where it receives communications from the carotid plexus.

Upon entering the superior orbital fissure, the nerve courses to the lateral rectus muscle, supplying it with motor innervation. This is the sole function of the abducens nerve (Fig. 18-3 and Tables 18-1 and 18-5).

VII. FACIAL NERVE

 Summary Bite. SVE, GVE, SVA, GVA, and GSA are the modalities carried by the facial nerve.

The facial nerve exhibits several modalities because its branches serve structures within the temporal bone, deep face, oral cavity, and the superficial face. The modalities carried by the facial nerve include: special visceral efferent, general visceral efferent, special visceral afferent, general visceral afferent, and general somatic afferent (Figs. 18-8 and 18-9 and Tables 18-1, 18-2, and 18-5).

The components of the facial nerve and their functions are as follows (see Fig. 18-8 and Tables 18-1, 18-2, and 18-5):

■ **Special Visceral Motor component** serves all of the muscles derived from the second pharyngeal arch, including the muscles of facial expression, the buccinator, platysma, and those of the scalp and external ear, the stapedius, posterior belly of the digastric, and stylohyoid muscles.
■ **General sensory component** supplies the external acoustic meatus.
■ **Visceral sensory component** supplies the soft palate and some of the pharynx.
■ **Special sensory component** is for taste to the anterior two thirds of the tongue.
■ **Parasympathetic component** effecting secretomotor function is supplied to the lacrimal, nasal, pala-

tine, submandibular, and sublingual glands (see Table 18-2).

The nerve possesses two roots, a large motor root and a smaller root, termed the **nervus intermedius**, containing the special sensory fibers for taste, parasympathetic fibers, and general sensory fibers. The two roots emerge from the brain between the pons and the inferior cerebellar peduncle.

These roots enter the internal acoustic meatus along with the vestibulocochlear nerve, but separate from it as the two roots enter the petrous portion of the temporal bone in a chamber of its own, the **facial canal** (Fig. 18-9).

Near the tympanic cavity, the facial nerve takes an abrupt turn inferiorly to exit the skull through the stylomastoid foramen. Located at this turn where the two roots fuse is the **geniculate ganglion**, the sensory ganglion of the facial nerve (Fig. 18-8 and Table 18-1).

Several branches arise from the nerve as it courses through the temporal bone, including the greater petrosal nerve from the geniculate ganglion, the nerve to the stapedius muscle, and the chorda tympani nerve.

Greater Petrosal Nerve

Arising from the geniculate ganglion is the greater petrosal nerve, which carries preganglionic parasympathetic fibers destined for the pterygopalatine ganglion along with sensory fibers for the soft palate and pharynx (Tables 18-1 and 18-2). The facial nerve leaves the petrous portion of the temporal bone via the **hiatus of the facial canal** near the foramen lacerum and then enters the pterygoid canal (vidian canal) of the sphenoid bone. Here it is joined by the **deep petrosal nerve**, a postganglionic sympathetic nerve arising from the carotid plexus whose cell bodies are located in the superior cervical ganglion. The combined nerve, known as the **nerve of the pterygoid canal (vidian nerve)**, passes through the same-named canal in the sphenoid bone to gain access to the

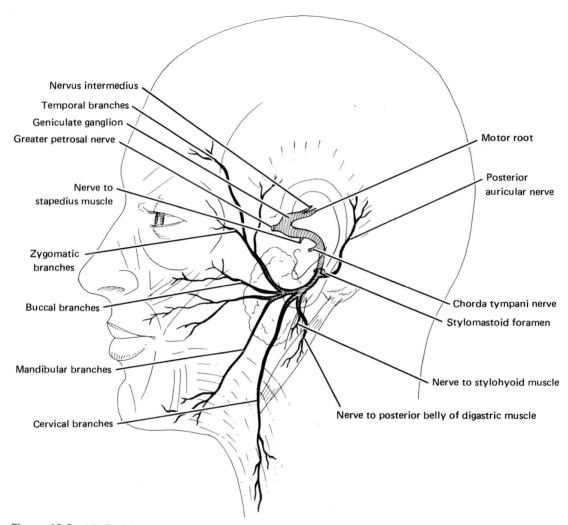

Figure 18-8. VII. Facial nerve.

pterygopalatine fossa, where it joins the pterygopalatine ganglion.

Preganglionic parasympathetic fibers synapse on postganglionic parasympathetic cell bodies housed within the pterygopalatine ganglion.

Fibers of these postganglionic parasympathetic neurons are communicated to nerves branching from the maxillary division of the trigeminal nerve for distribution to the lacrimal gland, as well as to small glands of the nasal cavity, pharynx, and palate.

The sympathetic component of the vidian nerve does not synapse in the pterygopalatine ganglion; instead, these postganglionic fibers are distributed in the same fashion as the postganglionic parasympathetic fibers.

The parasympathetic fibers are secretomotor in function, whereas the sympathetic fibers function mainly in vasoconstriction.

Some visceral sensory fibers from the geniculate ganglion travel along with the greater petrosal nerve to be distributed ultimately by branches of the maxillary division of the trigeminal nerve to the area of the soft palate via the lesser palatine nerve.

Nerve to the Stapedius Muscle

The nerve to the stapedius muscle, arising from the facial nerve as it descends across the tympanum, provides motor fibers to that muscle.

Chorda Tympani Nerve

The chorda tympani nerve arises from the facial nerve trunk just before the trunk's exit from the stylomastoid foramen. The chorda tympani courses cranialward in a canal of its own, diverging away from

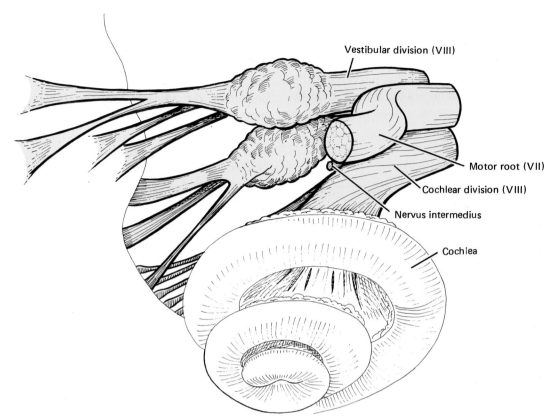

Vestibular division (VIII)

Motor root (VII)

Cochlear division (VIII)

Nervus intermedius

Cochlea

Figure 18-9. VIII. Vestibulocochlear nerve. Note the nervus intermedius and motor portion of the facial nerve accompanying the vestibular and cochlear divisions into the ear.

the main nerve, bending to pass over the tympanic membrane and across the manubrium of the malleus. It leaves the tympanic cavity to enter a canal in the petrotympanic fissure, then exits the skull at the spine of the sphenoid bone. The chorda tympani nerve, which may receive a communication from the otic ganglion, joins the lingual branch of the mandibular division of the trigeminal nerve for distribution. It contains special sensory fibers destined for taste buds on the anterior two thirds of the tongue and preganglionic parasympathetic fibers destined for the submandibular ganglion (see Figs. 18-7 and 18-8 and Tables 18-1 and 18-2).

The **submandibular ganglion**, suspended by short nerve filaments from the lingual nerve as it passes the hyoglossus muscle, receives the preganglionic parasympathetic fibers of the chorda tympani nerve via the parasympathetic root (Fig. 18-7). Postganglionic parasympathetic fibers from the submandibular ganglion pass to the submandibular gland or reenter the lingual nerve to be distributed to the sublingual gland and minor salivary glands in the floor of the mouth, providing them with secretomotor innervation. Sympathetic stimulation of the salivary glands is accomplished by postganglionic sympathetic fibers

accompanying the arteries serving the glands. The function of this stimulation is generally to elicit vasoconstriction.

Beyond the origin of the chorda tympani nerve, the facial nerve exits the skull through the stylomastoid foramen. There, it gives rise to the posterior auricular nerve and the nerves to the posterior digastric and stylohyoid muscles. It then passes into the retromandibular fossa to enter the substance of the parotid gland to form the parotid plexus.

Posterior Auricular Nerve

As the facial nerve exits the stylomastoid foramen, the posterior auricular nerve arises from it to pass superiorly between the auricle and the mastoid process. It divides into occipital and auricular branches after communicating with the auricular branch of the vagus nerve and great auricular and lesser occipital nerves of the cervical plexus. The **auricular branch** supplies motor innervation to the posterior auricular muscle of the ear and to some of its intrinsic muscles. The **occipital branch** courses posteriorly to supply the occipitalis muscle with motor innervation (Fig. 18-8).

Nerve to the Posterior Belly of the Digastric Muscle

The nerve to the posterior belly of the digastric muscle arises from the trunk of the facial nerve near the stylomastoid foramen and enters the muscle near its midbelly, providing it with motor innervation (Fig. 18-8).

Nerve to Stylohyoid Muscle

The nerve to the stylohyoid muscle arises from the facial nerve in a similar fashion to or in common with the nerve to the posterior digastric. The nerve to the stylohyoid muscle then enters the muscle at midbelly, providing it with motor innervation (Fig. 18-8).

Parotid Plexus

After entering the parotid gland, the facial nerve divides into **temporofacial** and **cervicofacial** divisions, which form the parotid plexus. From there emerge the branches supplying motor innervation to the muscles of facial expression. These terminal branches are named for the regions they supply, usually dividing into five major branches from the plexus: **temporal**, **zygomatic**, **buccal**, **mandibular**, and **cervical branches** (Fig. 18-8). Space does not permit a repeat of the complete descriptions of each branch's distribution or of the muscles served by each branch, other than to state that, generally, the branch serves facial muscles originating in the area of the nerve branch. The interested reader is referred back to Chapter 8 for a discussion of the distribution of the branches of the parotid plexus.

Note that branches of the facial nerve communicate freely with all of the terminal branches of the trigeminal nerve. These communications, for example, those between the auriculotemporal nerve and the facial nerve, apparently serve to facilitate distribution of the sensory branches of the trigeminal nerve about the face.

VIII. VESTIBULOCOCHLEAR NERVE

Summary Bite. SSA and SP (special proprioception within the vestibular mechanism for body balance) are the modalities carried in the vestibulocochlear nerve.

The nerve of hearing and balance, the vestibulocochlear nerve, is composed of two separate sets of fibers. The **vestibular nerve** for balance and the **cochlear nerve** for hearing are joined as a common nerve entering the internal acoustic meatus with the facial nerve (Fig. 18-9).

These two cranial nerves separate after entering the meatus as the vestibulocochlear nerve approaches the area of its destination within the inner ear. The vestibulocochlear nerve divides, sending the cochlear nerve into the laterally oriented cochlear apparatus and the vestibular nerve medially into the vestibular apparatus.

Cochlear Nerve

The cochlear nerve has its peripheral processes in the **organ of Corti**, located in the membranous labyrinth,

Clinical Considerations

Bell Palsy

Damage to the facial nerve (or its accidental analgesia during dental procedures) results in paralysis of the muscles of the affected side. Damage may occur during surgical involvement of the parotid gland, infection of the middle ear, knife wounds, or at birth during forceps delivery. Paralysis of the facial muscles results in ptosis of the eye (upper eyelid drooping); depression of the corner of the mouth with accompanying oozing of saliva; speech disorder (especially involving labial sounds); lack of muscle tone; and a sagging, distorted face. Bell palsy affects all of the ipsilateral muscles about the face as well as other muscles that developed from the second pharyngeal arch. Because of this fact, patients affected with Bell palsy have hyperacusis (loss of corneal blink) as well as loss of taste from the ipsilateral side of the anterior tongue.

Clinical Considerations

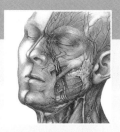

Conductive Hearing Loss

Conductive hearing loss results from a defect in the conduction of sound waves from the tympanic membrane through the bony ossicles to the oval window of the cochlea. Conditions that may contribute to conduction deafness include buildup of cerumen (ear wax), perforation of the tympanic membrane, otis media (middle ear cavity infection), and otosclerosis, excessive growth of bone around the oval window causing impaired movement of the stapes.

Nerve Deafness

Nerve deafness results from a lesion within the nerves transmitting impulses to the brain from the spiral organ of Corti. Other causes include certain diseases, drug abuse, and prolonged exposure to loud noises.

Ménière Disease

Ménière disease is related to excess fluid in the endolymphatic duct affecting the vestibular mechanism of the vestibulocochlear nerve. This disease is characterized by hearing loss, vertigo, nausea, tinnitus, and

vomiting. Drugs can be used for treatment, but in severe cases surgery is required.

Otitis Media

The auditory tube permits the spread of infection from the nasal cavity into the middle ear cavity. This condition (**otitis media**), resulting from acute infection, may result in the rupture of the eardrum and/or the infection may pass into the mastoid air cells. Antibiotics are used to treat this condition. Auditory tube obstructions often lead to middle-ear infections, especially in children.

Otosclerosis

Occasionally, the stapes becomes immobilized as a result of bony deposits around the oval window. This condition, known as **otosclerosis**, is a major cause of hearing loss, especially in older adults. It is usually correctable by surgical procedures. Both otitis media and otosclerosis, if left untreated, will result in deafness.

---

and its cell bodies are located in the **spiral ganglion of the cochlea**, which is housed in the modiolus of the cochlea (Fig. 18-9 and Tables 18-1 and 18-5). Central processes of the spiral ganglion become the cochlear division of the nerve responsible for the sense of hearing.

Vestibular Nerve

The vestibular nerve cell bodies are located in the **vestibular ganglion** within the internal auditory meatus of the temporal bone. Peripheral processes of these neurons divide to enter the vestibular mechanism, including the three semicircular canals.

Central processes of these neurons become the vestibular division of the vestibulocochlear nerve responsible for the sense of balance (Fig. 18-9 and Tables 18-1 and 18-5).

IX. GLOSSOPHARYNGEAL NERVE

 Summary Bite. SVA, GVA, GVE, GSA, and SVE are the modalities carried in the glossopharyngeal nerve.

The modalities within the glossopharyngeal nerve include: special visceral efferent, general visceral efferent, special visceral afferent, general visceral afferent, and general somatic afferent (see Fig. 18-10 and Tables 18-1, 18-2, and 18-5).

- **Special visceral efferent**. Because the glossopharyngeal nerve is the nerve of the third pharyngeal arch, it serves the only muscle derived from this arch, the stylopharyngeus muscle.

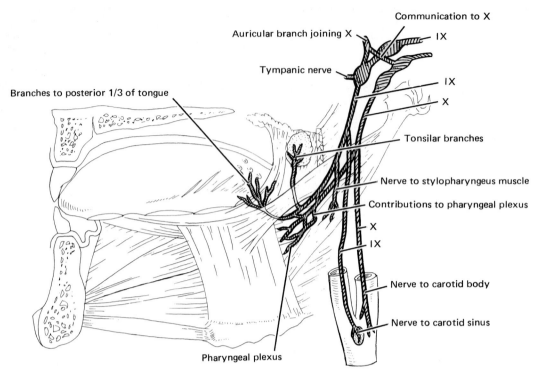

Figure 18-10. IX. Glossopharyngeal nerve. Observe the communications with the vagus nerve and the contributions of both to the pharyngeal plexus.

- **General visceral efferents (parasympathetic)** supply the parotid gland and other minor salivary glands in the mucous membrane in and about the posterior tongue and adjacent pharynx.
- **Special visceral afferents** are distributed to the taste buds located on the posterior one third of the tongue, as well as to those located in the circumvallate papillae.
- **General visceral afferents** supply the posterior one third of the tongue, the fauces, the palatine tonsils, and the pharynx. Other general visceral sensory fibers supply the carotid sinus with blood pressure receptors as well as to chemoreceptors located within the carotid body. The latter is a sensory function performed in conjunction with the vagus nerve.
- **General somatic afferents** supply cutaneous sensation about the ear.

The glossopharyngeal nerve leaves the brain as three or four rootlets adjacent to the vagus nerve along the medulla between the olive and the inferior cerebellar peduncle. The rootlets unite to exit the skull through the jugular foramen in company with the vagus and accessory nerves. Housed in the groove within the jugular foramen are the **superior and inferior ganglia** of the glossopharyngeal nerve, containing the cell bodies of the sensory fibers.

While passing through the jugular foramen, this nerve communicates with the facial nerve, the auricular branch and superior ganglion of the vagus nerve, and the superior cervical sympathetic ganglion.

Tympanic Nerve

The tympanic nerve arises from the inferior ganglion of the glossopharyngeal nerve (Fig. 18-10) and enters the petrous portion of the temporal bone, traveling to the tympanic cavity. Here it forms the **tympanic plexus** with fibers from the carotid plexus and the greater petrosal nerve. Branches from the tympanic plexus serve sensory functions to the mucous membranes of the eardrum, oval and round windows, mastoid air cells, and auditory tube.

The tympanic nerve emerges from the tympanic plexus as the **lesser petrosal nerve**, providing preganglionic parasympathetic fibers to the otic ganglion (see Tables 18-1 and 18-2), which it reaches by leaving the skull at the fissure between the petrous portion of the temporal bone and the greater wing of the sphenoid bone.

The **otic ganglion**, described in the section on the mandibular division of the trigeminal nerve, lies just outside the foramen ovale, immediately behind the mandibular nerve. This ganglion receives preganglionic parasympathetic fibers from the lesser petrosal

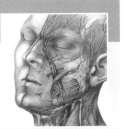

Clinical Considerations

Unilateral Lesion of the Glossopharyngeal Nerve Outside Brainstem

Unilateral lesion of the glossopharyngeal nerve outside of the brainstem will cause loss of taste from the posterior one third of the tongue, loss of salivation from the parotid gland on the ipsilateral side, loss of gag reflex, and loss of carotid sinus reflex.

---

nerve and possibly some fibers from the greater petrosal nerve communicated through the tympanic plexus. Postganglionic parasympathetic fibers leave the otic ganglion and are communicated to the auriculotemporal nerve for distribution to the parotid gland, providing it with secretomotor innervation.

Carotid Sinus Nerve

The nerve to the carotid sinus arises as a small filament from the glossopharyngeal nerve subsequent to nerve communications at the jugular foramen. This branch descends along the internal carotid artery, ending in the bifurcation of the common carotid artery (Fig. 18-10). This nerve functions as a baroreceptor within the carotid sinus. On its way to the carotid sinus, the nerve communicates with pharyngeal branch(es) of the vagus and branches from the superior cervical ganglion (postganglionic sympathetic fibers). Glossopharyngeal and vagus nerves transmit afferent fibers from the chemoreceptors within the carotid body.

Nerve to the Stylopharyngeus Muscle

As the glossopharyngeal nerve courses to the posterior pharyngeal wall, a nerve to the stylopharyngeus muscle arises to supply that muscle (Fig. 18-10).

Pharyngeal Branches

The main trunk of the glossopharyngeal nerve terminates as several pharyngeal branches to enter the posterior pharyngeal wall (Fig. 18-10). Some of these branches continue to the tongue as **lingual branches**, providing general sensation to the posterior one third of the tongue and special sensory fibers to the taste buds on that portion of the tongue as well as to those of the circumvallate papillae. Other branches penetrate the pharyngeal wall as **tonsillar branches**, communicating with the lesser palatine nerve of the maxillary division of the trigeminal nerve, to supply the soft palate, pharynx, and fauces with general sensation.

Pharyngeal Plexus

Other fibers of the glossopharyngeal nerve join with pharyngeal branches of the vagus nerve and branches from the superior cervical ganglion to form the **pharyngeal plexus**, located on the wall of the middle pharyngeal constrictor muscle (Fig 18-10). Branches from this plexus penetrate the wall of the pharynx and supply all of the muscles of the pharynx (except the stylopharyngeus) and soft palate (except the tensor veli palatini) with motor innervation and adjacent mucous membranes with sensory innervation.

Although the following information was presented in Chapter 16, it is appropriate to present it again because there is confusion related to the function of the individual nerves making up the pharyngeal plexus. Glossopharyngeal contributions to the pharyngeal plexus are sensory, whereas the vagal branches are motor. However, these motor branches are believed to consist mainly of fibers from the cranial portion of the accessory nerve (cranial nerve XI), which are contributed to the vagus nerve before it exits the skull. Postganglionic sympathetic fibers contributed from the superior cervical ganglion to the pharyngeal plexus are vasomotor in function.

X. VAGUS NERVE

 Summary Bite. GVE, SVE, GVA, and GSA are the modalities carried in the vagus nerve.

The cranial nerve having the most extensive distribution is the vagus nerve. In addition to its destinations within the head and neck, the vagus nerve also enters the thorax to serve the heart and lungs, and continues into the abdomen to supply most of the abdominal viscera (Figs. 18-10 and 18-11 and Tables 18-1 and 18-5).

The vagus nerve possesses five modalities, namely, special visceral efferent general somatic afferent, general visceral afferent, special visceral afferent, general visceral efferent.

- **Special visceral efferent**. The vagus is the nerve of the fourth pharyngeal arch, and its recurrent laryngeal branch is the nerve of the sixth pharyngeal arch. Consequently, the vagus nerve supplies muscles developed from those arches. Muscles developing from the fourth arch include the pharyngeal constrictors and the cricothyroid muscles. Muscles developed from the sixth arch include the intrinsic muscles of the larynx.

- **General somatic afferent** fibers are provided to the skin about the ear and external acoustic meatus.
- **General visceral afferent** supplies the mucous membranes of the pharynx, larynx, esophagus, bronchi, lungs, heart, and much of the abdominal viscera.
- **General visceral efferent** supplies the smooth muscles and glands of the digestive tract from the esophagus to (and including) most of the intestines, plus the bronchi and trachea.
- **Special visceral afferent** is supplied to the base of the tongue, aryepiglottic fold, and larynx.

The vagus nerve exits the brain at the medulla, between the olive and the inferior cerebellar peduncle just posterior to the glossopharyngeal nerve, via a cluster of 8 to 10 rootlets that unite to exit the skull

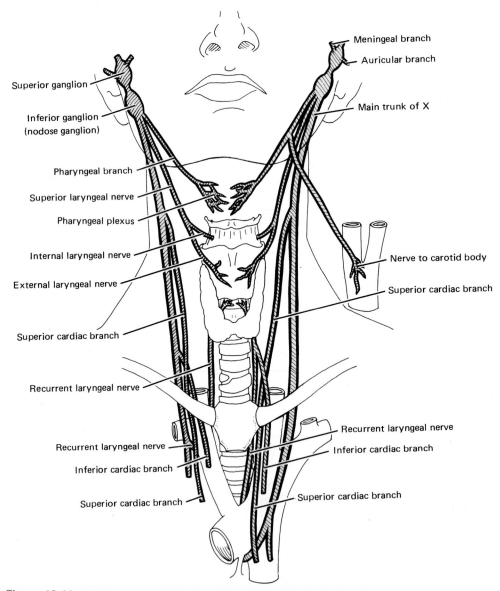

Figure 18-11. X. Vagus nerve. Only those branches arising in the head and neck are illustrated.

through the jugular foramen along with the glossopharyngeal and accessory nerves.

This nerve possesses two sensory ganglia: the **superior ganglion**, housed in the jugular fossa, and the **inferior (nodose) ganglion**, appearing as a swelling on the nerve just after it exits the jugular foramen (Figs. 18-10 and 18-11).

Peripheral processes of the neurons in these ganglia are distributed with the vagus nerve as the sensory component. These ganglia receive communications from the glossopharyngeal, facial, accessory, and hypoglossal nerves. The sympathetic nervous system communicates via a filament from the superior cervical ganglion, and a communication also exists between the vagal ganglia and the first and second cervical nerves.

The cranial root of the accessory nerve joins the vagus nerve just proximal to the inferior ganglion. Thus, the motor component to the muscles arising from the fourth and fifth pharyngeal arches, generally described as arising from the vagus nerve, are actually from this contribution to the vagus nerve by the accessory nerve. However, autonomic motor innervation to the esophagus and the structures within the thorax and abdomen attributed to the vagus arise from the dorsal motor nucleus of the vagus nerve.

Before its exit from the jugular fossa the vagus nerve gives off two branches: the meningeal and auricular branches.

Meningeal Branch

The meningeal branch of the vagus nerve returns to the cranial vault to supply the dura in the posterior cranial fossa (Fig. 18-11).

Auricular Branch

An auricular branch arises from the superior vagal ganglion, communicates with the glossopharyngeal nerve, and then enters the mastoid canal coursing to the facial canal. Here it communicates with the facial nerve, then exits through the tympanomastoid suture to communicate with the posterior auricular nerve before distributing to the skin of the posterior aspect of the ear and the external acoustic meatus.

Vagal Branches in the Neck

The following sections describe the branches and distributions of the vagus nerve as it courses through the neck. Branches arising from the vagus in the neck include the pharyngeal, superior laryngeal, and superior cardiac nerves. Also located in the neck is the recurrent laryngeal nerve that arises from the vagus nerve at the thoracic inlet to recur back into the neck.

Pharyngeal Branches

Pharyngeal branches of the vagus arise from the inferior vagal ganglion and pass over the internal carotid artery to the pharyngeal constrictor muscles, providing input to the pharyngeal plexus (Fig. 18-11). From this plexus, motor innervation is supplied to the pharyngeal but not the stylopharyngeus, as well as to all muscles of the soft palate except the tensor veli palatini. Mucous membranes of the pharynx are also supplied by the pharyngeal plexus.

Usually, the **nerve to the carotid body** originates from the pharyngeal branches. This nerve descends along the internal carotid artery to terminate in the carotid body housed in the bifurcation of the common carotid artery (Fig. 18-11). Chemoreceptors detect changes in oxygen and carbon dioxide tension as well as hydrogen ion concentration in the blood at this site.

As previously described, sensory fibers from the carotid body are also transmitted in the glossopharyngeal nerve.

Superior Laryngeal Nerve

The superior laryngeal nerve arises from the vagus at the inferior end of the inferior ganglion and passes deep to the internal carotid artery, descending to the thyroid cartilage, where it divides into external and internal branches (Fig. 18-11).

The smaller **external branch** continues to descend beneath the sternothyroid muscle to enter the cricothyroid and inferior pharyngeal constrictor muscles, which it supplies with motor innervation.

The larger **internal branch** courses over and pierces the thyrohyoid membrane. This branch supplies sensory innervation to the mucous membranes superiorly, to the base of the tongue, and to the epiglottis and the larynx as far inferiorly as the vocal folds. It is with this branch that the sensation of taste is transmitted to the brain from the base of the tongue, epiglottis, and larynx.

The internal laryngeal branch also contains parasympathetic fibers to the glands associated with the mucous membranes of the regions just described. Preganglionic fibers synapse on ganglionic plexuses within the walls of the viscera served, and from there the postganglionic fibers distribute secretomotor fibers to the glands.

Superior Cardiac Branches

As the trunk of the vagus nerve descends in the neck within the carotid sheath, between and posterior to the internal jugular vein and the internal carotid artery, superior cardiac branches are given off and descend

Clinical Considerations

Unilateral Lesion of the Vagus after Leaving Brainstem

Pharynx

Such a lesion results in flaccid paralysis or weakness in the muscles of the pharynx that bring about dysphagia (difficulty in swallowing); paralysis or weakness of the muscles of the larynx, resulting in dysphonia (hoarseness); paralysis or weakness in the soft palate; loss of sensation from pharynx and larynx, and the loss of the gag reflex. **Bilateral lesion of the vagus nerve** is not compatible with life.

Larynx

The intrinsic laryngeal musculature is served by two branches of the vagus nerve, the inferior laryngeal branch of the recurrent laryngeal nerve and the external branch of the superior laryngeal nerve. Because these two nerves are prone to damage, it is essential that they

be protected from injury during surgical procedures. The external laryngeal nerve, passing deep to the superior thyroid artery, supplies only a single muscle, the cricothyroid. Its section does not cause excessive damage to phonation. It will, however, affect the ability to tense the vocal cords and the ability of the patient to produce high-pitched sounds. In addition, damage to it causes some hoarseness and easy tiring of the voice.

Damage to the recurrent laryngeal or the inferior laryngeal nerves will result in serious complications, whose severity depends on the degree of damage and whether the injury is bilateral. Involvement may range from slight hoarseness to complete inability to vocalize and breathe, necessitating performance of a tracheotomy.

---

into the thorax (Fig. 18-11). Their function is not described here because it is outside the realm of this text.

Recurrent Laryngeal Nerve

At the root of the neck, the recurrent laryngeal nerve arises from the vagus and ascends back into the neck. On the right side, the nerve recurs around the subclavian artery, whereas on the left side the nerve recurs around the arch of the aorta (Fig. 18-11).

Upon reentering the neck, each recurrent laryngeal nerve follows a similar course deep to the carotid artery, along a groove between the trachea and the esophagus, to enter the larynx as **inferior laryngeal nerves**, piercing the cricothyroid membrane to supply all of the intrinsic muscles of the larynx, except the cricothyroid muscle, with motor innervation.

In the recurrent laryngeal nerve's path to the larynx, branches to the trachea and the esophagus supply those structures with sensory and parasympathetic innervation in much the same manner as the fibers of the internal branch of the superior laryngeal nerve but more distally. In addition, **pharyngeal branches** are supplied to the inferior pharyngeal constrictor muscle. Although they serve a minor role, sensory branches of the inferior laryngeal nerve provide sensory fibers to the larynx and overlap sensory fibers of the external laryngeal nerve.

The remaining branches and distributions of the vagus nerve within the thorax and abdomen are not described here. Those interested in this subject are referred to general textbooks in gross anatomy and neuroanatomy, as suggested in the Selected Readings.

XI. ACCESSORY NERVE

Summary Bite. SVE (communicated to the vagus nerve for the muscles of the pharynx and larynx) and SVE (assuming branchomeric origins for the sternocleidomastoid and trapezius muscles) are the modalities carried by the accessory nerve.

The accessory nerve arises from two sources: the brain and the spinal cord. This nerve is described as a motor nerve, serving the sternocleidomastoid and trapezius muscles, and its cranial root is regarded as the motor portion of the vagus nerve within the head and neck, including the contribution that the vagus nerve makes to the pharyngeal plexus.

The spinal portion arises from motor neurons in the first five (or more) spinal cord segments. This portion of the nerve emerges on the surface of the

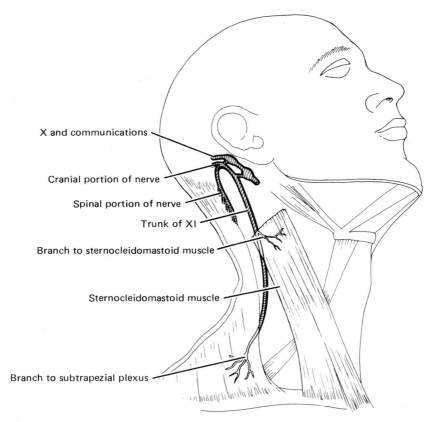

X and communications

Cranial portion of nerve

Spinal portion of nerve

Trunk of XI

Branch to sternocleidomastoid muscle

Sternocleidomastoid muscle

Branch to subtrapezial plexus

Figure 18-12. XI. Accessory nerve. Note the spinal portion ascending into the cranium to join the cranial portion before exiting the jugular foramen.

spinal cord to ascend into the skull via the foramen magnum to join or communicate with the cranial portion of the nerve before exiting the jugular foramen along with the vagus and glossopharyngeal nerves (Figs. 18-10 and 18-12 and Tables 18-1 and 18-5). The cranial portion leaves the brain very close to the vagus nerve and travels along with it to the jugular foramen. After communicating with the spinal portion, the cranial portion joins the vagus, and the spinal portion continues on to descend through the foramen.

The spinal portion descends posterior to the stylohyoid and digastric muscles to enter the sternoclei-domastoid muscle, which it pierces and serves before passing obliquely over the posterior triangle to terminate in and supply the trapezius muscle. Along its way, the nerve communicates with the second, third, and fourth cervical nerves.

XII. HYPOGLOSSAL NERVE

 Summary Bite. GSE is the modality carried by the hypoglossal nerve.

Clinical Considerations

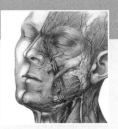

Accessory Nerve Injury

The accessory nerve, as it progresses subcutaneously through the neck, is subject to injury, (e.g., during lymph node biopsy, carotid artery and/or internal jugular vein surgical procedures). Injury produces weakness in the sternocleidomastoid and trapezius muscles, impairing neck movement and resulting in a drooping of the shoulder.

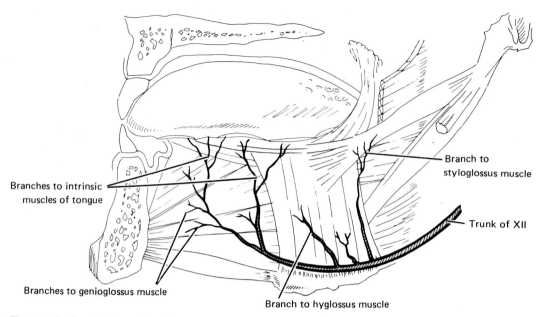

Figure 18-13. XII. Hypoglossal nerve.

The most caudal and the last of the cranial nerves is the hypoglossal nerve. This nerve is the motor nerve of the tongue.

It arises as several rootlets from the medulla between the olive and the pyramid and, passing through the hypoglossal canal, the rootlets unite to form a single nerve. It descends deep to the internal jugular vein and internal carotid artery, and then becomes superficial to them as it crosses them at the mandible.

The hypoglossal nerve then courses over the external carotid and lingual arteries deep to the digastric and stylohyoid muscles. It enters the muscles of the tongue, which it supplies, proceeding to the ventral tip of the tongue.

With the exception of the palatoglossus (innervated by the vagus via the pharyngeal plexus), the hypoglossal nerve innervates the hyoglossus, styloglossus, genioglossus, and intrinsic muscles of the tongue (Fig. 18-13 and Tables 18-1 and 18-5).

The hypoglossal nerve communicates with several nerves in its route, including the pharyngeal plexus, the lingual, and the first and second cervical spinal nerves. Branches from the first and second ventral cervical spinal nerves join the hypoglossal later to exit, forming the descending loop (superior root) of the ansa cervicalis, which innervates the infrahyoid muscles.

Some of the fibers from the first cervical nerve continue on to exit from the hypoglossal nerve near the posterior border of the hyoglossus muscle and enter the thyrohyoid and geniohyoid muscles, supplying them with motor innervation.

Clinical Considerations

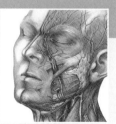

Hypoglossal Nerve Injury

Difficult third molar extractions and/or fractures of the mandible may damage the hypoglossal nerve (cranial nerve XII), causing paralysis of the tongue on the affected side. When the mouth is opened and the tongue is protruded, the genioglossus of the unaffected side will cause the tongue to deviate to the affected side. If the damage is prolonged, the tongue muscles will atrophy.

Anatomic Basis for Local Anesthesia

19

Key Terms

Aspiration minimizes the possibility of injecting anesthetic solution into a blood vessel; it must be carried out by the operator prior to injecting anesthetic solution into any target area. Aspiration is accomplished by developing a negative pressure at the needle tip of the syringe. If the needle tip has punctured the vascular wall, blood will be forced back into the syringe and become visible to the operator. *Any* blood returned is termed a positive aspiration and anesthetic solution should not be deposited. The syringe should be removed and a new site is

to be selected. Anesthetic solution inadvertently injected into a blood vessel may have an immediate toxic effect that involves the cardiovascular system, nervous system, and/or the tissue in the immediate vicinity of the injection. In fact, it has been shown that almost half of the mortality in dental offices is due to the administration of local anesthesia to sensitive patients or injection into a blood vessel. If the needle penetrates a blood vessel, the lesion may cause a localized extraoral swelling of hemorrhaging blood within a few minutes. It may also spread

into the neck before it can be brought under control.

Plexus Anesthesia is the technique of delivering anesthetic solution to the connective tissues overlying the periosteum to produce anesthesia in and about a limited number of teeth. Plexus anesthesia may be used to advantage in regions of the oral cavity where bony tissues surrounding the roots of the teeth are thin enough to permit adequate diffusion of the anesthetic agent. Thus, this method of delivery is commonly used for anesthetizing certain teeth in the maxillary arch and their supporting tissues. Even the maxillary buccal cortical plate is sufficiently thin (with the exception of the first molar region) so that plexus anesthesia in this area is advantageous.

Subperiosteal Injections may occur in maxillary plexus anesthesia. This can happen when the anesthetic solution is incorrectly delivered deep to the periosteum. Extreme care should be exercised to avoid subperiosteal injections because such injections can cause the fluid to tear the periosteum and its blood vessels from the bone, resulting in subperiosteal hematomas and considerable pain.

Trunk Anesthesia, also known as nerve block anesthesia, is the technique of delivering anesthetic solution close to the nerve trunk so that structures distal to the injections site are anesthetized. Most of the mandibular cortical plate is too thick for plexus anesthesia. Hence, for mandibular procedures, trunk anesthesia is the method of choice.

ANESTHESIA

Anesthesia is the loss of sensation due to injury, disease, or drug administration. Local anesthetics may be applied topically or injected either in the vicinity of the area to be anesthetized or into a conveniently accessible region in the proximity of the nerve or nerves supplying the area of interest.

These anesthetic substances are pharmacologic agents that stabilize cell membranes, thereby blocking or reducing the excitability of the membrane. When a region of a nerve fiber is exposed to an anesthetic solution, that fiber cannot relay impulses through the affected region; hence, nerve conduction is blocked.

Small, unmyelinated fibers (i.e., most pain fibers) are affected first, whereas larger, myelinated fibers (i.e., proprioception, touch, and motor) are blocked last.

Because the effects of local anesthetics are temporary, recovery of excitability occurs in the reverse order, that is, large, myelinated fibers become conductive first and small, unmyelinated fibers become conductive last. Because pain and temperature fibers are usually small, the anesthetic can be applied in quantities that interfere mostly with these sensations while only minimally affecting proprioception, sensation of touch, or motor functions.

Anesthetic agents may be introduced to anesthetize nerve endings, a process known as **infiltration**. Another process, known as a nerve block, can be employed to interfere with nerve conduction at a distance from the nerve ending. Infiltration is usually restricted to mucous membranes and is of limited use in the oral cavity. **Nerve blocks**, however, are important and are considered in two separate anesthesia categories: plexus anesthesia, restricted to a single tooth or a few teeth, and trunk anesthesia, involving blocking of pain sensation over a relatively large area. This chapter addresses anesthesia of the teeth and their adnexa (see Tables 19-1 and 19-2).

PLEXUS ANESTHESIA

Summary Bite. Plexus anesthesia in dentistry represents delivery of an anesthetic agent into the connective tissue overlying the periosteum. This anesthetic procedure is used to advantage where the cortical plate of the bone surrounding the dentition is thin and sufficiently cancellous to permit diffusion of the anesthetic agent.

Plexus anesthesia involves the delivery of anesthetic agent into the connective tissue overlying the periosteum. Plexus anesthesia may be used to advantage in regions of the oral cavity where bony tissues surrounding the roots of the teeth are relatively thin and sufficiently cancellous to permit adequate diffusion of the anesthetic agent.

The maxillary buccal cortical plate is sufficiently thin (with the exception of the first molar region) so that plexus anesthesia in this area is advantageous.

Maxillary Plexus Anesthesia

Summary Bite. Plexus anesthesia is the mode of anesthetic administration used for most of the anesthesia sites in the maxillary arch.

The maxillary teeth are supplied by the anterior superior, middle superior, and posterior superior alveolar nerves. The anterior superior and middle superior alveolar nerves are branches of the infraorbital nerve, whereas the posterior superior alveolar nerve is a branch of the trunk of the maxillary division of the trigeminal nerve.

Proper accomplishment of plexus anesthesia should occur deep to the alveolar mucosa at or slightly above the mucogingival junction, below the fornix. Otherwise, the anesthetic agent will be injected in a region of loose connective tissue, permitting rapid dilution and removal of the anesthetic

Table 19-1 Anesthesia of the Teeth and Supporting Tissues in the Maxillary Arch

Tooth and Supporting Tissues

Anesthetic Technique	Central Incisor	Lateral Incisor	Canine	First Premolar	Second Premolar	First Molar	Second Molar	Third Molar
Anterior Superior Alveolar	P X F X PL	P X F X PL	P X F X PL	P B PL	P B PL	P B PL	P B PL	P B PL
Middle Superior Alveolar	P F PL	P F PL	P F PL	P X B X PL	P X B X PL	P B PL	P B PL	P B PL
Posterior Superior Alveolar	P F PL	P F PL	P F PL	P B PL	P B PL	P X* B X PL	P X B X PL	P X B X PL
Greater Palatine	P F PL	P F PL	P F PL	P B PL X	P B PL X	P B PL X	P B PL X	P B PL X
Nasopalatine	P F PL X	P F PL X	P F PL X	P B PL	P B PL	P B PL	P B PL	P B PL
Infraorbital	P X F X PL	P X F X PL	P X F X PL	P X B X PL	P X B X PL	P B PL	P B PL	P B PL

B, buccal; *F*, facial; *P*, pulp; *PL*, palatal.
* In about 27% of the population, the mesialbuccal root of the first molar is not innervated by the posterior superior alveolar nerve, but by the middle superior alveolar nerve. Thus, for complete anesthesia of the first molar, it is suggested that both the PSA and MSA nerves be anesthetized.

Table 19-2 Anesthesia of the Teeth and Supporting Tissues in the Mandibular Arch

Tooth and Supporting Tissues

Anesthetic Technique	Central Incisor	Lateral Incisor	Canine	First Premolar	Second Premolar	First Molar	Second Molar	Third Molar
Inferior Alveolar Nerve Block *	P X F X L X	P X F X L X	P X F X L X	P X B X L X	P X B X L X	P X B L X	P X B L X	P X B L X
Buccal Nerve Block	P F X L	P F X L	P F L	P B L	P B L	P B X L	P B X L	P B X L
Mental Nerve Block	P X F X L	P X F X L	P F X L	P B X L	P B X L	P B L	P B L	P B L
Incisive Nerve Block	P X F X L	P X F X L	P X F X L	P X B X L	P X B X L	P B L	P B L	P B L

B, buccal; *F*, facial; *L*, lingual; *P*, pulp.
* Although the inferior alveolar (mandibular) nerve block is described to anesthetize the lingual supporting tissues of the mandibular teeth, clinical dental procedures affecting the lingual gingiva (especially in the molar region) may require anesthetizing the lingual nerve, which may be accomplished at the conclusion of administering the inferior alveolar nerve block.

Clinical Considerations

Aspiration

Aspiration must always be carried out by the operator prior to injecting anesthetic solution into any target area. The aspiration procedure minimizes the possibility of injecting anesthetic solution into a blood vessel. Aspiration is accomplished by developing a negative pressure at the needle tip by simply pulling back slightly on the thumb ring of the syringe (only 1 to 2 mm). If the needle tip has punctured the vascular wall, blood will be forced back into the syringe and become visible to the operator. Some clinicians aspirate several times during a slow injection because a single aspiration does not preclude penetration of the vessel by the bevel of the needle. *Any* blood returned is termed a positive aspiration and anesthetic solution should not be deposited. The syringe should be removed and a new site is to be selected. Anesthetic solution inadvertently injected into a blood vessel may have an immediate toxic effect that involves the cardiovascular system, nervous system, and/or the tissue in the immediate vicinity of the injection. In fact, it has been shown that almost half of the mortality in dental offices is due to the administration of local anesthesia to sensitive patients or injection into a blood vessel. If the needle penetrates a blood vessel, the lesion may cause a localized extraoral swelling of hemorrhaging blood within a few minutes. It may also spread into the neck before it can be brought under control.

solution. Therefore, the anesthetic agent is to be deposited at or coronal to the apex of the tooth, permitting the drug to penetrate the periosteum and thin cortical plate.

Anesthesia of the two premolars and the mesial buccal root of the first molar is achieved by depositing the anesthetic agent in the area just below the apex of the second premolar (this procedure anesthetizes the middle superior alveolar nerve, when present, and/or the dental plexus) (Fig.19-1).

When the palatal mucosa is involved in the operative procedures, the greater palatine nerve must also be blocked as it emerges from the greater palatine foramen.

Anesthesia of the canine as well as the lateral and central incisors may be accomplished by one of two procedures. One technique involves an anterior superior alveolar nerve block, a plexus anesthesia, accomplished by depositing anesthetic solution above the roots of the anterior teeth (Fig. 19-2).

Another technique involves an infraorbital nerve block, discussed in the next section, known as trunk anesthesia.

Anesthetizing the nasopalatine nerve in the vicinity of the incisive papilla (a particularly painful injection) will result in complete anesthesia on both sides of the anterior palatal region.

Clinical Considerations

Subperiosteal Injections

Anesthesia in most regions of the maxilla can be achieved by plexus anesthesia. This method places the anesthetic solution into the connective tissue overlying the periosteum. It is important to avoid subperiosteal injections because such injections cause tearing of blood vessels as the fluid detaches the periosteum from the bone, resulting in subperiosteal hematomas and considerable pain on recovery.

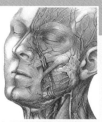

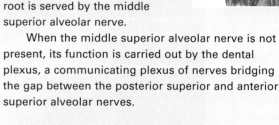

Middle Superior Alveolar Nerve Block

Although the middle superior alveolar nerve is reported to be present in only about 28% of the population, when present it innervates the premolar teeth of the upper arch and assists in the sensory innervation of the first maxillary molar.

Anesthesia of the three molars is achieved by injection in the region of the second molar and the second premolar. The latter site is essential only if anesthesia of the mesial buccal root of the first molar is desired, because this particular root is served by the middle superior alveolar nerve.

When the middle superior alveolar nerve is not present, its function is carried out by the dental plexus, a communicating plexus of nerves bridging the gap between the posterior superior and anterior superior alveolar nerves.

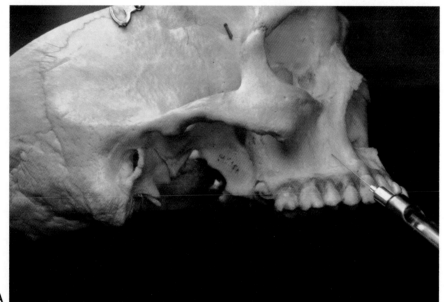

A

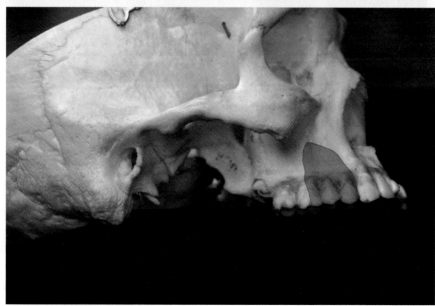

B

Figure 19-1. **(A)** Illustrates needle placement of anesthesia of the middle superior alveolar nerve. **(B)** Illustrates the area anesthetized.

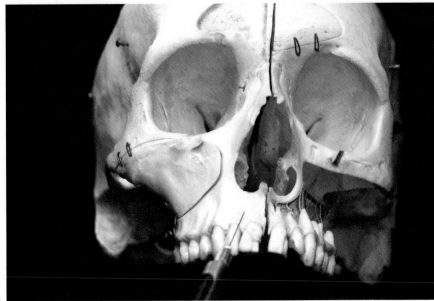

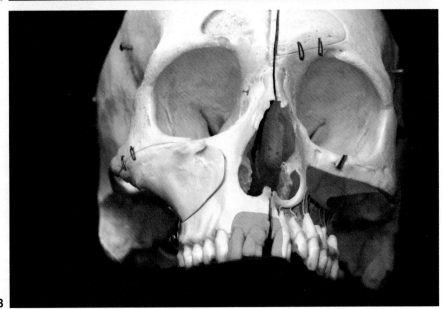

Figure 19-2. **(A)** Illustrates needle placement of anesthesia of the anterior superior alveolar nerve. **(B)** Illustrates the area anesthetized.

Mandibular Plexus Anesthesia

Summary Bite. Plexus anesthesia for the mandibular dentition is restricted to the region of the incisors. This is necessary because the cortical bone of much of the mandible is thick, thus prohibiting diffusion of the anesthetic agent.

Plexus anesthesia of mandibular teeth is usually accomplished only in the region of the incisors. However, most of the mandibular cortical plate is too thick for plexus anesthesia. Hence, for mandibular procedures, trunk anesthesia is the method of choice.

Plexus anesthesia of the mandibular incisors is accomplished by delivering anesthetic solution into the vestibular mucosa inferior to the root of the incisors. When manipulation of the lingual gingiva is planned, block anesthesia of the lingual nerve is necessary.

TRUNK ANESTHESIA

Summary Bite. Trunk anesthesia (nerve block) is a mode of anesthesia where the anesthetic solution is deposited in the immediate vicinity the nerve or nerve trunk proximal to the area to be treated.

Maxillary Teeth

Summary Bite. Several nerves serving the teeth and/or their supporting tissues within the maxillary arch are accessible for nerve blocks via trunk anesthesia.

Posterior Superior Alveolar Nerve Block

The posterior superior alveolar nerve (PSA) is accessible on the maxillary tuberosity as the nerve enters the small posterior superior alveolar foramen.

A block of the posterior superior alveolar nerve will anesthetize the three molars. However, during a posterior superior alveolar nerve block, anesthesia of the mesial buccal root of the first molar fails in about 28% of the patient population. Therefore, if profound dental procedures are to be performed on the maxillary first molar, the middle superior alveolar nerve should also be anesthetized.

It must be kept in mind that the posterior superior alveolar nerve block will not anesthetize the labial gingival (Fig.19-3).

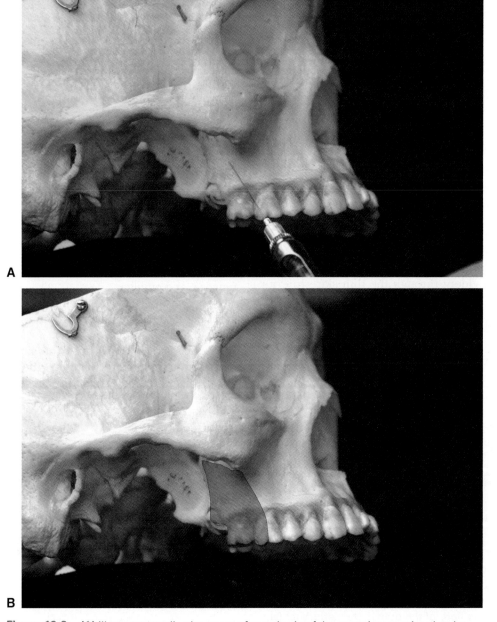

Figure 19-3. **(A)** Illustrates needle placement of anesthesia of the posterior superior alveolar nerve. **(B)** Illustrates the area anesthetized.

Clinical Considerations

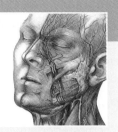

Posterior Superior Alveolar Nerve Block

Anesthetic solution for a posterior superior alveolar nerve block should be delivered through the mucosa of the fornix at the level of the second molar, following the maxilla very closely to circumvent penetration of the pterygoid plexus of veins. Although the veins are easily avoided, the posterior superior alveolar artery is not. If the artery is accidentally penetrated, a large hematoma will quickly result. The bleeding may be controlled by exerting pressure on the maxilla at the anterior border of the masseter muscle, just inferior to the zygomatic arch.

Even with following the rules of aspiration, this is one area where extreme care is important in preventing an anesthetic needle from penetrating the posterior superior alveolar artery just before it enters the bone.

Infraorbital Trunk Block

Although the infraorbital nerve block (sometimes called an IO nerve block) is less popular than the PSA nerve block, it provides profound anesthesia from the central incisor through the canine in every patient, and through the second premolar in about 72% of the patient population. Thus, this procedure is advantageous when two or more of those teeth are to be treated.

The infraorbital nerve may be reached in the infraorbital canal, where it gives rise to the anterior (and, sometimes, middle) superior alveolar nerves. The canal is accessible via the infraorbital foramen. The position of the foramen may be located by palpation of the orbital rim, where the zygomaticomaxillary suture is evident through the thin skin. Inferior to this suture, the bony ledge is felt to curve under, indicating the infraorbital foramen (Fig. 19-4).

Greater Palatine Nerve Block

The greater palatine nerve exits the same-named foramen to innervate the hard palate as far anteri-orly as the canine region, where it communicates with the nasopalatine nerve. Anesthesia may be accomplished by piercing the palatal mucosa midway between the roof of the mouth and the gingival margin of the third molar. Should the first premolar be involved, a nasopalatine block also must be performed (Fig. 19-5).

Mandibular Teeth
Nasopalatine Nerve Block

The nasopalatine nerve supplies the anterior portion of the hard palate, lingual alveolar bone of the six anterior teeth, as well as the entire anterior palatal mucosa, and gingiva.

The nasopalatine nerve exits the incisive foramen just posterior to the interdental papilla between the two central incisors.

Access is simple because the site of injection is just deep to the incisive papilla. When the premolars are involved, a greater palatine block should also be performed (Fig. 19-6).

Clinical Considerations

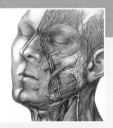

Infraorbital Nerve Block

Caution must be exercised in performing an infraorbital nerve block so that the thin, bony roof of the canal is not perforated.

If perforation occurs, the anesthetic solution will be deposited on the floor of the orbit in the periorbital fat, temporarily paralyzing the inferior rectus and inferior oblique muscles.

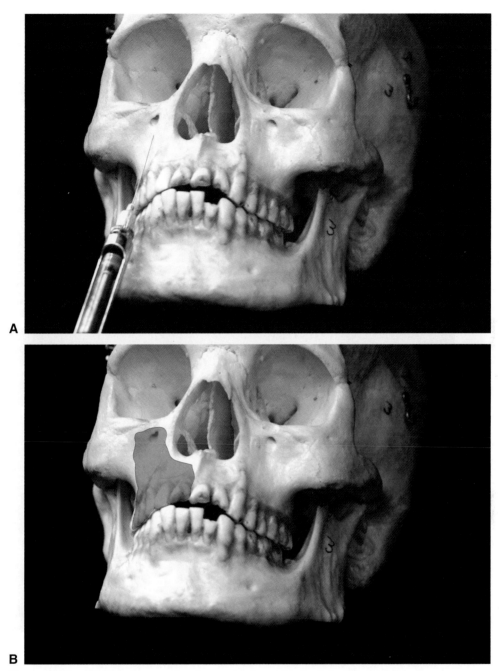

Figure 19-4. **(A)** Illustrates needle placement of anesthesia of the infraorbital nerve. **(B)** Illustrates the area anesthetized.

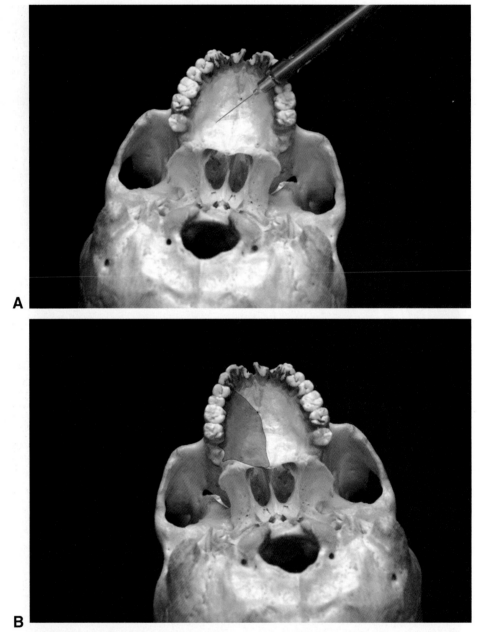

Figure 19-5. **(A)** Illustrates needle placement of anesthesia of the greater palatine nerve. **(B)** Illustrates the area anesthetized.

Clinical Considerations

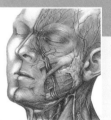

Greater Palatine Nerve Block

Care must be exercised in delivering a greater palatine nerve block. The anesthetic solution must not be injected into the greater palatine foramen or even close to it, because the lesser palatine nerves overlap the region. In the case where the anesthesia affects both the greater and lesser palatine nerves, both the soft and hard palates will be anesthetized, causing the patient to gag.

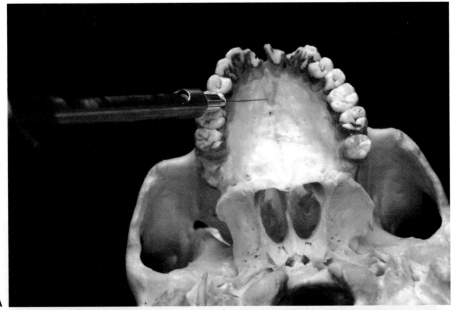

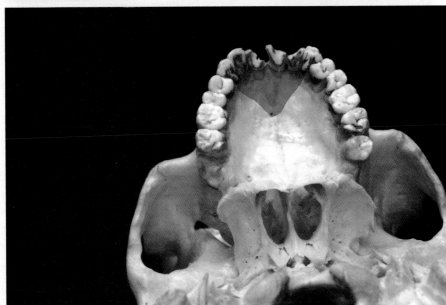

Figure 19-6. **(A)** Illustrates needle placement of anesthesia of the nasopalatine nerve. **(B)** Illustrates the area anesthetized.

Clinical Considerations

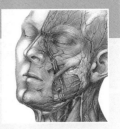

Nasopalatine Nerve Block

Both right and left nasopalatine nerves are anesthetized by this block; thus, the entire anterior palate from the right first premolar to left first premolar is anesthetized. Because the palatal mucosa is tightly bound to the maxillary bone, the nasopalatine nerve block is painful; therefore, the solution should be delivered slowly, in advance of the needle, and in small quantities.

Numbness to the anterior palate is somewhat discomforting to the patient.

Inferior Alveolar and Lingual Nerve Blocks

Block of the inferior alveolar nerve, also known as a **mandibular block**, occurs at the mandibular foramen just before the inferior alveolar nerve enters it.

The mandibular foramen is situated on the medial aspect of the ramus of the mandible, in close association with the lingula and the sphenomandibular ligament.

The anesthetic agent should be delivered to this point by piercing the mucosa between the retromolar pad and the pterygomandibular fold, at the level of the occlusal plane of the three mandibular molars. Most of the anesthetic solution should be deposited here.

To anesthetize the lingual nerve, which lies close by, it is necessary to deposit solution just anterior and medial to the bony landmark. Anesthesia of the inferior alveolar and lingual nerves desensitizes the mandibular teeth and gingiva on that side.

Occasionally, the buccal nerve must also be blocked to provide anesthesia of the mandibular buccal mucosa and gingiva (Fig. 19-7).

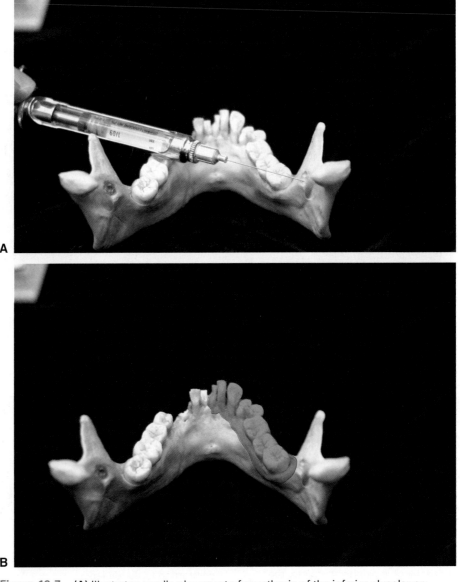

Figure 19-7. **(A)** Illustrates needle placement of anesthesia of the inferior alveolar or mandibular nerve. **(B)** Illustrates the area anesthetized.

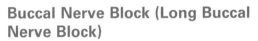

Clinical Considerations

Mandibular Nerve Block

One advantage to the mandibular nerve block is that it provides a wide area of anesthesia for working on more than one tooth during one appointment because it anesthetizes the inferior alveolar nerve, the incisive, mental, and commonly the lingual nerve on the mandibular quadrant. This would include the buccal mucoperiosteum anterior to the first molar. The buccal mucosa of the molars must be anesthetized with a buccal nerve block.

Disadvantages to the mandibular block include inadequate anesthesia (15%–20%); positive aspiration (10%–15%), highest of all intraoral anesthesia techniques; partial anesthesia due to inferior alveolar nerve/foramen anatomy; accessory innervation of the mandibular teeth; oral landmarks not consistent; and lower lip and tongue anesthesia discomforting to patients and dangerous for certain individuals.

Buccal Nerve Block (Long Buccal Nerve Block)

The buccal nerve crosses the anterior border of the ramus of the mandible at the level of the occlusal plane of the maxillary molars. Hence, this nerve may be anesthetized just lateral to the mandibular ramus. It is not necessary to anesthetize the buccal nerve unless anesthesia of the molar buccal gingiva is desired (Fig. 19-8).

Mental Nerve Block

The mental nerve exits the mandibular canal via the mental foramen, located on the lateral aspect of the mandibular body. The foramen is located just below the second premolar, halfway between the gingival margin and the inferior border of the mandible.

Anesthetic solution should be introduced deep to the mucosa at the level of the second mandibular premolar, approximately at the fornix. Successful block of the mental nerve will anesthetize the facial periodontium of the mandibular premolars, canine, and incisors on one side, including adjacent gingival and alveolar tissues and the periodontal ligament. It should be remembered that if pulpal tissue is to be anesthetized, it will be necessary to block the incisive nerve at the mental foramen (Fig.19-9).

Mandibular Incisive Nerve Block

The mandibular incisive nerve block is not frequently used because, when the inferior alveolar or mandibular block is performed, the anterior mandibular teeth are anesthetized. Also, when a mental nerve block is performed, the incisive nerve (the other terminal of the inferior alveolar nerve) may also anesthetized. The technique for administering the incisive block is very similar to that of a mental block, with the target area being the same. The major difference is that slightly more anesthesia is deposited at the mental foramen and, after retracting the needle, finger pressure is applied to force the anesthetic solution into the mental foramen (see Fig 19-9 for placement of the anesthetic).

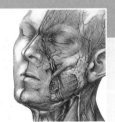

Clinical Considerations

Buccal Nerve Block

The success rate for buccal nerve anesthesia is nearly 100%; however, it can be uncomfortable if the needle penetrates the periosteum.

Because the tendon of the temporalis muscle may be penetrated, care must be exercised in depositing the anesthetic agent. Block anesthesia of the buccal nerve will anesthetize the buccal gingiva and mucosa of the mandibular molars.

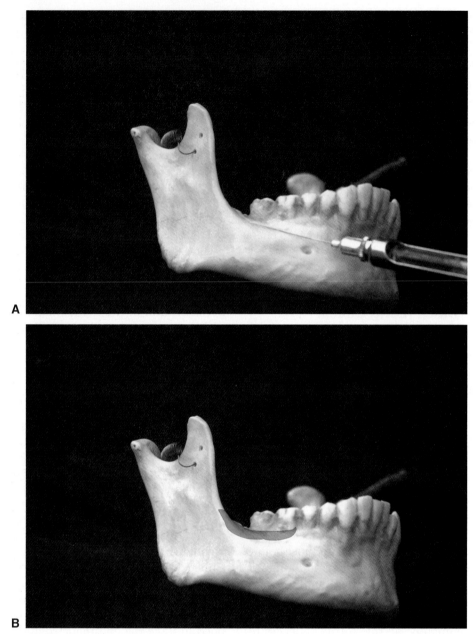

Figure 19-8. **(A)** Illustrates needle placement of anesthesia of the buccal nerve. **(B)** Illustrates the area anesthetized.

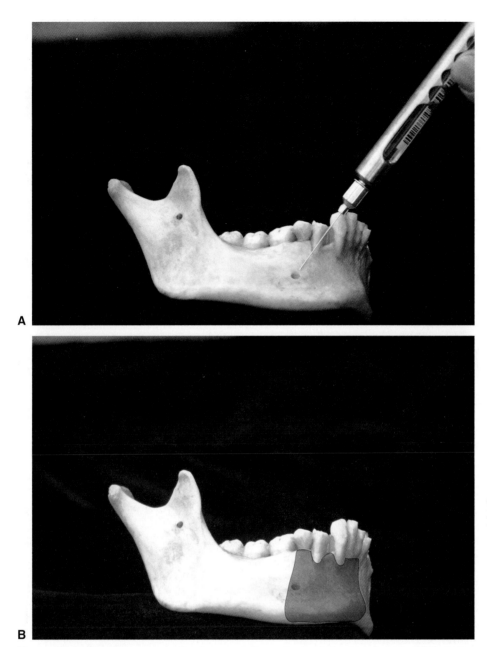

Figure 19-9. **(A)** Illustrates needle placement of anesthesia of the mental nerve. **(B)** Illustrates the area anesthetized.

Clinical Considerations

Mental Nerve Block

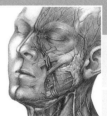

The mental nerve and the incisive nerve are the terminals of the inferior alveolar nerve. The mental nerve serves the buccal mucosa anterior to the buccal foramen to the midline, and also the skin on the lower lip and chin. Hence, it is used most often when buccal soft tissue requires anesthesia for a dental procedure. As such, the mental nerve block is infrequently utilized in dental procedures.

Clinical Considerations

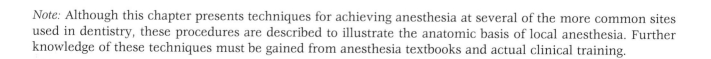

Mandibular Incisive Block

The incisive block in the mandible is not often utilized because an inferior alveolar (mandibular) block will anesthetize the anterior teeth in the mandibular arch. However, the mandibular incisive block will permit the oral professional to work on multiple anterior teeth at one appointment. It must be remembered that only the pulp of these anterior teeth will be anesthetized and, if lingual gingiva is to be involved, that region should also be anesthetized.

Note: Although this chapter presents techniques for achieving anesthesia at several of the more common sites used in dentistry, these procedures are described to illustrate the anatomic basis of local anesthesia. Further knowledge of these techniques must be gained from anesthesia textbooks and actual clinical training.

Lymphatics of the Head and Neck

20

Key Terms

Lymph is the term applied to the extra-cellular fluid that bathes the cells of the interstitial spaces. This fluid exits the capillary beds and the venules of the circulatory system and, because its pressure within the tissue is less than the venous pressure of the blood, it is unable to enter the venous system. Lymph contains proteins, fats, large particulate matter, and cells that find their way to lymphatic vessels, which deliver their contents to lymph nodes located along their course.

Lymph eventually returns to the circulatory system as it is collected first by small lymphatic vessels passing to larger and larger vessels, finally to enter the right lymphatic duct, or its counterpart on the left side, the thoracic duct. Lymph from these two ducts is emptied into the corresponding right and left subclavian veins.

Lymph Nodes are fairly constant in their location and the regional lymph that they filter. Lymph flows through at least one lymph node (but usually several) before returning to the circulatory system. In the lymph nodes foreign substances are phagocytosed and lymph is filtered. Lymph nodes are constant structures and their positions should be clearly understood by health professionals because these structures become swollen during infections and inflammations.

By understanding these facts, a health professional can sometimes pinpoint the region of a disease process simply by knowing the route of lymph flow through the node field when one or more nodes are involved.

For these reasons, the jugulodigastric and the omoclavicular lymph nodes are especially important to oral health professionals.

327

Extracellular fluid is constantly being produced in excess by the circulatory system. Consequently, the interstitial spaces of the body receive more fluid from the arterial end of a capillary network than that which returns at the venous end. The excess extracellular fluid, as well as proteins, fats, large particulate matter, and cells, find their way to lymphatic vessels, which deliver their contents to lymph nodes located along their course. Here, foreign substances are phagocytosed and lymph is filtered. Lymph nodes are constant structures and their positions should be clearly understood by health professionals because these structures become swollen during infections and inflammations. Because specific nodes receive lymph from relatively specific areas of the body, the clinician should be able to deduce the general location of the infection by knowledge of lymphatic drainage. This chapter includes the names and locations of the principal lymph nodes of the head and neck, and the areas they drain.

LYMPH NODES OF THE HEAD AND NECK

Lymph Nodes of the Head

Summary Bite. Because the central nervous system possesses no lymph vessels, the lymph nodes of the head are extracranial and regionalized into several groups about the scalp.

Lymph nodes of the head are all extracranial because the central nervous system possesses no lymph vessels or lymph nodes. The general pattern of lymph nodes about the head is that they are regionalized into several groups to drain the posterior and anterolateral scalp as well as the superficial and deep aspects of the face (Fig. 20-1 and Table 20-1).

- **Occipital lymph nodes** (two to four in number) are located on the back of the head, lying on the semispinalis capitis muscle just inferior to the attachment of the trapezius muscle.
- **Mastoid (postauricular) lymph nodes** (one to three in number) are located behind the ear on the mastoid process, superficial to the insertion of the sternocleidomastoid muscle.
- **Preauricular (superficial parotid) lymph nodes** (two to three in number) lie anterior to the ear, superficial to and sometimes deep to the capsule of the parotid gland. Those located deep to the capsule are sometimes grouped with the deep parotid lymph nodes described with those of the face.

Lymph Nodes of the Face

Summary Bite. Lymph nodes of the face are subdivided into those of the parotid, superficial face, and the deep face.

- **Parotid lymph nodes** (10 to 15 in number) form two groups: those lying embedded within the substance of the gland and those lying deep to the gland adjacent the pharyngeal wall.
- **Superficial facial lymph nodes** (up to 12 in number), disposed along the course of the facial artery and vein, are the:
  - **Maxillary (infraorbital) lymph nodes** in the vicinity of the infraorbital foramen;
  - **Buccal lymph node(s)** on/in the buccal fat pad over the buccinator muscle; and
  - **Mandibular lymph nodes** (two to three in number) along the facial artery and vein adjacent the masseter muscle.
- **Deep facial lymph nodes** follow the course of the maxillary artery in the infratemporal fossa superficial to the lateral pterygoid muscle. Two additional groups of deep nodes are important:
  - **Lingual lymph nodes** (numbering two to three) lying on the superficial aspect of the hyoglossus muscle; and
  - **Retropharyngeal lymph nodes** (two to three in number) located in the buccopharyngeal fascia behind the pharynx at the level of the atlas.

Lymph Nodes of the Neck

Summary Bite. Lymph nodes of the neck are disposed in several groups: the anterior cervical, submental, submandibular, superficial cervical, and deep cervical lymph nodes.

- **Anterior cervical lymph nodes** are inconsistent and are located in two groups, superficial and deep, in front of the viscera of the neck.
  - The **superficial group** is located in an irregular row along the course of the anterior jugular vein.
  - The **deep group** is subdivided into four small chains: the paratracheal lymph nodes of the tracheoesophageal groove; the infrahyoid lymph nodes, lying superficial to the thyrohyoid membrane; the pretracheal nodes, situated between the investing layer of the deep cervical fascia and the trachea; and the prelaryngeal nodes, which lie on the cricothyroid ligament.
- **Submental lymph nodes** are located between the anterior bellies of the right and left digastric muscles.

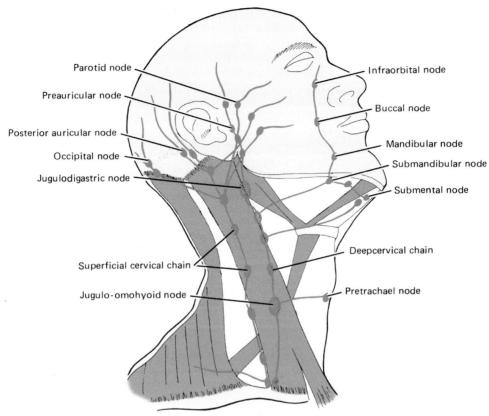

Parotid node
Preauricular node
Posterior auricular node
Occipital node
Jugulodigastric node
Superficial cervical chain
Jugulo-omohyoid node

Infraorbital node
Buccal node
Mandibular node
Submandibular node
Submental node
Deepcervical chain
Pretrachael node

Figure 20-1. Diagrammatic representation of lymphatic drainage of the head and neck.

- **Submandibular lymph nodes** are located in the same-named triangle in close proximity to the submandibular gland. Although these constitute a chain of three to six lymph nodes, the only constant node is the one at the facial groove of the mandible in close association with the facial artery.
- **Superficial cervical lymph nodes** may be found lying adjacent the external jugular vein as it passes superficial to the sternocleidomastoid muscle.
- **Deep cervical lymph nodes** are numerous and form a chain along the carotid sheath. These nodes are most important because, ultimately, they receive all of the lymph from the head and neck. Their efferent vessels form the **jugular trunk**, which delivers the collected lymph to the right lymphatic duct (or to the thoracic duct on the left side) to be returned to the circulatory system. These deep cervical lymph nodes parallel the carotid sheath along its entire length. The lymph nodes of this group may conveniently be organized into two subgroups: the superior and inferior deep cervical lymph nodes.
  - **Superior deep cervical lymph nodes**, some of which are large, form a chain, surrounding the internal jugular vein, extending from the mastoid process to the superior border of the subclavian triangle. The most superior node of this group is the large **jugulodigastric (tonsillar) lymph node**, located between the posterior belly of the digastric muscle and the internal jugular vein. This node is of particular importance in physical diagnosis.
- **Inferior deep cervical lymph nodes** reside in the subclavian triangle. Nodes of this group are in close association with the brachial plexus, the subclavian artery and vein, and the omohyoid muscle. A large, constant node of this group, located in the vicinity of the intermediate tendon of the omohyoid muscle, is the **jugulo-omohyoid lymph node**. (This node is located in a border zone between the superior and inferior deep cervical nodes; therefore, reference to its group association varies.)

Accompanying the deep chain in the posterior cervical triangle are the **accessory lymph nodes** (numbering two to six) lying alongside the accessory nerve, and the **transverse cervical lymph nodes** (1 to 10 in number) accompanying the transverse cervical vessels.

Table 20-1 Lymph Nodes of the Head and Neck

Node	Location	Afferent	Efferent
Superficial Lymph Nodes of the Head			
Occipital (2–4)	Superior nuchal line between sternocleidomastoid and trapezius	Occipital part of scalp	Superficial cervical lymph nodes Accessary lymph nodes
Mastoid (1–3)	Superficial to sternocleidomastoid insertion	Posterior parietal scalp Skin of ear, posterior external acoustic meatus	Superior deep cervical nodes Accessary lymph nodes
Preauricular (2–3)	Anterior to ear over parotid fascia	Drains areas supplied by superficial temporal artery Anterior parietal scalp Anterior surface of ear	Superior deep cervical lymph nodes
Parotid (up to 10 or more)	About parotid gland and under parotid fascia Deep to parotid gland	External acoustic meatus Skin of frontal and temporal regions Eyelids, tympanic cavity Cheek, nose (posterior palate)	Superior deep cervical lymph nodes
Facial Superficial (up to 12) Maxillary Buccal Mandibular	Distributed along course of facial artery and vein	Skin and mucous membranes of eyelids, nose, cheek	Submandibular nodes
Deep	Distributed along course of maxillary artery lateral to lateral pterygoid muscle	Temporal and infratemporal fossa Nasal pharynx	Superior deep cervical lymph nodes
Superficial Cervical Lymph Nodes			
Anterior cervical Superficial	Anterior jugular vein between superficial cervical fascia and infrahyoid fascia	Skin, muscles, and viscera of infrahyoid region of neck	Superior deep cervical lymph nodes
Deep	Between viscera of neck and investing layer of deep cervical fascia	Adjoining parts of trachea, larynx, thyroid gland	Superior deep cervical lymph nodes
Submental (2–3)	Submental triangle	Chin Medial part of lower lip Lower incisor teeth and gingiva Tip of tongue Cheeks	Submandibular lymph node to jugulo-omohyoid lymph node and superior deep cervical lymph nodes
Submandibular (3–6)	Submandibular triangle adjacent submandibular gland	Facial nodes Chin Lateral upper and lower lips Submental nodes Cheeks and nose, anterior nasal cavity Maxillary and mandibular teeth and gingiva Oral palate Lateral parts of anterior 2/3 of tongue	Superior deep cervical lymph nodes and jugulo-omohyoid lymph nodes

(continued)

Table 20-1 Lymph Nodes of the Head and Neck

Node	Location	Afferent	Efferent
Superficial cervical (1–2)	Along external jugular vein superficial to sternocleidomastoid muscle	Lower part of ear and parotid region	Superior deep cervical lymph nodes
Deep Cervical Lymph Nodes			
Superior deep cervical	Surrounding internal jugular vein deep to sternocleidomastoid and superior to omohyoid muscle	Occipital nodes Mastoid nodes Preauricular nodes Parotid nodes Submandibular nodes Superficial cervical nodes Retropharyngeal nodes	Inferior deep cervical nodes or separate channel to jugulo-subclavian junction
Jugulodigastric	Junction of internal jugular vein and posterior digastric muscle	Palatine and lingual tonsils Posterior palate Lateral portions of the anterior 2/3 of tongue	Inferior deep cervical lymph nodes
Jugulo-omohyoid	Above junction of internal jugular vein and omohyoid muscle	Posterior 1/3 of tongue Submandibular nodes Submental nodes	Inferior deep cervical lymph nodes
Inferior deep cervical	Along internal jugular vein below omohyoid muscle deep to the sternocleidomastoid muscle	Transverse cervical nodes Anterior cervical nodes Superior deep cervical nodes	Jugular trunk
Retropharyngeal (1–3)	Retropharyngeal space	Posterior nasal cavity Paranasal sinuses Hard and soft palate Nasopharynx, oropharynx Anditory tube	Superior deep cervical nodes
Accessory (2–6)	Along accessory nerve in posterior triangle	Occipital nodes Mastoid nodes Lateral neck and shoulder	Transverse cervical nodes
Transverse cervical (1–10)	Along transverse cervical blood vessels at level of clavicle	Accessory nodes Apical axillary nodes Lateral neck Anterior thoracic wall	Jugular trunk or directly into thoracic duct or right lymphatic duct or independently into junction of internal jugular vein and subclavian vein

LYMPHATIC DRAINAGE OF THE HEAD AND NECK

Summary Bite. Lymph within the superficial and deep regions of the head and neck passes through one to several lymph nodes via minor lymph vessels, and from there into major lymph vessels. The lymph is eventually emptied into either the right or left subclavian veins to be returned to the cardiovascular system.

Superficial Tissues

The back of the scalp is drained by the occipital lymph nodes, whose efferent vessels empty into the superficial cervical lymph nodes. The lymph vessels of the medial surface of the ear, the lateral aspects of the eyelids, the temporal region, and most of the forehead drain into the mastoid, preauricular, and parotid lymph nodes. Efferents from these nodes then pass into the superior deep cervical lymph nodes. The remainder of the eye and middle ear are drained by

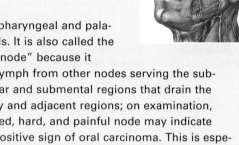

Clinical Considerations

Jugulodigastric Lymph Node

The jugulodigastric lymph node is a large node of the superior deep cervical lymph node chain that extends along the surface of the internal jugular vein. The jugulodigastric lymph node lies between the tendon of the posterior belly of the digastric muscle and the internal jugular vein. It is readily palpable, especially when it is swollen, hard, or painful to touch. This lymph node is sometimes called the "principal node of the tongue" because it receives lymph from the lateral portions of the anterior two thirds of the tongue. Sometimes it is called the "tonsillar node" because it receives lymph from the pharyngeal and palatine tonsils. It is also called the "sentinel node" because it receives lymph from other nodes serving the submandibular and submental regions that drain the oral cavity and adjacent regions; on examination, an enlarged, hard, and painful node may indicate the first positive sign of oral carcinoma. This is especially true of this node because drainage to this node comes from areas difficult to observe in an oral examination.

the preauricular (parotid lymph nodes), which then drain into the superior deep cervical lymph nodes.

Submandibular lymph nodes receive lymph from the nose, cheek, and lip, either directly or via the buccal lymph nodes. The lateral aspect of the cheek and the skin over the bridge of the nose are partially drained also by the parotid lymph nodes.

Lymph from the mucosa over the floor of the mouth, the tip of the tongue, and the central portion of the lower lip is drained into the submental lymph nodes, whence it empties into the jugulo-omohyoid lymph node of the inferior deep cervical chain.

Superficial tissues of the neck are drained by the deep cervical lymph nodes directly or indirectly. Lymph from the posterior cervical triangle may first enter the superficial cervical and occipital nodes, from which the lymph flows to the deep cervical lymph nodes. Lymph from the anterior cervical triangle, above the hyoid bone, is drained into the submental and submandibular lymph nodes, whereas lymph collected from the region inferior to the hyoid bone drains into the anterior cervical lymph nodes, whose efferents deliver it to the inferior deep cervical lymph nodes.

Deep Tissues

Most of the lymph of the nasal cavity, paranasal sinuses, and nasopharynx drains into the retropharyngeal lymph nodes or passes directly to the inferior deep cervical lymph chain. The thyroid gland is drained by the pretracheal, prelaryngeal, and paratracheal lymph nodes, whence lymph flows to the deep cervical lymph nodes.

Frequently, some of the lymph from this endocrine gland passes directly into the deep cervical lymph nodes. The tracheal, esophageal, and laryngeal lymph in the region of the neck also passes either directly or indirectly, via the prelaryngeal or paratracheal lymph nodes, into the deep cervical chain. Tonsillar lymph is drained into the jugulodigastric lymph node of the superior deep cervical chain.

Lymph drainage from the gingiva, teeth, and tongue deserves special attention. Gingival lymph is gathered on the lingual and vestibular surfaces by submucosal plexuses of lymph vessels, which are consolidated into a series of vessels behind the molars. From here the lymph passes either to the submandibular lymph nodes or, occasionally, into the deep cervical lymph nodes.

Lymph vessels of the pulp and those of the periodontal ligament of the same tooth are drained by a common vessel. Lack of agreement exists concerning the precise path of lymph drainage of teeth, but a reasonable case may be made for the following description.

The mandibular incisors are drained by the submental lymph nodes, and the remaining teeth (both maxillary and mandibular) are drained by the submandibular lymph nodes. Generally, lymphatic drainage is ipsilateral, although for structures near the midline it is both ipsilateral and contralateral.

Lymphatic drainage of the tongue is complex because the tongue has a rich lymphatic plexus of vessels that is drained by three vessel groups: the marginal, dorsal, and central vessels. In addition, drainage from the two sides is intermingled to a large extent, and the base of the tongue is drained by lymph nodes situated more cranially than those that receive lymph from the tip of the tongue. Vessels from the tip of the tongue pass to the submental nodes along with those of the region of the lingual frenulum.

The lateral aspect of the anterior two thirds of the tongue is also drained by marginal vessels, into the jugulodigastric lymph nodes. The central vessels drain the medial region of the anterior two thirds of the tongue, delivering the lymph to the jugulo-omohyoid lymph nodes. In addition, dorsal vessels drain the region of the sulcus terminalis and the posterior one third of the tongue, delivering lymph to the marginal lymph vessels that are drained by the jugulo-omohyoid lymph nodes.

Accessory lymph nodes located about the accessory nerve in the posterior cervical triangle may drain occipital and mastoid nodes in addition to areas of the lateral neck and shoulder. The transverse cervical nodes, located in the posterior cervical triangle, drain the accessory chain of nodes, the lateral neck, the anterior thoracic wall, the mammary gland, and, occasionally, the upper limb. Efferents from this group may pass into the jugular lymphatic trunk, the thoracic duct, or the right lymphatic duct, or they may enter the internal jugular or subclavian veins independently.

Clinical Considerations

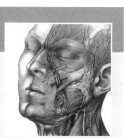

Lymph Node Examination

Lymph nodes of a healthy individual are soft, nonpalpable structures. However, infection, inflammation, and carcinomatous involvement of areas drained by lymph nodes cause these structures to become palpable, swollen, hard, and maybe even painful.

Implications of the Disease State from Lymph Node Examinations

The health professional dealing with the oral cavity should examine patients for swollen, painful lymph nodes, especially the submental, submandibular, and superficial and deep cervical chains. The last group may be palpated with relative ease by manipulation of the relaxed sternocleidomastoid muscle.

Diseased states of the oral cavity will most probably be reflected in the submental and submandibular lymph nodes. Remembering that, in the process of lymph drainage, the fluid passes through a series of lymph nodes before emptying into the thoracic or right lymphatic ducts, it becomes evident that each lymph node group is a "barrier" where the disease agent is being combated. The first such site is known as the **primary node**, which drains into a **secondary node** that may be drained by a **tertiary node**. The more nodes that are interposed in the disease agent's route of spread before reaching the major lymphatic channels, the better the chance of successfully combating the disease. Hence, a knowledge of lymphatic drainage of the head and neck assists the health professional dealing with this region in determining the site of disease manifestation.

Treatment of cervical metastases may involve a radical surgery, that is, a "block resection" of the cervical lymph nodes. It is essential that all lymph nodes of the particular side of the neck be removed. To ensure that this is the case, connective tissues, muscles, glands, and even nerves of the area are frequently sacrificed.

Vascular Supply of the Head and Neck

21

Key Terms

Arterial Supply to the head and neck arises primarily from branches originating from three sources: the subclavian artery and the external and internal carotid arteries.

Common Carotid Artery, similar to the subclavian artery origins, differs between the left and right sides. The right common carotid artery originates from the brachiocephalic trunk, whereas the left common carotid artery originates from the arch of the aorta. The common carotid arteries possess no branches in the neck; rather, each common carotid artery bifurcates at the level of the thyroid cartilage into the internal and external carotid arteries.

External Carotid Artery is the other terminal of the common carotid artery arising at the bifurcation of the common carotid artery. The external carotid artery has six collateral and two terminal branches. The branches serve structures in the neck and the head, including the face, oral cavity, and nasal cavity. The two terminal arteries serve the oral cavity, deep face and the structures about it, and the side of the head.

External Jugular Vein drains the face and the neck. Veins draining the face are divided into superficial and deep veins. Small veins drain a particular area and then these veins drain into larger veins. and still larger named veins become

regional veins receiving contributions from many areas. There are many direct communications between veins of areas and regions. These form venous plexuses in many regions within the head and neck as well as within the cranium. Thus, these plexuses are possible avenues for the spread of infection.

Internal Carotid Artery possesses no branches in the neck. Instead, it enters into the cranial vault via the carotid canal to serve the structures within the cranium.

Internal Jugular Vein drains the cranium before exiting the cranial cavity via the jugular foramen. Most of the veins draining the cranium are detailed in Chapter 17.

Subclavian Artery origins differ on the left and right sides of the body. The right subclavian artery is the terminal of the brachiocephalic trunk, whereas the left subclavian artery arises from the arch of the aorta. Both of the subclavian arteries ascend into the neck deep to and in a specific relationship with the anterior scalene muscle. Thus, the first part of the subclavian artery lies medial to the anterior scalene muscle; the second part of the subclavian artery lies behind the anterior scalene muscle; whereas and the third part of the artery lies lateral to the anterior scalene muscle. The several branches arising from the subclavian artery are described as arising from one of these three parts. Most of the neck structures are vascularized by branches of the subclavian arteries.

Venous Drainage from the head and neck is collected into two major venous trunks: the internal and external jugular veins.

The head and neck receive most of their vascular supply from branches of the external and internal carotid arteries, as well as from certain branches of the subclavian artery. Most of the blood within the internal carotid artery and the vertebral branch of the subclavian artery is destined for the brain, whereas all of the blood carried by the external carotid artery and some branches of the subclavian artery supplies the remainder of the region. Drainage of this area is accomplished by the tributaries of the internal and external jugular veins, as well as those of the vertebral vein. This chapter discusses the branches and tributaries of these major vessels and their locations, sources, and destinations in a systemic fashion. However, vessels whose primary concerns are the brain and the internal base of the skull will not be detailed here; instead, that material may be found in Chapter 17.

COMMON CAROTID ARTERY

The **common carotid arteries** of the two sides have different origins. The right common carotid artery is a branch of the brachiocephalic trunk, whereas the left arises directly from the arch of the aorta. Consequently, the right common carotid artery is contained wholly within the neck, whereas the left common carotid artery begins in the upper thorax and enters the neck in the vicinity of the sternoclavicular joint. Once in the neck, both vessels are enclosed in their own compartment of the carotid sheath and ascend approximately to the level of the thyroid cartilage (although this is variable), where each bifurcates into an **external** and an **internal carotid artery** (Figs. 21-1 and 21-2). Because these vessels are considered terminal branches, the common carotid artery is said to have no branches in the neck. The common carotid artery presents a slight dilation at its bifurcation, the **carotid sinus**, a modified region of the vessel. It is innervated by the glossopharyngeal nerve, whose function is to monitor blood pressure. An additional structure, the **carotid body**, is also associated with the region of bifurcation. This small, oval, reddish-brown structure, lying within the wall of the carotid artery and innervated by branches of the glossopharyngeal and vagus nerves, is a chemoreceptor, monitoring oxygen and carbon dioxide tensions as well as hydrogen ion concentration.

Clinical Considerations

Carotid Sinus Syndrome

Carotid sinus syndrome may result in loss of consciousness due to simple head movements. The syndrome relates to the hypersensitivity of the carotid sinus due to an unknown etiology. Sudden slight pressure changes, such as that occasioned by movement of the head, may result in stimulation of the carotid sinus. Impulses relayed by the sinus reduce blood pressure and slow the pumping action of the heart, thus decreasing blood supply to the brain and resulting in sudden loss of consciousness.

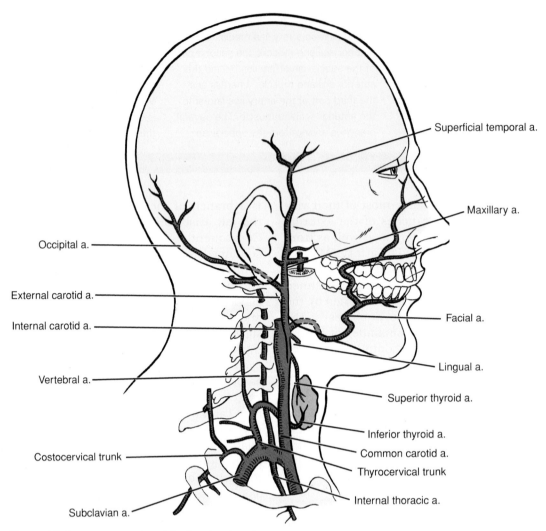

Figure 21-1. Major arteries of the head and neck.

External Carotid Artery

The **external carotid artery** has six collateral and two terminal branches. They are described in the order of their origins from inferior to superior.

Superior Thyroid Artery

The **superior thyroid artery** is the first branch of the external carotid artery, arising from its ventral aspect, just superior to the bifurcation of the common carotid artery (Figs. 21-1 and 21-2). The superior thyroid artery descends in the neck, accompanied by the same-named vein and the external laryngeal nerve, reaches the superior pole of the thyroid gland, and divides into its terminal branches, some of which anastomose with their counterparts of the other side and with branches of the inferior thyroid artery. The superior thyroid artery has four named branches—the infrahyoid, sternocleidomastoid, superior laryngeal,

and cricothyroid arteries—as well as its terminal anterior, posterior, and occasionally lateral glandular branches serving the thyroid gland.

▨ The **infrahyoid artery (branch)** is a small vessel, passing, as its name implies, inferior to the hyoid bone to anastomose with its counterpart on the other side. Along its path, it supplies muscular branches to the infrahyoid muscles in its vicinity.

▨ The **sternocleidomastoid artery (branch)** passes ventral to the carotid sheath, supplying the same-named muscle on its deep surface and sends small twigs to structures in its vicinity.

▨ To distribute to the larynx, the **superior laryngeal artery** passes superficial to the inferior pharyngeal constrictor muscle and pierces the thyrohyoid membrane, accompanied by the internal laryngeal nerve. Within the larynx, it serves its muscles, glands, and mucosa.

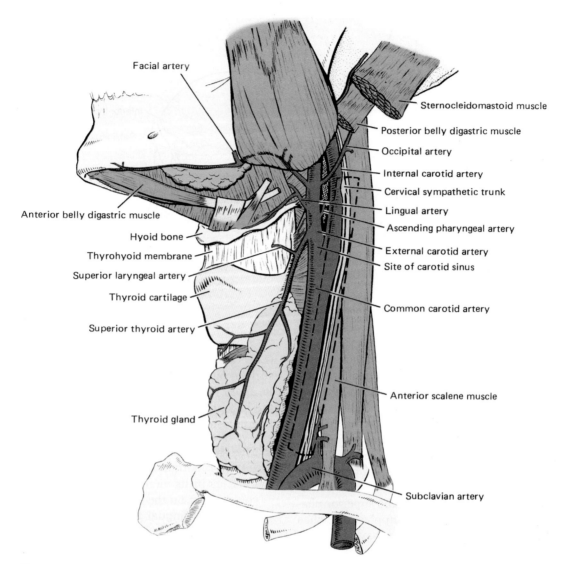

Facial artery

Sternocleidomastoid muscle

Posterior belly digastric muscle

Occipital artery

Internal carotid artery

Cervical sympathetic trunk

Lingual artery

Ascending pharyngeal artery

External carotid artery

Site of carotid sinus

Anterior belly digastric muscle

Hyoid bone

Thyrohyoid membrane

Superior laryngeal artery

Thyroid cartilage

Superior thyroid artery

Common carotid artery

Anterior scalene muscle

Thyroid gland

Subclavian artery

Figure 21-2. The carotid artery and its branches. The *dashed outline* indicates the relative position of the internal jugular vein.

The small **cricothyroid artery** courses along the cricothyroid ligament, supplying the muscle of the same name and additional structures in its vicinity.

The **glandular branches** of the superior thyroid artery are the anterior, posterior, and, occasionally, lateral branches. The **anterior branch** follows the superior border of the lateral lobe, distributes to its anterior surface, and forms an anastomosis with its opposite across the isthmus. The **posterior branch** follows a similar course on the deep aspect of the lateral lobe, ramifies on that surface, and forms an anastomosis with the **inferior thyroid artery**, also supplying the parathyroid gland. Occasionally a **lateral branch** is present, which supplies the lateral aspect of the lateral lobe.

Ascending Pharyngeal Artery

The **ascending pharyngeal artery**, the smallest branch of the external carotid artery, arises on the medial aspect of that artery, shortly after the bifurcation of the common carotid artery (Fig. 21-2). Along its ascent, between the pharynx and the internal carotid artery, it provides unnamed muscular branches to the prevertebral muscles, as well as branches to structures in the vicinity of its path. This artery has four named branches: pharyngeal, meningeal, inferior tympanic, and palatine.

The **pharyngeal branches** are variable in number (two to four) and supply the stylopharyngeus and middle pharyngeal constrictor muscles as well as the region of the pharyngeal mucosa in its vicinity.

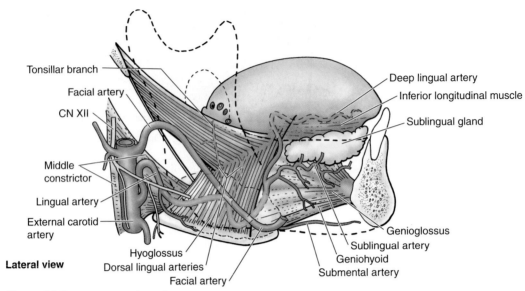

Tonsillar branch

Facial artery

CN XII

Middle constrictor

Lingual artery

External carotid artery

Lateral view

Hyoglossus

Dorsal lingual arteries

Facial artery

Deep lingual artery

Inferior longitudinal muscle

Sublingual gland

Genioglossus

Sublingual artery

Geniohyoid

Submental artery

Figure 21-3. Blood supply to the tongue.

The **meningeal arteries** enter the cranial cavity via the jugular foramen **(posterior meningeal branch)**, hypoglossal canal, and foramen lacerum to serve the dura mater.

The **inferior tympanic artery** gains access to the tympanic cavity via the petrous portion of the temporal bone, to vascularize that cavity's medial wall. It is accompanied by the tympanic branch of the accessory nerve.

The **palatine artery** courses along the superior pharyngeal constrictor muscle and supplies branches to the tonsils, auditory tube, and soft palate, anastomosing with other arteries of this region.

Lingual Artery

The **lingual artery** often arises in common with the facial artery, then becoming the linguofacial trunk. The lingual artery originates near the posterior extent of the greater cornu of the hyoid bone, passes deep to the hypoglossal nerve, then between the middle pharyngeal constrictor and hyoglossus muscles

(Figs. 21-1 through 21-3). The artery enters the deep surface of the tongue and extends as far anteriorly as its apex. The lingual artery has four named branches: the suprahyoid, dorsal lingual, sublingual, and deep lingual arteries.

The slender **suprahyoid artery** courses along the superior border of the hyoid bone, serving the muscles in its vicinity, and anastomosing with its counterpart on the other side.

The **dorsal lingual artery** arises deep to the hyoglossus muscle. It ascends to the posterior dorsum of the tongue to supply the palatoglossal arch, mucous membrane of the tongue, palatine tonsil, and some of the soft palate, freely anastomosing with other arteries in its vicinity.

The **sublingual artery** arises at the border of the hyoglossus muscle to course between the genioglossus and mylohyoid muscles on its way to the sublingual gland, which it supplies along with adjacent muscles in addition to the mucous membrane of the

Clinical Considerations

Sublingual Artery Damage

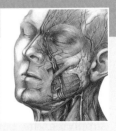

The sublingual artery, occasionally injured during dental procedures, may present problems to the surgeon attempting to ligate its source because it may arise from the submental branch of the facial artery rather than from the lingual artery.

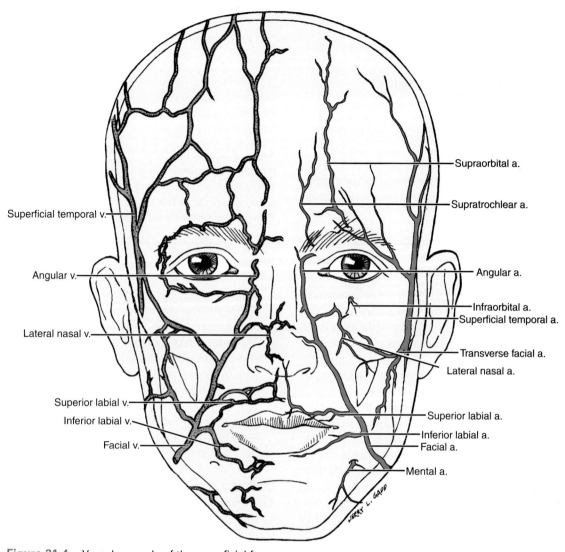

Figure 21-4. Vascular supply of the superficial face.

floor of the mouth and gingiva. Branches of this artery anastomose with the submental branch of the facial artery.

- The terminus of the lingual artery, known as the **deep lingual artery**, passes along the ventral aspect of the tongue, immediately deep to the mucous membrane, accompanied by the lingual nerve, to its apex, where it will anastomose with its counterpart of the other side.

Facial Artery

The **facial artery** arises just above (or in common with) the lingual artery and ascends, deep to the stylohyoid and posterior belly of the digastric muscles, to lie in a groove on the posterior aspect of the submandibular gland. The vessel enters the face by crossing the base of the mandible, just anterior to the masseter muscle, in the groove for the facial artery (Figs. 21-1, 21-2, and 21-4). In the face, the facial artery travels superficially, just under the cover of the platysma muscle. It passes, via a tortuous path, deep to the zygomaticus major, risorius, and levator anguli oris muscles, to the corner of the mouth. Here, it ascends lateral to the nose to terminate as the angular artery at the medial corner of the eye. The branches of the facial artery are the ascending palatine, tonsillar, glandular, and submental arteries in the neck and the inferior labial, superior labial, lateral nasal, and angular arteries in the face.

- The **ascending palatine artery** originates near the tip of the styloid process. It ascends between

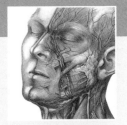

Clinical Considerations

Facial Artery Compression

Applying pressure to the facial artery as it passes over the inferior border of the mandible just anterior to the angle will diminish blood flow to that side. However, it must be remembered that because of the many anastomoses on the face, the flow cannot be completely stopped in an area where one of its branches may have been lacerated.

Pulse rates

Rather than use the radial artery for determining pulse rate, anesthesiologists use either the superficial temporal artery, accessed anterior to the ear just superior to the zygomatic arch, or the facial artery just as it crosses the mandible anterior to the masseter muscle.

that process and the superior pharyngeal constrictor muscle, then between the stylopharyngeus and styloglossus muscles, to supply the levator veli palatini, superior pharyngeal constrictor and neighboring muscles, soft palate, tonsils, and auditory tube, finally anastomosing with other arteries in its vicinity.

- The **tonsillar artery** passes between the styloglossus and medial pterygoid muscles and pierces the superior pharyngeal constrictor muscle to supply the palatine tonsil and the posterior tongue.

- The **glandular arteries** distribute as three or four vessels to the submandibular gland to supply it and the adjacent area.

- The **submental artery** arises from the facial artery near the anterior border of the masseter muscle. It follows the base of the mandible in an anterior direction and turns onto the chin at the anterior border of the depressor anguli oris muscle. The submental artery supplies the muscles it encounters along its passage and forms anastomoses with several arteries in its vicinity, including the mental and sublingual arteries.

- The **inferior labial artery** originates near the corner of the mouth, passes deep to the depressor anguli oris muscle, and pierces the orbicularis oris muscle. The artery courses superficial to that muscle, supplying it as well as the substance of the lip. It forms an anastomis with its counterpart of the other side and with branches of the mental and submental arteries.

- The **superior labial artery** arises just above and follows the same pattern as the inferior labial artery. It passes superficial to the orbicularis oris muscle in the upper lip to serve that muscle as well as the substance of the upper lip. It sends a small twig, the septal branch into the nasal septum, and another

one, the alar branch, into the wing of the nose. The terminus of the vessel will anastomose with its counterpart of the opposite side.

- The **lateral nasal artery** is a small branch arising at and passing into the wing and bridge of the nose, which it supplies. This vessel will anastomose with various other arteries in its vicinity.

- The **angular artery** is the terminal continuation of the facial artery, supplying the tissues in the vicinity of the medial corner of the eye and anastomosing with arteries of that region.

Occipital Artery

The **occipital artery** originates on the posterior aspect of the external carotid artery, approximately at the same level as the origin of the facial artery. It passes superficial to the hypoglossal nerve, the sternocleidomastoid muscle, and the posterior belly of the digastric muscle and lodges in the groove for the occipital artery on the medial aspect of the mastoid process (Figs. 21-1 and 21-2). It passes between the splenius capitis and semispinalis capitis muscles and pierces the superficial layer of the deep cervical fascia at the region of attachment of the trapezius and sternocleidomastoid muscles, just inferior to the superior nuchal line. The artery ramifies in the superficial fascia of the scalp, serving the back of the head. The occipital artery has the following branches: sternocleidomastoid, mastoid, auricular, muscular, descending, meningeal, and occipital arteries.

- The **sternocleidomastoid artery** originates near or at the origin of the occipital artery, or occasionally directly from the external carotid artery. It courses across the hypoglossal nerve and enters the deep aspect of the sternocleidomastoid muscle, which it serves. Frequently, this artery exists as two separate upper and lower branches, where the latter accompanies the accessory nerve into the muscle.

▨ The **mastoid artery** is a small branch that gains access to the cranial cavity via the mastoid foramen. Along its path, it supplies the mastoid air cells, dura mater, and additional structures in its vicinity.

▨ The **auricular branch** passes superficial to the mastoid process to reach and supply the back of the auricle.

▨ The several unnamed **muscular branches** of the occipital artery distribute to the digastric, stylohyoid, longissimus, and splenius capitis muscles.

▨ The **descending artery**, the longest of all of the branches, originates while the occipital artery is still deep to the splenius capitis muscle. Shortly after its origin, the descending artery bifurcates into a superficial and a deep branch, serving the trapezius muscle and the deep muscles of the back of the head and neck, respectively. The superficial branch anastomoses with the transverse cervical artery, whereas the deep portion will anastomose with the vertebral and deep cervical arteries, providing a collateral circulation between the subclavian and external carotid systems of arteries.

▨ The **meningeal artery branches** gain access to the cranial vault via the condyloid canal and jugular foramen to vascularize the dura mater and the bones of the posterior cranial fossa.

▨ **Occipital branches**, which are usually two in number (medial and lateral), follow the course of the greater occipital nerve to serve the muscles and tissues of the scalp. Small branches may traverse the parietal foramen to supply the parietal meninges.

Posterior Auricular Artery

The **posterior auricular artery** arises from the posterior aspect of the external carotid artery near the level of the distal end of the styloid process. In passing through the substance of the parotid gland, it provides glandular and muscular branches to several muscles along its course. Its three named branches are the stylomastoid, auricular, and occipital arteries.

▨ The **stylomastoid artery** ascends to enter the stylomastoid foramen, accompanying the facial nerve, where it provides a twig, the **posterior tympanic artery**, that will follow the chorda tympani nerve to vascularize the tympanic membrane. The stylomastoid artery serves the mastoid air cells, stapedius muscle, and structures in its vicinity.

▨ The **auricular branch** reaches the back of the auricle to supply it and its anterior aspect either by piercing the cartilage or by coursing around its free edge.

▨ The **occipital artery** crosses superficial to the insertion of the sternocleidomastoid muscle to supply it

and the scalp in the vicinity. Its branches anastomose with branches of the superficial temporal and occipital arteries.

Superficial Temporal Artery

The **superficial temporal artery**, one of the terminal branches of the external carotid artery, arises near the level of the earlobe within the substance of the parotid gland, which it supplies. The vessel branches profusely at its cranial-most aspect to supply the region superficial to the zygomatic arch as far medially as the lateral corner of the eye, as well as the temple and the lateral aspect of the scalp (Figs. 21-1, 21-4 through 21-6). The branches of the superficial temporal artery include the transverse facial, middle temporal, zygomatico-orbital, anterior auricular, frontal, and parietal arteries.

▨ The **transverse facial artery** arises near the level of the mandibular condyle within the substance of the parotid gland. It accompanies and supplies the parotid duct in its path across the masseter muscle. In addition, it sends branches to the parotid gland, masseter muscle, and other tissues in its vicinity.

▨ The **middle temporal artery** pierces the temporalis fascia near its origin to supply the temporalis muscle and anastomoses with branches of the deep temporal arteries.

▨ The **zygomatico-orbital artery**, occasionally a branch of the middle temporal artery, follows the zygomatic arch to the lateral corner of the eye. Subsequent to supplying the orbicularis oculi muscle, it will anastomose with branches of the ophthalmic artery.

▨ The **anterior auricular branches** serve the anterior aspect of the ear, the ear lobe, and the proximal region of the ear canal. This vessel will anastomose with branches of the posterior auricular artery.

▨ The **frontal branch** follows a tortuous path deep to the integument of the forehead, where it ramifies, supplying the frontalis and orbicularis oculi muscles as well as additional tissues of the region. It will anastomose with branches of the supraorbital and supratrochlear arteries.

▨ The **parietal branch** passes posterosuperiorly behind the auricle, supplying it and the side and back of the scalp. It will anastomose with branches of the occipital and posterior auricular arteries and its counterpart of the other side.

Maxillary Artery

The **maxillary artery**, the large terminal branch of the external carotid artery, originates deep within the body of the parotid gland. It courses anteriorly,

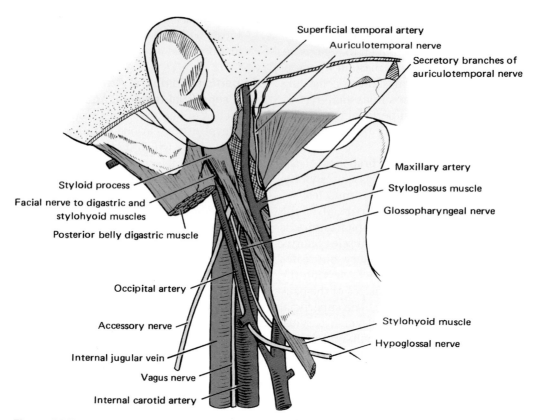

Figure 21-5. Arteries and nerves deep to the parotid bed.

medial to the ramus of the mandible near the level of the condylar process but superficial to the spheno-mandibular ligament (Figs. 21-1, 21-6, and 21-7). Passing along the superficial or deep surface of the lateral pterygoid muscle, the maxillary artery reaches and enters the pterygopalatine fossa, where it divides into its terminal branches. The maxillary artery is described as consisting of three portions as it courses through the mandibular, pterygoid, and pterygopalatine regions. The first or **mandibular portion** courses deep to the mandible between the ramus and the sphenomandibular ligament. Its branches are the deep auricular, anterior tympanic, inferior alveolar, middle meningeal, and accessory meningeal arteries. The course of the second or **pterygoid portion** of the maxillary artery is inconsistent because it may be either superficial or deep to the lateral pterygoid muscle, and the artery enters the pterygopalatine fossa by passing between the two heads of this muscle. Branches of the pterygoid portion are the deep temporal, pterygoid, masseteric, and buccal arteries. The third or **pterygopalatine portion** of the maxillary artery gains access to the pterygopalatine fossa via the pterygomaxillary fissure. Branches of the ptery-gopalatine portion are the posterosuperior alveolar, infraorbital, greater palatine, artery of the pterygoid canal, pharyngeal, and sphenopalatine arteries.

Branches of the Mandibular Portion

▨ The small **deep auricular artery** passes medial to the temporomandibular joint, which it supplies to penetrate the wall of the external acoustic meatus, serving its lining and the tympanic membrane.

▨ The **anterior tympanic artery** is also small and may arise as a common trunk with the deep auricular artery. It ascends to enter the petrotympanic fissure to reach the tympanic cavity, where it serves the tympanic membrane and associated structures.

▨ The **inferior alveolar artery** arises from a point between the condylar process of the mandible and the sphenomandibular ligament. It passes inferiorly to enter, along the inferior alveolar nerve and vein, the mandibular foramen. Within the mandibular canal, in the vicinity of the first premolar tooth, it bifurcates to form the **incisive** and **mental arteries**. Additional branches of the inferior alveolar artery are the mylohyoid and dental arteries. The **mylohyoid artery** arises from its parent vessel before that artery enters the mandibular foramen. It passes along the mylohyoid groove, accompanied by the mylohyoid nerve, to serve the muscle of the same name. **Dental branches** enter the alveolus, periodontal ligaments, and roots of the molar and premolar teeth. The **incisive branch** continues anteriorly within the mandible to serve

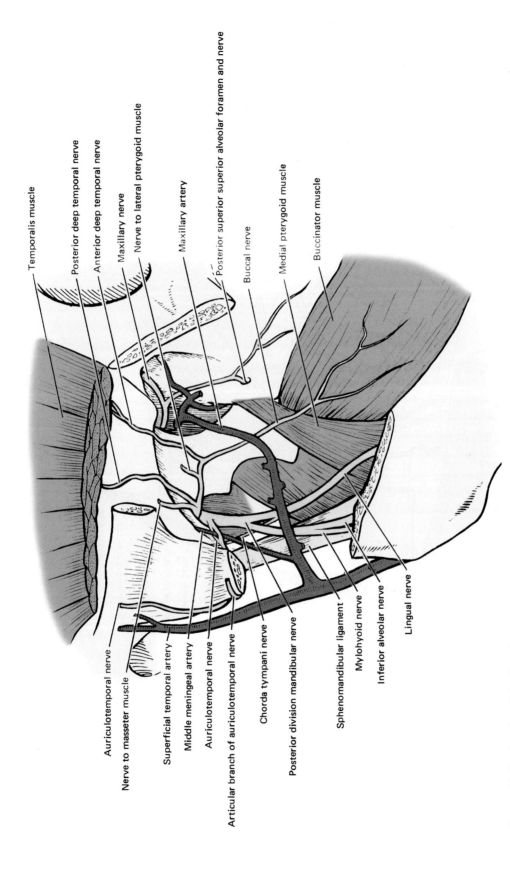

Temporalis muscle

Posterior deep temporal nerve

Anterior deep temporal nerve

Maxillary nerve

Nerve to lateral pterygoid muscle

Maxillary artery

Posterior superior superior alveolar foramen and nerve

Buccal nerve

Medial pterygoid muscle

Buccinator muscle

Auriculotemporal nerve

Nerve to masseter muscle

Superficial temporal artery

Middle meningeal artery

Auriculotemporal nerve

Articular branch of auriculotemporal nerve

Chorda tympani nerve

Posterior division mandibular nerve

Sphenomandibular ligament

Mylohyoid nerve

Inferior alveolar nerve

Lingual nerve

Figure 21-6. Arteries of the deep face.

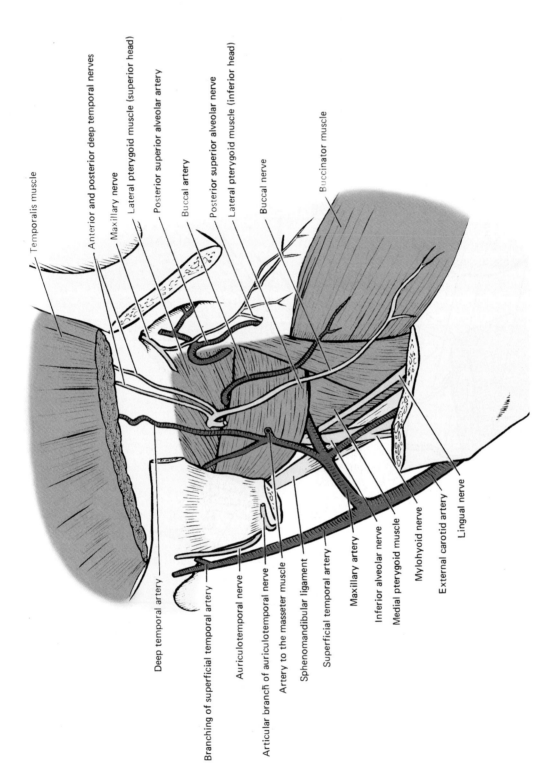

Figure 21-7. Arteries of the deep face. Note the maxillary artery diving beneath the lateral pterygoid muscle.

the canine, lateral, and central incisor teeth and to anastomose with its counterpart of the other side. The **mental artery**, accompanied by the mental nerve and veins, exits the mandibular canal via the mental foramen to vascularize the chin and lower lip. Its branches anastomose with those of the inferior labial and submental arteries.

- The **accessory** and **middle meningeal arteries** arise from the superior aspect of the maxillary artery or by a common trunk from the same artery. As the middle meningeal artery ascends to enter the foramen spinosum, it is engirdled by the two roots of the auriculotemporal nerve. The **accessory meningeal artery** traverses the foramen ovale. The distribution of these arteries is detailed in Chapter 17.

Branches of the Pterygoid Portion

- The **anterior** and **posterior deep temporal arteries** pass superiorly, deep to the temporalis muscle that they supply. They anastomose with the middle temporal and lacrimal arteries.
- The short **pterygoid arteries** arise from this portion to vascularize the medial and lateral pterygoid muscles.
- The **masseteric artery**, accompanied by the same-named nerve, passes through the mandibular notch to serve the masseter muscle. Some of its branches anastomose with branches of the transverse facial and facial arteries.
- The **buccal artery** accompanies the buccal nerve and passes in close association to the tendon of the temporalis muscle. It arborizes on the buccinator muscle to supply it and the mucous membrane of the mouth. Branches of the buccal artery anastomose with those of the infraorbital and facial arteries.

Branches of the Pterygopalatine Portion

- The **posterior superior alveolar artery** branches from the maxillary artery as that vessel enters the pterygomaxillary fissure. It travels along the maxillary tuberosity and enters the posterior superior alveolar foramen in conjunction with the like-named nerve. The vessel ramifies within the maxilla to serve the maxillary sinus, molar and premolar teeth, and neighboring gingiva.
- The **infraorbital artery** appears as the continuation of the maxillary artery; however, it may originate in common with the posterior superior alveolar artery. It enters the floor of the orbit through the inferior orbital fissure, lies in the infraorbital groove, then leaves the orbit via the infraorbital canal to enter the face by way of the infraorbital foramen. Branches of the infraorbital artery are the **orbital branches**, serving the inferior oblique and inferior

rectus muscles, as well as the lacrimal gland. The **anterior superior alveolar branches** vascularize the maxillary sinus, maxillary canine, and incisor teeth as well as their respective gingiva. The **facial branches** enter the face via the infraorbital foramen deep to the levator labii superioris muscle, where they provide **labial**, **nasal**, and **palpebral branches** to serve the lacrimal sac, nose, and upper lip. The various branches anastomose with branches of the angular, dorsal nasal, buccal, transverse facial, and facial arteries.

- The descending palatine artery descends in the pterygopalatine canal then gives rise to the **greater palatine artery** and its branch, the **lesser palatine artery**, which gain entrance to the palate via the greater palatine and lesser palatine foramina, respectively (Fig. 21-8). The greater palatine artery courses in an anterior direction on the lateral aspect of the hard palate to supply the palatal mucosa, gingiva, and glands and then proceeds to anastomose with the nasopalatine artery in the incisive canal. The lesser palatine artery vascularizes the soft palate and tonsil. It will anastomose with the ascending palatine branch of the facial artery as well as the tonsillar branches of the facial, lingual, and ascending pharyngeal arteries.
- The small **artery of the pterygoid canal** passes through the posterior wall of the pterygopalatine fossa by way of the pterygoid canal to supply part of the auditory tube, pharynx, middle ear, and sphenoidal sinus.
- The small **pharyngeal branch** passes dorsally, through the pharyngeal canal, to vascularize the auditory tube, sphenoidal sinus, and portions of the pharynx.
- The **sphenopalatine artery** leaves the pterygopalatine fossa via the sphenopalatine foramen on its medial wall to enter the nasal fossa, where it vascularizes portions of the nasal conchae and meatuses by its **posterior lateral nasal branches** as well as the posterior segment of the median nasal septum by its **posterior septal branches**. The longest branch of this vessel is the **nasopalatine artery**, which descends along the vomer bone to enter the incisive canal. It is here that it will anastomose with branches of the greater palatine artery.

Internal Carotid Artery

The **internal carotid artery** has no branches in the neck. It ascends deep to the parotid gland, digastric muscle, and muscles attached to the styloid process in its own compartment of the carotid sheath (Fig. 21-2). The internal carotid artery gains access to the cranial cavity via the carotid canal of the petrous

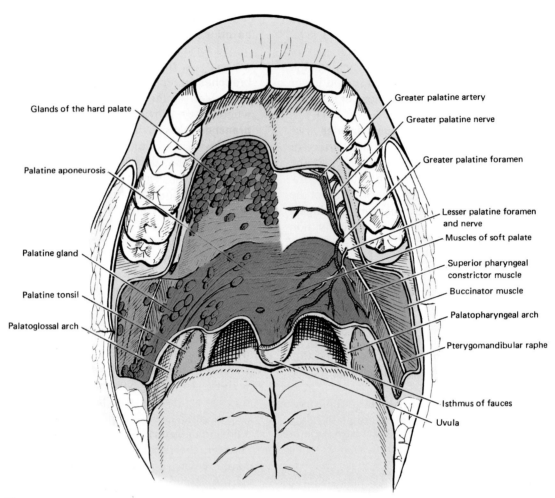

Figure 21-8. Arteries and nerves of the palate.

Glands of the hard palate

Palatine aponeurosis

Palatine gland

Palatine tonsil

Palatoglossal arch

Greater palatine artery

Greater palatine nerve

Greater palatine foramen

Lesser palatine foramen and nerve

Muscles of soft palate

Superior pharyngeal constrictor muscle

Buccinator muscle

Palatopharyngeal arch

Pterygomandibular raphe

Isthmus of fauces

Uvula

Clinical Considerations

Epistaxis (Nosebleed)

Bleeding from the nose subsequent to injury of the nose is a common occurrence and is usually relatively easy to control. Normally. the source of blood flow is the **Kiesselbach area**. the mucosa of the anteroinferior region of the nasal septum, where the septal branch of the superior labial, anterior ethmoidal, nasopalatine, and greater palatine arteries anastomose.

The bleeding is controlled by pressure or by packing the nose with cotton. Occasionally bleeding is from higher up in the nose, where control may require more heroic action. When the injury is from a direct blow, the cribiform plate of the ethmoid bone may be fractured.

temporal bone to vascularize regions of the brain, orbit, portions of the nasal cavity, and forehead. Associated with the artery is the carotid plexus of nerves, composed of postganglionic sympathetic nerve fibers derived from the superior cervical sympathetic ganglion. The internal carotid artery is described as having four portions: cervical, petrous, cavernous, and cerebral, referring to its termination in the vicinity of the lateral cerebral fissure. The **cervical portion** of the artery has no branches. The **petrous portion**, located entirely within the carotid canal of the petrous temporal bone, has four branches: the caroticotympanic, artery of the pterygoid canal, cavernous, and hypophyseal arteries. The **cavernous portion**, located within the cavernous sinus (but isolated from the cavernous blood by the endothelially lined fibrous sheaths), gives rise to the ganglionic, anterior meningeal, ophthalmic, and anterior and middle cerebral arteries. The **cerebral portion** gives rise to the ophthalmic and anterior and middle cerebral arteries. Its terminal branches are the posterior communicating and anterior choroidal arteries.

Petrous Portion

Because the arteries of the petrous portion are small, they will be treated as a single unit. The **caroticotympanic branch** leaves the carotid canal to gain access to the tympanic cavity, part of which it vascularizes. The **artery of the pterygoid canal** is not always present; when it is, it will anastomose with the same-named branch of the maxillary artery within the pterygoid canal. The several **cavernous** and **hypophyseal branches** supply the trigeminal ganglion, pituitary gland, and dura mater in their vicinity.

Cavernous Portion

The small **ganglionic** and **anterior meningeal branches** supply the trigeminal ganglion and the dura mater of the anterior cranial fossa, respectively.

Cerebral Portion

Ophthalmic Artery

The **ophthalmic artery** originates a few millimeters dorsal to the optic foramen (canal) through which it gains access to the orbit accompanied by the optic nerve, which is superior and medial to it. Within the orbit, the artery crosses superior to the nerve, but inferior to the superior rectus muscle, to reach the medial wall of the orbit. The ophthalmic artery serves the orbit as well as the eyeball, and its muscles and its branches are described accordingly. The **orbital group** consists of the lacrimal, supraorbital, posterior and anterior ethmoidal, medial palpebral, supratrochlear, and dorsal nasal arteries. The **ocular group** is composed of the central artery of the retina, short and long posterior ciliary, anterior ciliary, and muscular arteries.

- The **lacrimal artery** arises on the lateral aspect of the ophthalmic artery and passes, accompanied by the lacrimal nerve, to the lacrimal gland, which it supplies. The **lateral palpebral branches** of the lacrimal artery serve the upper and lower eyelids. Additional named branches include the **zygomatic** and **recurrent branches**. The former, passing through the zygomaticotemporal and zygomaticofacial foramina, serves the contents of the temporal fossa and the substance of the cheek, whereas the latter supplies the dura mater, reaching it via the superior orbital fissure.
- The **supraorbital artery** courses forward in the orbit on the medial margin of the superior rectus muscle and then travels with the frontal nerve, superficial to the levator palpebrae superioris muscle (serving both muscles), to reach and enter the supraorbital foramen. The artery distributes on the forehead and will anastomose with branches of the superficial temporal and supratrochlear arteries, as well as with its counterpart of the other side.
- The small **posterior ethmoidal artery** leaves the orbit via the same-named foramen, accompanying the same-named nerve, supplies the posterior ethmoidal air cells, the dura mater of the cribriform plate, and regions of the nasal cavity.
- The **anterior ethmoidal artery** is larger than the previous vessel. It leaves the orbit by way of the anterior ethmoidal foramen, accompanying the same-named nerve. It vascularizes the frontal sinus, all of the ethmoidal air cells (except for the posterior), and a region of the dura mater of the anterior cranial fossa. Its large **nasal branch** enters the nasal cavity along a hiatus by the crista galli to serve the walls of the nasal cavity. A cutaneous twig of the nasal branch serves the bridge of the nose.
- The **superior** and **inferior medial palpebral arteries** each form an arch in the upper and lower eyelids, respectively. The inferior palpebral artery also sends a twig to the nasolacrimal sac and duct. These vessels form extensive anastomoses with other arteries of the region and with each other.
- The **supratrochlear artery**, a terminal branch of the ophthalmic artery, leaves the orbit medial to the supraorbital foramen. It serves the forehead and will anastomose with the supraorbital artery and its counterpart of the other side.
- The **dorsal nasal artery**, the inferiorly positioned terminal branch of the ophthalmic artery, leaves the orbit at its medial angle to serve the bridge and side of the nose. Its lacrimal branch supplies the nasolacrimal sac and duct.
- The small **central artery of the retina** passes within the optic nerve to supply it as well as the retina of the bulb.

Clinical Considerations

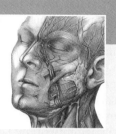

Blockage—Central Artery of the Retina

Because branches of the central artery of the retina are very small, obstructions such as small emboli may cause instant and total blindness. This condition is usually unilateral and occurs mostly in older individuals.

- The several **short posterior ciliary arteries** pass to the eyeball around the periphery of the optic nerve. They pierce the sclera to serve it and the ciliary processes.
- The two **long posterior ciliary arteries** pass lateral and medial to the optic nerve to supply the ciliary muscle and iris, subsequent to piercing the sclera.
- The **anterior ciliary arteries** pass deep to the conjunctiva and penetrate the sclera just posterior to the corneoscleral junction to serve the ciliary muscles.
- The **superior** and **inferior muscular branches** serve all of the extrinsic muscles of the eyeball, as well as the levator palpebrae superioris.

The **anterior cerebral, middle cerebral, posterior communicating**, and **anterior choroidal arteries** are discussed in Chapter 17.

SUBCLAVIAN ARTERY

The **subclavian artery** is a short vessel extending as far laterally as the outer border of the first rib. The origins of the right and left subclavian arteries differ in that the left one arises directly from the arch of the aorta, whereas the right is one of the terminal branches of the brachiocephalic trunk (Figs. 21-1, 21-2, and 21-9).

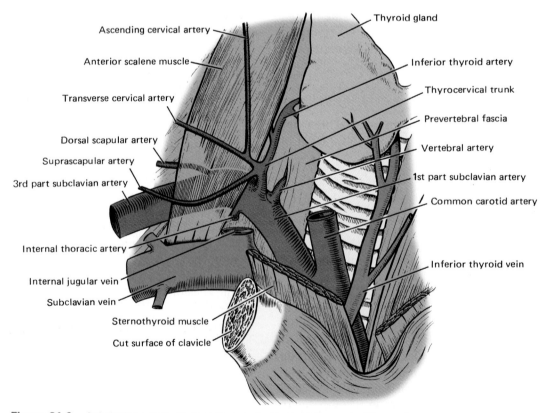

Figure 21-9. Subclavian artery, its branches, and vessels at the root of the neck.

The right subclavian artery originates deep to the sternoclavicular joint, and the left originates behind the common carotid artery around the third or fourth thoracic vertebra. Both right and left subclavian arteries travel superiorly to the root of the neck and posterior to the anterior scalene muscle, emerging into the posterior triangle through the interval between the anterior and middle scalene muscles on their way to the lateral border of the first rib, where each artery becomes known as the axillary artery. This passage, deep to the anterior scalene muscle, permits a convenient division of the subclavian artery into three parts. The first part is from the origin of the vessel to the medial border of the anterior scalene muscle; the second part lies deep to this muscle; and the third part extends from the lateral border of the anterior scalene to the lateral border of the first rib. The branches of the subclavian artery are the vertebral artery, internal thoracic artery, and thyrocervical trunk from the first part, the costocervical trunk from the second part, and the dorsal scapular artery from the third part.

First Part of the Subclavian Artery

Vertebral Artery

The **vertebral artery** takes its origin from the posterosuperior aspect of the first part of the subclavian artery. It ascends behind the anterior scalene muscle, along the transverse process of the seventh cervical vertebra, and enters the foramen transversarium of the sixth cervical vertebra (Fig. 21-9). The artery travels through the foramina transversaria of the upper six cervical vertebrae and enters the suboccipital triangle, from where it traverses the foramen magnum. Branches of the vertebral artery are described according to the region occupied by the vessel, namely, cervical and cranial branches. The cervical branches are the spinal and muscular arteries, whereas the cranial branches are five in number: the meningeal, posterior spinal, anterior spinal, posteroinferior cerebellar, and medullary arteries. Only the cervical branches will be discussed here because the cranial branches were treated in Chapter 17.

■ The numerous **spinal arteries** gain access to the vertebral canal via the intervertebral foramina to serve the spinal meninges, spinal cord, and bony vertebral column. The unnamed **muscular branches** provide numerous twigs to supply the deep muscles of the neck. Branches of these vessels anastomose with other vessels in their vicinity.

Internal Thoracic Artery

The **internal thoracic artery** originates from the inferior aspect of the first part of the subclavian artery. This artery passes directly inferiorly on the internal anterior thoracic wall just lateral to the margin of the sternum to the sixth or seventh rib, where it bifurcates to form the medially placed **superior epigastric** and laterally positioned **musculophrenic arteries**. Because the internal thoracic artery is a vessel whose distribution is limited to the thorax and abdomen, its branches will not be discussed.

Thyrocervical Trunk

The **thyrocervical trunk** is a short vessel arising from the superior aspect of the first part of the subclavian artery. This trunk lies just medial to the anterior scalene muscle, where it trifurcates to form three major branches: the suprascapular, transverse cervical, and inferior thyroid arteries.

■ The **suprascapular artery** travels obliquely across the anterior surface of the anterior scalene muscle and deep to the sternocleidomastoid muscles, which it supplies. It passes deep to the inferior belly of the omohyoid muscle to reach the scapular notch. Occasionally, the suprascapular artery is a branch of the third part of the subclavian artery.
■ The **transverse cervical artery** crosses the neck in a fashion similar to but above the suprascapular artery. It crosses the floor of the subclavian triangle, accompanied by the spinal accessory nerve, to burrow under the anterior border of the trapezius muscle, supplying it and other muscles in the vicinity.
■ The **inferior thyroid artery** travels superiorly in front of the medial border of the anterior scalene muscle. It then passes deep to the carotid sheath and approaches the inferior aspect of the thyroid gland, which it supplies. The inferior thyroid artery has several small branches, including the **ascending** and **descending branches** ending in the body of the thyroid gland, as well as **muscular branches** and the **ascending cervical artery** supplying anterior vertebral muscles of the neck. In addition, branches are also distributed to the larynx (the **inferior laryngeal artery**), trachea (**tracheal artery**), and esophagus.

Second Part of the Subclavian Artery

Costocervical Trunk

The **costocervical trunk** has different origins on the two sides of the body. On the left, it springs from the posterior aspect of the first part of the subclavian artery, whereas on the right it springs from the posterior aspect of the second part of that artery. This trunk has two terminal branches: the superior intercostal and deep cervical arteries.

- The **superior intercostal artery** serves the first and second intercostal spaces.
- The **deep cervical artery** is interposed between the first rib and the transverse process of the seventh cervical vertebra. It passes between the semispinalis cervicis and semispinalis capitis muscles, supplying these as well as adjacent muscles, finally anastomosing with the occipital and vertebral arteries.

Third Part of the Subclavian Artery

Dorsal Scapular Artery
The **dorsal scapular artery** is the only branch arising from the third part of the subclavian artery, although frequently it is a branch of the second part. The dorsal scapular artery passes among the trunks of the brachial plexus, anterior to the middle scalene muscle, to reach the superior angle of the scapula, where it supplies muscles in the vicinity.

VEINS OF THE HEAD AND NECK

The veins serving the region of the head and neck are subdivided, for descriptive purposes, into three major groups: the veins of the face, cranium, and neck. Most of the veins of the cranium are detailed in Chapter 17 and will not be discussed at this point.

Veins of the Face

The veins of the face are subdivided into two categories, namely, superficial and deep veins. The named superficial veins are the facial, superficial temporal, posterior auricular, occipital, and retromandibular veins (Fig. 21-4), and the named deep veins are the maxillary and pterygoid plexus of veins.

Facial Vein
The **facial vein** serves as the principal venous vessel of the superficial face. It begins in the medial corner of the eye as the **angular vein**, by the confluence of the supratrochlear and supraorbital veins, and passes inferiorly, following the course of the facial artery deep to the zygomaticus major and zygomaticus minor muscles, where it parts company with the artery to empty into the internal jugular vein. The facial vein communicates with the pterygoid plexus of veins and with the ophthalmic veins, both of which present possible passageways to the cavernous sinus due to lack of directional valves. Tributaries of the facial vein include the **deep facial vein**, which connects it to the pterygoid plexus of veins; the **frontal vein**, which drains a region of the forehead; and the **supraorbital** and **supratrochlear veins**. In addition, the superior palpebral, external nasal, masseteric, anterior parotid, superior and inferior labial, and submental veins also join the facial vein.

Superficial Temporal Vein
The **superficial temporal vein** follows the course of the same-named artery to drain the scalp, temple, and part of the forehead and ear. This vessel begins

Clinical Considerations

Thrombophlebitis of the Facial Vein

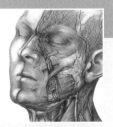

The facial vein does not contain valves; thus, blood flow may pass in either direction and into other venous vessels that may be connected to the cavernous sinus located in the dural venous sinus deep within the cranium. These connections include the superior ophthalmic vein, pterygoid venous plexus, inferior ophthalmic vein, and/or the deep facial vein. Infections in the face, especially in the "triangular danger zone of the face" bordered by the upper lip, lateral aspect of

the nose, and lateral corners of the eyes above the supraorbital ridge, may cause inflammation of the facial vein and development of thrombophlebitis (clot formation) of the facial vein. Pieces of the infected clot may become free to eventually pass into the cavernous sinus, giving rise to thrombophlebitis of the cavernous sinus—a life-threatening situation if left untreated.

as a plexus of small veins on the side and top of the head. Among the tributaries of the superficial temporal vein are the **transverse facial vein, middle temporal vein,** and **anterior auricular veins**.

Posterior Auricular Vein

The **posterior auricular vein**, one of the two veins participating in the formation of the **external jugular vein**, begins as a plexus of small veins behind the ear and courses in an anteroinferior direction, passing superficial to mastoid attachment of the sternocleidomastoid muscle. Its tributaries include the **stylomastoid vein**.

Occipital Vein

The **occipital vein** enters the suboccipital triangle to join a plexus of veins drained by the vertebral vein. Tributaries of the occipital vein include the **mastoid, emissary vein**. Occasionally, the occipital vein joins either the internal jugular or the posterior auricular veins.

Retromandibular Vein

The **retromandibular vein**, one of the two veins participating in formation of the **external jugular vein**, is frequently formed within the substance of the parotid gland. It is formed when the maxillary vein joins the superficial temporal vein. Tributaries of this short vessel include the common facial, middle temporal, and anterior auricular veins.

Maxillary Vein

The relatively short **maxillary vein** follows the mandibular portion of the same-named artery deep to the mandibular ramus to participate in conjunction with the superficial temporal vein, in the formation of the **retromandibular vein**. The maxillary vein arises from the pterygoid plexus of veins.

Pterygoid Plexus of Veins

The **pterygoid plexus of veins** is a massive network of venous channels lying on or about the surfaces of the lateral and medial pterygoid muscles and extending into the spaces of the deep face within the infratemporal fossa (Fig. 21-10). This plexus is in direct or indirect communication with a vast area, including the cranial cavity and cavernous sinus, the nasal cavity, orbit, paranasal sinuses, and superficial face. Some of its tributaries include the middle meningeal veins, posterior superior and inferior alveolar veins, veins that serve the muscles of mastication, as well as the infraorbital vein, buccal veins, and sphenopalatine

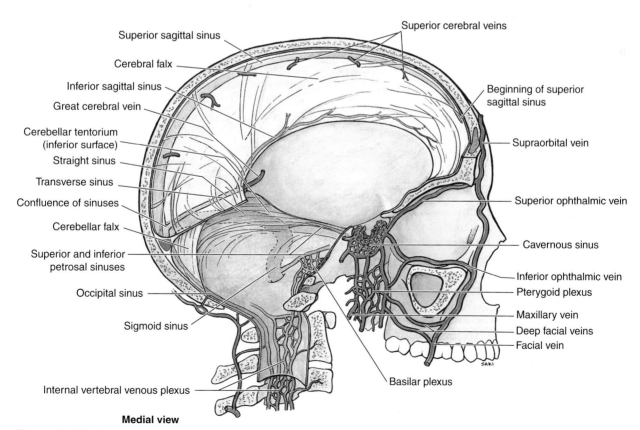

Medial view

Figure 21-10. Venous sinuses of the dura mater and their communications.

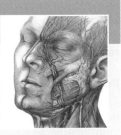
vein. In addition, it receives emissary veins and a communication from the inferior ophthalmic vein. Moreover, numerous smaller named and unnamed veins join the pterygoid plexus of veins.

Veins of the Cranium

Although most of the **veins of the cranium** were detailed in Chapter 17, the superior and inferior ophthalmic veins of the orbit will be treated in this section.

Superior Ophthalmic Vein

The **superior ophthalmic vein** is formed by the nasofrontal vein, which communicates with the **angular** (derived from the supraorbital and supratrochlear) **veins**. It enters the cranial cavity via the superior orbital fissure and empties its contents into the **cavernous sinus**. Its tributaries include the posterior and anterior ethmoidal, lacrimal, ciliary, and a branch of the inferior ophthalmic veins. In addition, numerous smaller named and unnamed veins join the superior ophthalmic vein.

Inferior Ophthalmic Vein

The **inferior ophthalmic vein** is formed by the confluence of several small veins in the anterior floor of the orbit, among which are unnamed inferior muscular branches and the **anterior ciliary vein**. The inferior ophthalmic vein bifurcates into a superior portion that usually joins the superior ophthalmic vein (or drains directly into the cavernous sinus), and an inferior portion that becomes a tributary of the pterygoid plexus of veins, which it reaches by way of the inferior orbital fissure.

Veins of the Neck

The veins of the neck include the external jugular, internal jugular, vertebral, and subclavian veins (Figs. 21-10 and 21-11).

External Jugular Vein

The **external jugular vein** is formed by the union of the **posterior auricular** and **retromandibular veins** just posterior to the angle of the mandible, sometimes within the body of the parotid gland. It passes straight down the neck, under the cover of the platysma muscle and associated superficial fascia, superficial to the fleshy belly of the sternocleidomastoid muscle. Along its path it crosses this muscle at an oblique angle. Once it reaches the subclavian triangle, the external jugular vein pierces the investing fascia, parallels the posterior border of the sternocleidomastoid muscle, and dives deep to the clavicle to deliver its blood into the **subclavian vein**, which it joins (Figs. 21-10 and 21-11). The external jugular vein has two pairs of incompetent valves just before it empties into the subclavian vein. Several tributaries join the external jugular vein, namely, the **posterior external jugular vein**, which drains the superficial aspect of the back of the neck, and two others, the **transverse cervical** and **suprascapular veins**. The last two veins drain the region of the shoulder. Another superficial vessel, the **anterior jugular vein**, occasionally empties into the external jugular vein, but usually it joins the subclavian vein directly. The anterior jugular vein is variable, but normally it begins at the level of the body of the hyoid bone and descends parallel to the anterior midline of the neck. Inferiorly, near the origin of the medial head of the sternocleidomastoid muscle, the anterior jugular vein pierces the superficial lamina of the investing layer and turns laterally, pierces the posterior lamina, and joins the subclavian (or occasionally, the external jugular) vein. While it is between the two laminae of the investing facia, the anterior jugular vein communicates with its corresponding vein of the other side via a venous connection, the **jugular arch**, which occupies the suprasternal space.

The external jugular, posterior external jugular, and anterior external jugular veins have numerous smaller named and unnamed tributaries, which drain the areas in their immediate vicinity.

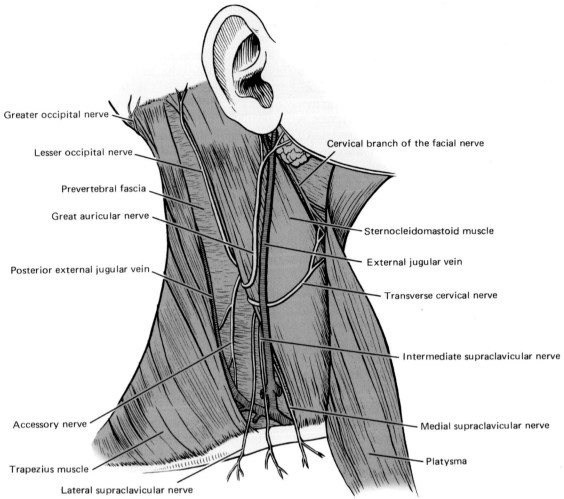

Greater occipital nerve

Lesser occipital nerve

Prevertebral fascia

Great auricular nerve

Posterior external jugular vein

Accessory nerve

Trapezius muscle

Lateral supraclavicular nerve

Cervical branch of the facial nerve

Sternocleidomastoid muscle

External jugular vein

Transverse cervical nerve

Intermediate supraclavicular nerve

Medial supraclavicular nerve

Platysma

Figure 21-11. Venous vessels of the posterior triangle of the neck.

Clinical Considerations

Venous Manometer

The **external jugular vein** may be used as a venous manometer because in a supine patient the venous blood pressure is not high enough to engorge this vessel much above the clavicle. During failure of the right side of the heart, constriction of the superior venae cavae and increased pressure in the thorax induces a pressure buildup in the venous side of the circulatory system, and this is evidenced by engorgement of the external jugular vein.

Under severe conditions, the vessel may be filled as high as the base of the mandible. This extremely important sign should be recognized by dental professionals using reclining chairs in their practice; the patient should be referred immediately for possible cardiac care.

Internal Jugular Vein

The **internal jugular vein** is the principal vessel responsible for collecting blood from the brain, superficial aspects of the face, and neck. The vessel extends from its dilated origin, the **superior jugular bulb** housed in the jugular foramen, to its inferior dilation, the **inferior jugular bulb** terminating in the brachiocephalic vein (Fig. 21-9). The internal jugular vein is enclosed in the carotid sheath as it travels the length of the neck, and its tributaries pierce this fascia to deliver their blood to the vessel. The internal jugular vein receives blood from the following tributaries: dural venous sinus drainage from with the cranium; the facial vein from the superficial face; the lingual vein from the tongue and floor of the mouth; and pharyngeal, superior and middle thyroid, and, occasionally the occipital veins from the neck. The dural venous sinuses and their drainage into the superior bulb of the internal jugular vein are described in Chapter 17. The facial and occipital veins are detailed in this chapter under the heading "Veins of the Face"; therefore, only the lingual, pharyngeal, and superior and middle thyroid veins are discussed here.

The **lingual vein** receives several tributaries that drain the tongue and floor of the mouth—the **sublingual, dorsal lingual,** and **deep lingual veins,** which follow the paths of their corresponding arteries. The small **pharyngeal veins** communicate with the pharyngeal plexus of veins and sometimes deliver their blood to the superior thyroid, lingual, or facial veins instead of to the internal jugular vein. The **superior** and **middle thyroid veins** both drain the thyroid gland and join the internal jugular vein at its superior and inferior aspects, respectively. Both vessels receive smaller named and unnamed tributaries. The inferior thyroid vein usually delivers its blood into the brachiocephalic trunk.

Vertebral Veins

Unlike their arterial counterpart, the **vertebral veins** do not traverse the foramen magnum; instead, they are formed from the confluence of many small tributaries within the suboccipital triangle. The vertebral veins enter the foramen transversarium of the axis and form a plexus of veins surrounding the vertebral artery, and descend with it within the foramina transversaria of the remaining cervical vertebrae except the last. They end in the brachiocephalic vein or occasionally in the subclavian vein. Tributaries of the vertebral veins include the **anterior** and **accessory vertebral veins** and the **deep cervical vein**.

Subclavian Vein

The **subclavian vein** is short because it is the continuation of the axillary vein, and it joins the internal jugular vein to form the large brachiocephalic vein (Fig. 21-9). Thus, the subclavian vein extends from the external border of the first rib to the junction with the internal jugular vein, passing anterior to the anterior scalene muscle, which separates it from the subclavian artery. Here it lies in front of the subclavius muscle, which acts as a cushion, protecting the underlying vessels and nerves.

The main tributary of the subclavian vein is the **external jugular vein**, although frequently the subclavian may receive the **dorsal scapular** and **anterior jugular veins**. The left subclavian vein receives lymph from most of the body via the **thoracic duct**, whereas lymph from the right upper quadrant of the body is delivered to the right subclavian vein by the **right lymphatic duct**. These ducts pierce the superior aspects of the subclavian veins, just before these are joined by the internal jugular veins.

Fasciae of the Head and Neck

22

Key Terms

Cervical Fascia (fascia of the neck) is divided into superficial and deep cervical fascia. Superficial cervical fascia is simple, whereas deep cervical fascia is generally divided into investing, pretracheal, and prevertebral fasciae. It's interesting to note that some specialized areas of the deep cervical fascia assist in forming subcomponents of the deep fascia. Cervical fascial clefts are those spaces between fascial layers that may permit the invasion of infection even into the thoracic cavity, leading to grave results.

Fascia represents thickened condensations of fibroelastic connective tissue that surround and separate movable structures of the body from each other. This would include certain bony joints, individual muscles, muscle masses, and certain neurovascular components. Spaces between layers of the fascia are occupied with loose connective tissue that may permit the quick and easy spread of infection from one area to another. Thus, it is important for the clinician to be familiar with the locations and connections between fascia, and the intercommunications between facial spaces. With this knowledge, the clinician may be able to prevent the spread of infection and develop a sound therapeutic program of treatment.

Fasciae of the Face and Deep Face are continuations of the cervical fascia as it proceeds over the mandible and on to the scalp. The fascia of the face possesses superficial and deep components with many subdivisions. The many fascial layers and subdivisions of the fascia share fascial spaces and clefts, which makes the face and deep face an easy target for the spread of infection from one area to another and, if improperly treated, perhaps eventually into the thorax. Clinicians must be fully aware of how infection may be spread in and about the face, deep face, and oral cavity.

Fascial Names are frequently controversial because of their varied thicknesses, described limits, attachments, and interrelationships. Moreover, various authors are in disagreement and may assign different names to the same fascial layer. The student has to learn to live with this and, with some extra study, may be able to distinguish one name from another. Fascia and fascial spaces presented in this chapter are categorized based on boundaries and communications so that names will be less confusing to the clinician.

Fasciae are thickened condensations of fibro-elastic connective tissue that separate various movable structures from one another. Spaces between layers of fascia are filled with a loose type of connective tissue that permits infection to spread from one locale to another with relative ease.

Because infection may travel along these fascial sheets, the clinician should possess a working knowledge of their locations, extent, and intercommunications. Armed with this knowledge, one can anticipate possible complications that may arise from the various procedures that were performed and develop a sound therapeutic program for their prevention and treatment.

Because fasciae are merely sheets of connective tissue of various thicknesses, considerable controversy surrounds their limits, attachments, and interrelationships. Compounding these problems is that different authors frequently assign different names for the same fascial layer or suggest that some of the flimsier connective tissue sheets do not deserve to be classified as fascia.

The goal of this chapter is to present fascia and fascial spaces from a standpoint of boundaries and communications so that varying terminologies will be less confusing to the clinician.

CERVICAL FASCIA

 Summary Bite. Cervical fascia (fascia of the neck) is subdivided into superficial and deep cervical fascia.

Superficial Cervical Fascia

Summary Bite. Superficial cervical fascia, since it surrounds the neck, is cylindrical in shape. The platysma muscle, located in the anterior portion of the neck, is contained within this fascia, as are some of the superficial nerves of the cervical plexus.

The fascia of the neck is subdivided into superficial and deep layers. The **superficial cervical fascia** (tela subcutanea) surrounds the neck in a cylindrical fashion. It contains the platysma anterolaterally as well as the cutaneous branches of the cervical plexus. Inferiorly, the fascia is continuous with that over the pectoral and deltoid region anteriorly, and posteriorly it blends with the fascia over the back, where it becomes firmly attached to the deep fascia (Fig. 22-1). This thin fascia is freely attached anteriorly, thus

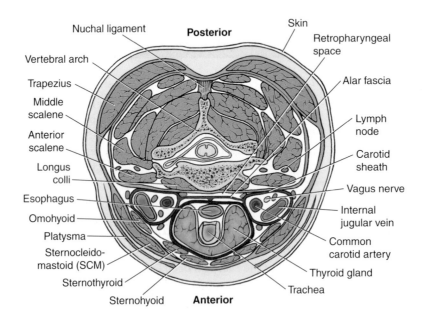

Figure 22-1. Cervical fascia and spaces. The view passes through the neck at the isthmus of the thyroid gland, approximately at the level of the seventh cervical vertebra.

facilitating movement unlike that in its thick, attached posterior region.

Superiorly, the superficial cervical fascia passes into the head posteriorly, and over the mandible and parotid gland anteriorly to cover the face and skull. The muscles of facial expression as well as nerves and vessels that serve these structures are located in this fascial layer.

The superficial fascia is separated from the deep fascia by a fascial plane permitting free movement of the skin in this region.

Deep Cervical Fascia

Summary Bite. Deep cervical fascia is generally described as composed of three layers: investing, pretracheal, and prevertebral.

The **deep cervical fascia** is, for descriptive purposes, usually divided into three layers: investing, pretracheal, and prevertebral, although this is not a completely accurate division. Actually, several other named fascial layers are of anatomic and clinical importance in the cervical region.

Investing Fascia

Investing fascia, known also as the **superficial** or **anterior cervical** layer of the **deep fascia,** surrounds the neck as a cylinder covering the anterior and posterior cervical triangles and investing the muscles forming the boundaries of these triangles (see Chapter 7 and Figs. 22-1 and 22-2).

This fascia arises from the spinous processes of the cervical vertebral column and ligamentum nuchae, and then encircles the neck. As it passes anteriorly, it divides into two laminae enveloping the trapezius muscle. The two layers unite before crossing over the posterior cervical triangle to form a single, thickened sheet. While there, it splits to surround the inferior belly of the omohyoid muscle and forms a ligament that fixes the intermediate tendon of that muscle in a constant position relative to the clavicle.

At the posterior border of the sternocleidomastoid muscle, the investing fascia divides once more to encompass that muscle. The two layers fuse again at the anterior border of the sternocleidomastoid before passing superficial to the anterior triangle as a single layer. As this fascia encounters the suprahyoid muscles, it envelops each muscle with a thin fascial covering that is attached to the mandible superiorly and the hyoid bone inferiorly.

As the investing fascia leaves the hyoid bone, it envelopes the infrahyoid muscles, surrounding each muscle with a thin fascial covering. Inferiorly, the fascia is attached to the acromion of the scapula and

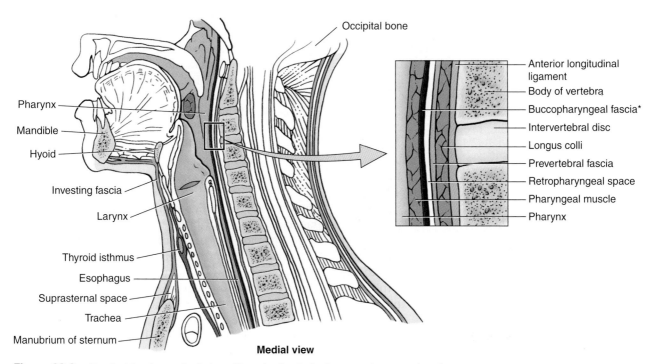

Figure 22-2. Cervical fascia, sagittal view. Note the fascia in the retropharyngeal region.

the clavicle. Subsequently, the investing fascia divides to become attached to the anterior and posterior surfaces of the manubrium, creating a space between the two layers known as the **suprasternal space**. This space usually contains the jugular arch, a venous connection between the two anterior jugular veins, and an occasional lymph node embedded in adipose tissue.

The superior extent of the investing layer of the deep cervical fascia attaches to the external occipital protuberance, the superior nuchal line, and the mastoid process of the temporal bone. Here it splits to enclose the adjacent parotid gland and continues superiorly as the **parotid fascia**.

The superficial lamina of the fascia attaches to the inferior margin of the zygomatic arch, and the deep lamina continues along the temporal bone to the carotid canal. It is from this deep lamina that the **stylomandibular ligament** is formed, coursing from the styloid process to the inferior border of the angle of the mandible. Thus, this ligament effectively separates the parotid from the submandibular gland.

Although the anterior and external jugular veins appear to course between the superficial and deep cervical fasciae, they actually course within the superficial layer of the investing fascia.

Pretracheal Fascia
Pretracheal fascia, or middle layer of the deep cervical fascia, encases the trachea, esophagus, pharynx, larynx, and thyroid gland.

Because most of the viscera of the neck is encased by this layer, it is sometimes referred to as the visceral fascia. The thin, filmy anterior lamina of this fascia lies deep to, but makes contact and blends with, the deep layer of the investing fascia covering the infrahyoid muscles. Because of this intimate relationship, the pretracheal fascia is sometimes described as being derived from the deep layer of the investing fascia.

The remainder of the pretracheal fascia completely invests the thyroid gland, and its deeper layer encircles the larynx and trachea as a tubular structure while being well developed on the pharynx and lateral aspects of the esophagus as the **buccopharyngeal fascia**, thus separating the esophagus from the prevertebral fascia (Fig. 22-2).

On covering the superior pharyngeal constrictor muscle, the buccopharyngeal fascia continues laterally over the buccinator muscle and attaches to the pterygoid hamulus and pterygomandibular raphe and is attached superiorly to the pharyngeal tubercle of the occipital bone.

The portion blanketing the medial pharyngeal constrictor muscle continues anteriorly, with the pretracheal fascia covering the hyoglossus and genioglossus muscles. Additional superior attachments include the hyoid bone and the stylohyoid ligament.

Inferiorly, the pretracheal fascia begins with the oblique line of the thyroid cartilage and descends to merge with the fascia covering the aorta and the fibrous pericardium and to the fascia of the posterior thoracic wall.

Prevertebral Fascia
Prevertebral fascia, the third major layer of the deep cervical fascia, encases the layers of musculature about the vertebral column. This fascia is described as originating from the ligamentum nuchae and the spinous processes of the cervical vertebrae. It covers those muscles of the back that extend the neck and, therefore, lies deep to the trapezius muscle and the investing fascia. Laterally, it blankets the scalene muscles and then turns medially to attach to the transverse processes, where it splits, forming a double lamina that fuses with its two layered counterparts of the opposite side. In its position, it forms the floor of the posterior cervical triangle (Fig. 22-3).

Superiorly, it is in contact with the investing fascia covering the trapezius muscle. Inferiorly, this fascia continues into the thorax to cover the muscles of the neck as they insert into the rim of the superior thoracic aperture.

A fascial space is evident in the posterior triangle housing the accessory nerve and a few lymph nodes. Near the base of the posterior triangle, the fascial space is enlarged as the prevertebral fascia passes over the scalene muscles. This permits passage of parts of the subclavian and external jugular veins, the transverse cervical and suprascapular vessels, supraclavicular and suprascapular nerves, and the inferior belly of the omohyoid muscle.

As the roots of the brachial plexus emerge from between the anterior and middle scalene muscles, the prevertebral fascia is reflected onto them, which blends with the axillary sheath. In covering the anterior scalene muscle, the fascia also overlies the phrenic nerve as it courses superficial to that muscle on its way to the thoracic cavity.

In addition, as the prevertebral fascia approaches the anterior tubercles of the vertebrae where it attaches, it also contributes to the formation of the posterior portion of the carotid sheath and covers the cervical sympathetic trunk. In continuing on its medial course from the anterior tubercle, the fascia splits into two laminae as it crosses the midline immediately deep to the buccopharyngeal fascia of the posterior visceral wall. The anterior lamina is called the **alar fascia**, which blends laterally with the carotid sheath and is loosely attached in the midline to the buccopharyngeal fascia. The alar fascia fuses with the

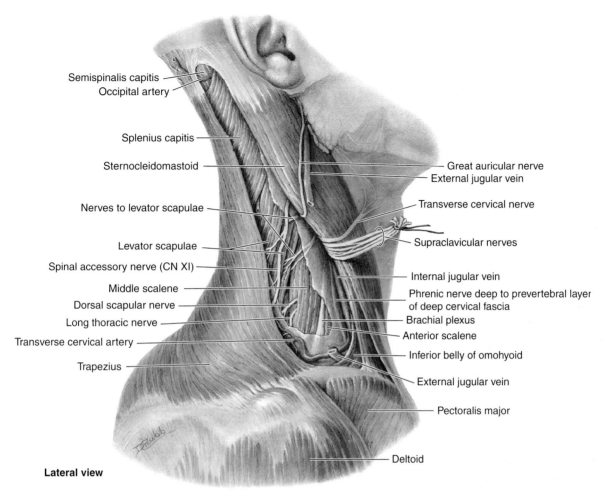

Semispinalis capitis
Occipital artery
Splenius capitis
Sternocleidomastoid
Nerves to levator scapulae
Levator scapulae
Spinal accessory nerve (CN XI)
Middle scalene
Dorsal scapular nerve
Long thoracic nerve
Transverse cervical artery
Trapezius

Great auricular nerve
External jugular vein
Transverse cervical nerve
Supraclavicular nerves
Internal jugular vein
Phrenic nerve deep to prevertebral layer of deep cervical fascia
Brachial plexus
Anterior scalene
Inferior belly of omohyoid
External jugular vein
Pectoralis major
Deltoid

Lateral view

Figure 22-3. Lateral cervical region. The investing fascia has been removed. Observe the deep cervical fascia overlying the cervical nerves and deep muscles.

buccopharyngeal fascia at about the level of the seventh cervical vertebra, or it may continue into the thorax before fusing with the visceral fascia. The posterior lamina, lying against the body of the vertebrae, remains known as the prevertebral fascia. Thus, the space formed between these two laminae is referred to as the **"danger space"** or **"Space 4,"** not to be confused with the retropharyngeal space, which is discussed later. The danger space is continuous from the base of the skull through the neck into the thorax, to end at the diaphragm.

Carotid Sheath

Summary Bite. The carotid sheath surrounds the common carotid artery, internal jugular vein, vagus nerve, and the internal carotid artery. The sheath is composed of contributions from the investing and pretracheal fasciae. Its posterior wall receives contributions from the investing fascia, thus completing the cylindrical sheath.

The fascial covering that surrounds the common carotid artery, internal jugular vein, vagus nerve, and internal carotid artery is the **carotid sheath** (Fig. 22-1).

This cylindrical structure lies between the investing and pretracheal fasciae anteromedially and between the investing and prevertebral fasciae posteromedially. The anterolateral portion of the sheath is formed by the investing fascia, with some contribution from the pretracheal fascia. The posterior wall is derived from a medial lamina of the investing fascia; thus, the medial wall of the sheath is formed as the two leaves of the forming sheath unite. In addition, the medial wall of the carotid sheath is attached to the prevertebral fascia. Superiorly, this sheath is attached to the skull around the jugular foramen, and inferiorly it is continuous with the fasciae of the great vessels and heart. The interior of the carotid sheath is compartmentalized to separate the arteries, vein, and nerve.

CERVICAL FASCIAL SPACES

> **Summary Bite.** Fascial spaces and clefts in the cervical fascia are important to the clinician because they can provide passageways for the spread of infections.

Potential spaces, spaces, and fascial clefts between fascial layers and the structures they cover are of clinical importance because they may afford passageways for the spread of infection. Although many of these spaces are inconsequential, several are worthy of description.

Visceral Compartment

> **Summary Bite.** The visceral compartment of the neck, as the word implies, refers to the viscera of the anterior neck, which includes the thyroid gland, trachea, esophagus, the pharyngeal constrictor muscles, bounded anteriorly by the deep layer of the infrahyoid and pretracheal fascia, part of the carotid sheath, and posteriorly by the the buccopharyngeal fascia.

The visceral compartment of the neck includes the area bounded anteriorly by the deep layer of the infrahyoid fascia and the pretracheal fascia surrounding the thyroid gland, trachea, esophagus, and pharyngeal constrictor muscles; laterally by the medial portion of the carotid sheath; and posteriorly by the buccopharyngeal fascia superiorly, blending with the visceral fascia inferiorly.

The anterior portion of this compartment surrounding and anterior to the trachea has been termed the pretracheal space, whereas that posterior to the trachea and surrounding the esophagus posteriorly is termed the retrovisceral space, often referred to as the retropharyngeal space. The retropharyngeal space is continuous inferiorly (caudal to the pharyngeal constrictors) with the retroesophageal space; thus, the term retrovisceral space is the more accurate and inclusive term.

Pretracheal Space

The **pretracheal space** located in the visceral compartment of the neck surrounds the trachea as it lies against the esophagus. It is limited superiorly by the infrahyoid attachments to the thyroid cartilage and hyoid bone, and inferiorly it continues into the mediastinum.

Retropharyngeal Space (Retrovisceral Space)

The **retropharyngeal space** lies in the posterior portion of the visceral compartment between the buccopharyngeal fascia covering the pharynx/esophagus and the alar fascia. It may not be restricted to the neck, however, because it extends superiorly to the base of the skull and inferiorly, depending on where it fuses with the visceral fascia. Infections of and about the oral cavity may dissect into this space and, if left untreated, may breach the rather flimsy alar fascia and enter the "danger space."

Danger Space (Space 4)

The **danger space** is often described as being synonymous with that of the retropharyngeal (retrovisceral) space when, in fact, it is not. The retropharyngeal space is bounded anteriorly by the buccopharyngeal fascia and posteriorly by the alar fascia. The danger space lies behind the alar fascia in the pocket formed between the alar fascia and the anterior leaf of the prevertebral fascia passing just anterior to the vertebral bodies from one transverse process across the midline to the other transverse process.

Clinical Considerations

Danger Space

The "danger space," extends from the base of the skull to the diaphragm and is a closed space. It appears, therefore, that infections located in the danger space result from infectious dissections through the alar fascia from the retropharyngeal (retrovisceral) space. Therefore, this space is of particular importance to the clinician because it is the pathway for the transmission of infections from the head and neck into the mediastinum. Spread of infection via this route can be life-threatening.

FASCIAE OF THE FACE AND DEEP FACE

> **Summary Bite.** The cervical fascia continues up over the mandible and to the remainder of the head, where it is specialized as the superficial and deep fascia.

The fasciae about the face, the deep face, and the remainder of the head are continuations of the fasciae of the neck, and in some areas are further specializations of the deep fasciae covering certain regions and structures of the deep face.

Superficial Fascia

> **Summary Bite.** Lying just deep to the skin of the face and scalp is the superficial fascia. This fascia contains the muscles of facial expression and their nerves, arteries, and veins.

The **superficial fascia** (tela subcutanea) of the face and scalp lies immediately deep to the skin and contains the muscles of facial expression, along with their nerves, arteries, and veins. This layer of fascia is closely applied to the skin except around the eyelids, about the buccal fat pad, and near the galea aponeurotica of the scalp. Except for a danger space, this fascia is without spaces.

Deep Fascia

> **Summary Bite.** The investing layer of the deep fascia extends from the hyoid bone and, as it reaches the mandible, it splits into medial and lateral leaflets to encase the bone. It then passes to the zygomatic area. The fascia covers the muscles of the floor of the mouth and also encapsulates the submandibular gland and encloses the masseter and medial pterygoid muscles as they insert into the mandible. Moreover, the fascia forms a capsule around the parotid gland and is known as the parotideomasseteric fascia.

The superficial layer of the deep cervical fascia (investing fascia) extends superiorly over the mandible from its attachment to the hyoid bone anteriorly, and from the vicinity of the sternocleidomastoid laterally, to reach the zygomatic area. In coursing across this region, the fascia covers the muscles forming the floor of the mouth, namely, the mylohyoid and anterior belly of the digastric muscles. As the fascia reaches the mandible, it forms two leaflets to attach to the medial and lateral aspects of this bone. Along its way, the fascia also splits and fuses to encapsulate the submandibular gland and to enclose the insertions of the masseter and the medial pterygoid muscles. Laterally, that portion of the fascia covering the masseter muscle also blankets the angle and ramus of the mandible before inserting on the zygomatic arch (Fig. 22-4). The other leaf of this fascia covers the inferior surface of

Clinical Considerations

Thrombophlebitis of the Facial Vein

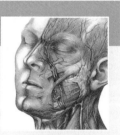

The facial vein does not contain valves; thus, blood flow may pass in either direction and enter other venous vessels that lead to the cavernous sinus located in the dural venous sinus deep within the cranium. These connections include the superior ophthalmic vein, pterygoid venous plexus, inferior ophthalmic vein, and/or the deep facial vein.

Face

Danger Area of the Face

The area bordered by the upper lip, the lateral aspect of the nose, and the lateral corner of the eye superior to the supraorbital ridge represents the danger area of the face. Squeezing pimples and tampering with boils in this region should be avoided because blood from this area may enter directly (or indirectly via the ophthalmic vein) into the cavernous sinus of the cranial fossa. Infection entering the cavernous sinus via this route may result in thrombosis, cerebral edema, and possibly death.

Lacerations and Facial Incisions

Because the skin of the face does not possess typical deep fascia, lacerations and facial incisions tend to gape open. Therefore, they must be carefully sutured to minimize scarring.

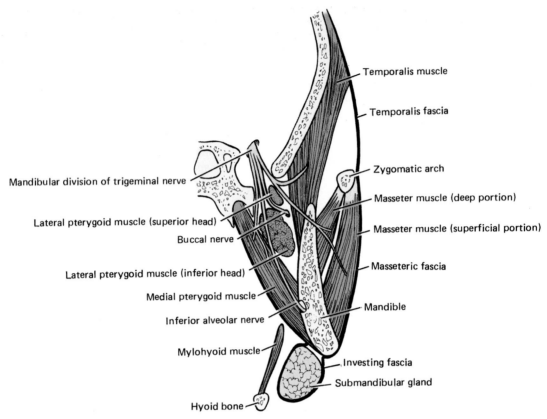

Figure 22-4. Masticator space. A frontal section through the temporal bone, zygomatic arch, and body of the mandible illustrating the muscles of mastication, their fascia, and the masticator space.

the medial pterygoid muscle and then inserts on the medial surface of the lateral pterygoid plate. Further posteriorly, that portion of the investing fascia surrounding the insertion of the sternocleidomastoid muscle separates to pass to the zygomatic arch, and in so doing forms a capsule (parotid fascia, parotideomasseteric fascia) surrounding the parotid gland.

This splitting of the superficial layer of the deep cervical fascia (investing fascia) as it passes superiorly from its attachment to the hyoid bone forms numerous potential spaces; however, because most are closed, they do not communicate with each other. As the fascia encompasses the submandibular gland it becomes the capsule of the gland. This fascia is thicker on the lateral than on the medial aspect; thus, dissecting infections in this area usually progress in a medial direction.

Masticator Space

Summary Bite. The masticator space contains the muscles of mastication, the maxillary artery and its branches, the mandibular nerve and its branches, connective tissue, and much of the buccal fat pad. The space is the result of the splitting of the investing fascia at the inferior

border of the mandible to enclose the medial and lateral pterygoid and masseter muscles as well as the inferior border of the temporalis muscle.

The **masticator space** is formed as the investing fascia splits at the inferior border of the mandible to cover the medial and lateral pterygoid and masseter muscles as they attach to the inferior border of the mandibular ramus (Fig. 22-4). Further superiorly, the fascia covers the inferior border of the temporalis muscle blending with its fascial covering.

The space is closed posteriorly as the two laminae of the fasciae fuse with each other. Anteriorly, the investing fascia fuses to the mandible in front of the masseter and temporalis muscles and then passes medially across the buccal fat pad to attach to the maxilla and to blend with the fascia covering the buccinator muscle.

The masticator space contains the muscles of mastication, the maxillary artery and its branches, the mandibular nerve and its branches, connective tissue, and much of the buccal fat pad.

The fascial space of the parotid gland contains that gland, several lymph nodes, the facial nerve, and several of its branches that will exit the space to supply the muscles of facial expression.

Clinical Considerations

Masticator Space Infection

The deep fascia splits at the mandible, forming two laminae around its inferior border. As a consequence, the muscles of mastication (the temporalis, masseter, medial and lateral pterygoid muscles) are thus enclosed by a compartment termed the masticator space (see Fig. 22-4). The two laminae of the deep fascia fuse again at the superior border of temporalis muscle where it originates from the skull. In addition to containing the muscles of mastication, this large space also contains the maxillary artery and many of its branches, and the mandibular division of the trigeminal nerve and many of its branches, as well as much of the buccal fat pad. The masticator space also communicates with many other spaces within the head and neck, which may contribute to the spread of infections and or neoplasms from the oral cavity.

Salivary gland tumors, abscesses, hemangiomas, and metastatic extensions of squamous cell carcinoma, especially from the floor of the mouth, tonsillar fossa, and nasopharynx, can extend into the masticator space. Persons suspected of having masticator space infections are very ill and need immediate medical attention.

Submandibular Space

Summary Bite. The submandibular space is bounded by the tongue and the mucous membrane of the floor of the mouth. The mylohyoid muscle divides the submandibular space into the sublingual and the submaxillary spaces that communicate at the inferior border of the mylohyoid muscle. Housed within the submandibular space are the submandibular gland and part of its duct; structures in the floor of the oral cavity, including the sublingual gland; the geniohyoid and genioglossus muscles; the lingual and hypoglossal nerves; and the lingual artery and some of its branches.

The **submandibular space** is larger than the space enclosed by the fascia covering the submandibular gland. Indeed, it is bounded superiorly by the tongue and mucous membrane of the floor of the mouth, and inferiorly by the superficial layer of the deep cervical fascia (investing fascia) covering the anterior belly of the digastric muscle, as well as the mylohyoid muscle and its attachment at the hyoid bone.

The mylohyoid muscle divides the submandibular space into the **sublingual space** superiorly and the **submandibular space** inferiorly. These two spaces communicate with each other at the posterior margin of the mylohyoid muscle.

The submandibular space contains the submandibular gland and part of its duct, as well as structures housed in the floor of the oral cavity, including the sublingual gland, the geniohyoid and genioglossus muscles, the lingual and hypoglossal nerves, and the lingual artery and some of its branches.

Although the submandibular space is described as being bilateral, because of its position in the vicinity of the midline and its relations to the mylohyoid muscle, communication normally occurs between the two sides. In addition, the submandibular space communicates with the lateral pharyngeal space via its subdivision, the sublingual space.

Peripharyngeal Spaces

Summary Bite. The peripharyngeal spaces are common space surrounding the pharyngeal wall and communicating with the submandibular space. These spaces freely communicate with several other spaces, including the masticator space; thus, the peripharyngeal spaces are readily available avenues for the spread of infection from such areas as the teeth, throat, nose, as well as from the mandible and maxillae.

Surrounding the pharyngeal wall posteriorly and laterally and communicating anteriorly with the submandibular space is a common space that is further subdivided into the **peripharyngeal spaces**. This space, encircling the perimeter of the pharynx, lies deep to all laminae of the superficial layer of the deep cervical fascia (investing fascia) and freely communicates with several other spaces. The peripharyngeal spaces (because of their relationships with other fascial spaces) and the masticator space are accessible avenues for the spread of infection by way of perforations through other fascial layers. Infections that may break into the peripharyngeal spaces include those of the teeth, nose, throat, mandible, maxillae, etc.

Retropharyngeal Space

The **retropharyngeal space** was described during the discussion of fascial spaces in the neck. The reader should recall that the retropharyngeal space lies behind the pharynx/esophagus covered by the buccopharyngeal fascia.

The retropharyngeal space extends from the base of the skull and, depending on where the buccopharyngeal and alar fasciae fuse, perhaps into the mediastinum. It is bounded posteriorly by the alar fascia, anteriorly by the buccopharyngeal fascia, and laterally by loose connective tissue separating it rather incompletely from the lateral pharyngeal space.

The retropharyngeal space is regarded as the primary route of the spread of infection from lesions in the head and neck into the danger space, and from there into the thorax because it is accessible to dissecting or perforating infections originating from numerous neighboring fascial spaces.

Lateral Pharyngeal Space

The retropharyngeal space extends laterally around the pharynx, with only loose connective tissue intervening between it and the space lateral to it, the **lateral pharyngeal space** (known also by various other names, including parapharyngeal, peripharyngeal, pharyngomaxillary, pterygomandibular, and pterygopharyngeal).

The lateral pharyngeal space is bounded medially by the buccopharyngeal fascia and laterally by the pterygoid muscles and the capsule of the parotid gland. Its superior extent is similar to that of the retropharyngeal space in that it reaches the base of the skull; however, inferiorly it extends only as far as the hyoid bone, being limited by the fascia of the submandibular gland, stylohyoid muscle, and posterior belly of the digastric muscle. Coursing through this space are the two other muscles originating from the styloid process: the styloglossus and stylopharyngeus muscles. The lateral pharyngeal space extends to the pterygomandibular raphe and, above the submandibular gland, communicates with the floor of the oral cavity. Because of its extent and association about the structures of the oral region, it is the most frequently infected secondary area from the primary areas of the masticator space, teeth, tongue, salivary glands, and tonsillar region.

Infections perforating into this space readily gain access to the retropharyngeal space and, eroding the alar fascia, pass into the mediastinum. Thus, the lateral pharyngeal space is of utmost importance to the clinician.

Glossary

Abducens nerve. Sixth cranial nerve.

Abduction. A motion that moves a structure away from the body centerline.

Accessory bone. A bone formed when ossification centers fail to unite during development.

Accessory nerve. Eleventh cranial nerve.

Adam's apple. Laryngeal prominence. A prominent protuberance of the thyroid cartilage in the anterior midline of the neck, especially in adult males.

Adduction. A motion that moves a structure closer to the body centerline.

Adenoids. Hypertrophy of the pharyngeal tonsil as a result of infection.

Aditus. An opening or inlet.

Afferent. Leading toward a specific area, as toward the central nervous system or a lymph node.

Agonists. Muscles whose contractions produce a desired motion.

Alveolar arch. Bony portions on the maxillae and mandible that surround the teeth.

Alveolus. A small cavity. The socket of a tooth.

Anastomosis. Direct communication between blood vessels and between nerves.

Anatomy. The science of the structure of the body.

Anesthesia. Loss of sensation as a result of injury, disease, or induction by drugs.

Ankyloglossia. "Tongue-tied." The lingual frenulum is attached too far anteriorly on the tongue, impeding speech.

Anomaly. Deviation from the normal.

Ansa cervicalis. Nerve loop derived from C1, C2, and C3 to supply the infrahyoid muscles.

Ansa subclavia. Loop around the subclavian artery connecting the middle and inferior cervical sympathetic ganglia.

Antagonists. Muscles that act in opposition to agonists.

Anterior. Front of the body.

Anterior triangle. Triangular area of the neck bounded by the sternocleidomastoid muscle, the anterior midline of the neck, and the inferior border of the mandible.

Aponeurosis. A flat, sheetlike tendinous muscle attachment.

Appendicular skeleton. Bony skeleton composed of the bones comprising the superior and inferior extremities.

Arachnoid. Intermediate layer of the meninges covering the brain and spinal cord.

Arachnoid granulations. Modified elements of the arachnoid that filter cerebrospinal fluid from the subarachnoid space into the lacunae lateralis.

Arrector pili. Involuntary smooth muscles arising in the dermis and inserting into the hair follicle. Contractions produce "goose bumps."

Articular disc. Meniscus. The disc intervening between the mandibular condyle and the temporal bone.

Atlas. First cervical vertebra. Articulates with the occipital bone of the skull.

Auditory tube. Eustachian tube. Opening of the middle ear cavity into the pharynx.

Autonomic nervous system. A functional system controlling cardiac and smooth muscles and glandular activity.

Axial skeleton. Bony skeleton composed of the skull, vertebral column, hyoid bone, ribs, and sternum.

Axis. The second cervical vertebra.

Basal ganglia. Subcortical nuclei associated with somatic motor functions.

Blind spot. Optic disc. The light-insensitive region of the retina where the optic nerve exits the bulb of the eye.

Blood–brain barrier. Pial-glial elements surrounding blood vessels of the central nervous system that control the entry of materials into the intercellular spaces of the central nervous system.

Bolus. A masticated (chewed) chunk of food ready for deglutition (swallowing).

Bony depressions. Intervals between bony elevations. Descriptions include pits, foveae, and fossae.

Bony elevations. Sites of attachment of structures to bone. Descriptions include lines, crests, ridges, processes, tubercles, tuberosities, and spines.

Brachial plexus. Plexus of nerves formed by the ventral primary rami of C5, C6, C7, C8, and T1, with contributions from C4 and T2.

Brainstem. The oldest part of the central nervous system, mainly responsible for vital functions.

Branchial arches. Pharyngeal arches.

Branchial grooves. Pharyngeal clefts.

Buccal glands. Minor salivary glands located in the mucosa of the buccal vestibule.

Buccopharyngeal fascia. Posterior lamina of the pretracheal fascia.

Bursae. Fluid-filled sacs overlying joints, functioning in lubrication.

Canal. A passageway or tunnel in bone.

Cardiac muscle. Heart muscle. A special striated involuntary muscle.

Carotid body. Structure located at the bifurcation of the common carotid artery to monitor oxygen tension and carbon dioxide in the bloodstream.

Carotid plexus. Postganglionic sympathetic fibers derived from the superior cervical ganglion, traveling on the internal carotid artery.

Carotid sheath. Fascial sheath, derived from the deep cervical fascia, enveloping the major neurovascular bundle of the neck.

Carotid sinus. Structure located in the wall of the internal carotid artery at its beginning, monitoring blood pressure.

Carotid triangle. One of the subdivisions of the anterior triangle of the neck, bounded by the posterior belly of the digastric, the superior belly of the omohyoid, and the sternocleidomastoid muscles.

Cartilaginous joint. A bony union or joint with cartilage interposed between the bones.

Caudal. Inferior. Toward the tail.

Cavernous sinus. A large, labyrinthine dural venous sinus located lateral to the sella turcica.

Central nervous system. CNS. Composed of the brain and spinal cord.

Cephalic. Rostral. Toward the rostral (head) end of the organism.

Cerebellum. Portion of the brain derived from the metencephalon. Responsible for balance and spatial orientation.

Cerebral arterial circle. Circle of Willis. Arterial anastomosis around the base of the brain.

Cerebral hemispheres. Largest portion of the brain, derived from the prosencephalon.

Cerebrospinal fluid. CFS. A clear, colorless, acellular fluid produced by the choroid plexus. Circulates in the ventricles of the brain, the central canal of the spinal cord, and the subarachnoid space.

Cervical plexus. Plexus of nerves formed by the ventral primary rami of C1, C2, C3, C4, and (sometimes) C5.

Cervical sympathetic trunk. Cervical continuation of the thoracic sympathetic trunk.

Chain ganglia. Sympathetic ganglia located along the vertebral column.

Choanae. Apertures of the nasal cavities opening into the nasopharynx.

Choroid plexus. Modified pial/ependymal elements located in the ventricles of the brain that function to elaborate cerebrospinal fluid.

Ciliary body. A portion of the middle coat of the eye, including the ciliary muscle and ciliary process.

Circle of Willis. Cerebral arterial circle.

Collateral ganglia. Sympathetic ganglia located away from the vertebral column, usually near the viscera, along major blood vessels.

Computed tomography. A radiographic procedure whereby cross-sectional images of the body are visualized.

Conchae. Turbinate bones. Three mucosa-covered, scroll-like bones on the lateral nasal wall that jut into the nasal fossa.

Condyle. The rounded articular end of a bone.

Cones. Light-sensitive cells of the retina specialized for color vision.

Confluence of sinuses. A region of dural sinuses, located at the internal occipital crest, receiving several major venous sinuses of the dura mater.

Cornea. Anteriorly placed, modified, transparent portion of the sclera of the eye.

Coronal plane. Frontal plane. A vertical plane at right angles to the sagittal plane.

Coronal suture. A skull suture located in the frontal plane, from temple to temple.

Cranial. Superior. In the direction of the head, craniad.

Cranial fossa. A deep depression in the internal base of the skull consisting of three regions: anterior, middle, and posterior.

Cranial outflow. Parasympathetic outflow from the brain in cranial nerves III, VII, IX, and X.

Craniosacral outflow. The combined parasympathetic outflow regions of origin for the entire body.

Crenated tongue. Indentations along the lateral margins of the tongue indicating impressions from the teeth.

Cricothyrotomy. A relatively safe emergency procedure for opening the airway by incising the cricothyroid membrane to relieve dyspnea.

Deep. Relative position from the surface of the body from any direction.

Deep cervical lymph nodes. Chain of lymph nodes following the carotid sheath. These ultimately receive all of the lymph from the head and neck.

Deep fascia. Connective tissue sheath surrounding and compartmentalizing many of the structures of the body, including the muscles.

Deglutition. The act of swallowing.

Dendrite. One of the cell processes of a neuron that conducts impulses toward the cell body.

Depress. To pull down or lower.

Dermal papillae. Projections of the dermis that interdigitate with epidermal pegs at the epidermis–dermis interface.

Dermis. Deep layer of the skin beneath the epidermis.

Developmental anatomy. The study of the growth and development of an organism from conception to birth.

Diaphragma sella. An incomplete covering composed of meningeal dura that acts as a membraneous lid over the sella turcica.

Diencephalon. Rostral-most portion of the brainstem.

Diploic veins. Veins traveling in and draining the diploë of the skull.

Distal. 1. Away from the origin. 2. Term used in describing relative positions of the teeth. Away from the midline anteriorly.

Dorsal. Equal to posterior but usually reserved for quadrupeds.

Dorsal horn. Gray matter of spinal cord containing cell bodies receiving sensory axons from the dorsal root.

Dorsal root. Sensory root carrying axons from dorsal root ganglion to the spinal cord.

Dorsal root ganglion. Sensory ganglion located on the dorsal root of each spinal nerve.

Duct of Bartholin. Large sublingual duct of the sublingual gland opening very near or with the submandibular duct at the sublingual caruncula.

Ducts of Rivinus. Small sublingual ducts of the sublingual gland opening along the surface of the plica sublingualis below the tongue.

Dura mater. The outer layer of the meninges covering the brain and spinal cord.

Efferent. Leading away from a specific area, as away from the central nervous system or a lymph node.

Elastic cartilage. Type of cartilage located in the external ear, auditory tube, epiglottis, and parts of the larynx.

Elevate. To lift up.

Emissary veins. Veins originating on the scalp, then emptying into the dural venous sinuses through like-named foramina in the skull.

Endochondral bone formation. Type of bone development on a cartilaginous template.

Epidermal pegs. Projections of the epidermis that interdigitate with the dermal papillae at the epidermis–dermis interface.

Epidermis. Surface layer of the skin.

Epiglottis. An unpaired, leaf-shaped piece of elastic cartilage of the larynx projecting above and anterior to the superior laryngeal aperture.

Eustachian tube. Auditory tube.

Extension. A motion that increases the joint angle.

External. Away from the center of the body.

External acoustic meatus. Opening in the temporal bone leading into the middle ear.

Extrinsic muscles of the eye. Muscles attached to and responsible for movement of the eyeball.

Extrinsic muscles of the tongue. Muscles that originate outside the tongue but inserting into it, thus making the tongue a highly moveable structure.

Facial nerve. Seventh cranial nerve.

Falx cerebelli. Meningeal reflection of the dura mater, on the caudal surface of the tentorium cerebelli, intervening between the two cerebellar hemispheres.

Falx cerebri. Sickle-shaped meningeal reflection of the dura mater intervening between the right and left cerebral hemispheres.

Fascia. Collagenous connective tissue that encloses structures and separates them into various groups.

Fibrocartilage. Type of cartilage in intervertebral discs, pubic symphysis, and mandibular symphysis, as well as on certain regions of the temporomandibular joint.

Fibrous joint. A bony joint connected by fibrous connective tissue.

Fissured tongue. Excessive fissures in the dorsum of the tongue.

Fixators. Muscles that act to stabilize a structure.

Flexion. A motion that reduces the joint angle.

Foramen. An opening or hole in bone, usually for passage of an artery, vein, and/or nerve.

Foramen cecum. Shallow, pitlike depression on tongue, just posterior to the sulcus terminalis, indicating the opening of the embryologic thyroglossal duct.

Fordyce granules. Ectopic sebaceous glands incorporated into the vestibular mucosa during development.

Frontal plane. Coronal plane. A vertical plane at right angles to the sagittal plane.

Ganglion. An accumulation of neuron cell bodies outside the central nervous system.

General somatic afferent. Sensation traveling to the central nervous system from the body.

General somatic efferent. Motor innervation from the central nervous system to the skeletal muscles.

General visceral afferent. Sensation traveling to the central nervous system from the viscera.

General visceral efferent. Motor innervation from the central nervous system to the smooth muscles of the viscera.

Gingiva. The gums. Specialized mucosa overlying the alveolar bone of each dental arch.

Glands of Blandin-Nuhn. Minor salivary glands located on either side of the lingual frenulum.

Glands of von Ebner. Minor serous salivary glands that empty into the vallate papillae.

Glaucoma. Condition of increased pressure in the anterior chamber of the eye.

Glossopharyngeal nerve. Ninth cranial nerve.

Gray matter. Region of the central nervous system consisting mainly of cell bodies.

Gray rami communicantes. Unmyelinated fibers (postganglionic) entering spinal nerve from a sympathetic ganglion.

Groove. A linear depression on a bone housing a structure.

Gross anatomy. Macroscopic anatomy. Study of the body with the unaided eye.

Gyrus. Convoluted elevation of the cerebral hemispheres, bounded by sulci.

Histology. The study of tissues. Used interchangeably with "microscopic anatomy."

Horizontal plane. Transverse plane. A plane passing through body at right angles to the sagittal and frontal planes.

Hyaline cartilage. Type of cartilage found on articular surfaces of bones. Forms a template for endochondral bone formation.

Hyoid arch. Second pharyngeal arch giving rise to the muscles of facial expression, in addition to some other structures.

Hypoglossal nerve. Twelfth cranial nerve.

Hypophysis. Pituitary gland.

Inferior. Tailward or caudal.

Inferior cervical ganglion. Inferior-most ganglion of the cervical sympathetic trunk. Located at the level of the seventh cervical vertebra.

Infrahyoid muscles. Strap muscles. Several muscles attached to the inferior aspect of the hyoid bone.

Infratemporal fossa. A region inferior to the zygomatic arch and deep to the mandible.

Insertion. Site on the bone or in skin where the muscle inserts.

Internal. Closer to the center of the body.

Intermaxillary segment. Merged medial nasal prominences that gives rise to the bulb and columella of the nose, medial portion of the upper lip, anterior palate with the four incisors, and a portion of the median nasal septum.

Intramembranous bone formation. Type of bone development within mesenchyme and without a cartilaginous model.

Intrinsic muscles of the eye. Smooth muscles located within the eyeball, responsible for accommodation and pupil size.

Intrinsic muscles of the tongue. Four muscles wholly within the tongue, responsible for altering its shape.

Investing fascia. Superficial layer of the deep cervical fascia.

Involuntary muscle. Smooth or nonstriated muscle and striated cardiac muscle. Contraction occurs without conscious control.

Iris. Colored, anteriorly placed portion of the intermediate tunic of the eye.

Isthmus faucium. Oropharyngeal isthmus.

Jugulodigastric lymph node. A large lymph node of the deep cervical chain located between the posterior belly of the digastric muscle and the internal jugular vein.

Jugulo-omohyoid lymph node. A large node of the deep cervical chain located near the intermediate tendon of the omohyoid muscle.

Kiesselbach area. Anteroinferior region of the nasal septum, a common site of nosebleed.

Labial commissure. Lateral connection of the upper and lower lip.

Labial frenula. Folds of tissue attaching the lips to the gingiva.

Labial glands. Minor salivary glands located in the mucosa of the labial vestibule.

Lacrimal puncta. Orifice of the lacrimal canaliculus located on each eyelid, in the vicinity of the medial commissure.

Lacuna lateralis. Meninx-lined depressions on either side of the superior sagittal sinus. These house the arachnoid granulations.

Lambdoidal suture. A suture of the skull separating the occipital bone from the parietal bones.

Lamina. A flat membranous or osseous plate.

Langer lines. Cleavage lines in skin used in surgery.

Laryngeal pharynx. Most inferior region of the pharynx surrounding the larynx.

Lateral. Away from the midline of the body.

Lingual frenulum. Tissue fold attaching the ventral surface of the tongue to the floor of the oral cavity.

Lingual tonsils. Tonsillar tissue located on the base of the tongue.

Lymphatic ring of Waldeyer. Clumps of lymphatic tissue surrounding the oropharynx.

Lymph nodes. Filtering bodies located along the lymphatic vessels. Lymphocytes are also propagated here.

Macroglossia. Large tongue.

Macroscopic anatomy. Study of the human body with the unaided eye.

Mandibular arch. First pharyngeal arch to form, which gives rise to the maxilla and mandible among other structures.

Mandibular fossa. Glenoid fossa. A concavity in the temporal bone that is the area of articulation with the mandible.

Mandibular torus. Bony exostosis on the lingual aspect of the mandible, protruding into the floor of the oral cavity proper.

Masticator compartment. A fascia-enclosed space on the lateral aspect of the face, containing the muscles of mastication.

Maxillary process. Superior-most developing segment of the mandibular arch in pharyngeal arch formation.

Meatus. A passageway or tunnel in bone.

Meatuses. Tunnels deep to the turbinate bones of the nasal cavity.

Meckel cartilage. A cartilage developed in the mandibular arch that later nearly disappears.

Medial. Toward the midline of the body.

Median lingual sulcus. A shallow groove on the dorsum of the tongue.

Median plane. Plane passing through body from anterior to posterior through the midline. Midsagittal plane.

Median rhomboid glossitis. An area devoid of papillae on the dorsum of the tongue.

Medulla. Medulla oblongata. The caudal-most portion of the brainstem. It contains the fourth ventricle.

Meninx. Meninges (plural). Membranes covering the central nervous system: the dura mater, arachnoid, and pia mater.

Meniscus. Articular disc. Disc intervening between the mandibular condyle and the temporal bone.

Mental symphysis. Mandibular symphysis. Area of fusion of the right and left halves of the mandible.

Mesencephalon. Midbrain. A short segment of the brainstem located between the diencephalon and the pons. It contains the third ventricle.

Mesial. Term used to describe relative positions of teeth nearest the midline, anteriorly.

Metencephalon. Part of the brainstem between the mesencephalon and myelencephalon surrounding the cerebral aqueduct.

Metopic suture. An inconstant suture, which may persist, between the developing halves of the frontal bone.

Microglossia. Small tongue.

Microscopic anatomy. Specialized study of cells, tissues, and organs of the body using a microscope.

Middle cervical ganglion. A small, inconstant cervical sympathetic ganglion located at the level of the sixth cervical vertebra.

Midsagittal plane. Median plane passing through the body from anterior to posterior through the midline.

Minor salivary glands. Small salivary glands located in the oral, palatal, and lingual mucosae.

Motor end plate. An axon terminal that participates in the formation of a myoneural junction.

Mucogingival junction. A sharp, scalloped line separating the gingival mucosa from alveolar mucosa.

Muscle fascicle. A bundle of muscle fibers surrounded by perimysium.

Muscles of facial expression. Muscle mass developed in the second branchial arch. These muscles arise in hypodermis or on bone and insert into the dermis of the face, scalp, and neck.

Muscles of mastication. Four muscles responsible for masticatory motions: the masseter, temporalis, external pterygoid, and internal pterygoid.

Muscular triangle. One of the subdivisions of the anterior triangle of the neck, bounded by the sternocleidomastoid and superior belly of the omohyoid muscles and the midline of the neck.

Nasal septum. Vertical midline structure of the nasal cavity, composed of the perpendicular plate of the ethmoid and vomer bones along with cartilage.

Nasopharyngeal tonsil. Tonsillar tissue located behind the lip of the auditory tube on the posterior pharyngeal wall.

Nasopharynx. Most superior region of the pharynx, ending inferiorly at the soft palate.

Neuroanatomy. The specialized study of the structure and function of the nervous system.

Neuron. Specialized cell of the nervous system able to perceive stimuli and conduct them along its processes.

Neurovascular bundles. Nerves and vessels traveling together, enwrapped in connective tissue.

Nodose ganglion. Inferior ganglion of the vagus nerve.

Notch. A greatly depressed region on a bone functioning as a passageway.

Nucleus. An accumulation of neuron cell bodies within the central nervous system.

Occipital triangle. One of the subdivisions of the posterior triangle of the neck, bounded by the inferior belly of the omohyoid, sternocleidomastoid, and trapezius muscles.

Oculomotor nerve. Third cranial nerve.

Olfactory bulb. An extension of the olfactory tract located on the cribriform plate of the ethmoid bone. It receives olfactory filaments.

Olfactory nerve. First cranial nerve.

Optic chiasma. Region of decussation of the two optic nerves resting on the chiasmatic groove of the sphenoid bone.

Optic nerve. Second cranial nerve.

Oral cavity proper. Area internal to the dental arches.

Origin. Site on a bone from which muscle arises.

Oropharyngeal isthmus. Posterior boundary of the oral cavity. Muscular aperture guarding pharynx.

Oropharynx. Middle portion of the pharynx, extending from the soft palate to the larynx.

Ossicles of the ear. Three small bones of the middle ear: the malleus, incus, and stapes.

Otitis media. Infection of the middle ear cavity.

Palatine torus. Bony exostosis of the palate, protruding into the oral cavity.

Palpebral fissure. Space between upper and lower eyelids.

Panniculus adiposus. Areas of the body containing large deposits of fat in the superficial fascia.

Paranasal sinuses. Four mucosa-lined cavities in the bones of the face. They communicate with the nasal fossae.

Parasympathetic nervous system. Division of the autonomic nervous system originating in the brain and sacral spinal cord. This system returns the body to homeostatic state.

Parotid fascia. Cranial continuation of the investing fascia that encloses the parotid gland.

Parotid papilla. Opening of the parotid duct (Stenson duct) in the buccal vestibule opposite the second maxillary molar.

Passavant bar. A ridge of tissue on the posterior wall of the pharynx, representing the contact zone between pharynx and palate when the pharynx is sealed off.

Peripheral nervous system. The portion of the nervous system located outside the skull and vertebral canal, and including the 12 pairs of cranial nerves and the 31 pairs of spinal nerves.

Pharyngeal arches. Branchial arches. Bulging bars of mesoderm observed in the head/neck of the developing embryo. Each gives rise to certain structures.

Pharyngeal clefts. Branchial grooves. Grooves on the surface of the developing head/neck region of an embryo between the pharyngeal arches.

Pharyngeal pouches. Branchial pouches. Outpocketings of the pharynx during development.

Pia mater. Inner-most delicate layer of the meninges covering the brain and spinal cord.

Posterior. Back of the body.

Posterior triangle. Triangular area of the neck, bounded by the sternocleidomastoid and trapezius muscles and the middle one third of the clavicle.

Postganglionic. Visceral motor neurons whose cell bodies are located in one of the autonomic ganglia.

Preganglionic. Visceral motor neurons of the autonomic system that have not yet synapsed in one of the autonomic ganglia.

Pretracheal fascia. Deep layer of the deep cervical fascia surrounding the viscera of the neck.

Pretrached fascia. Deep layer of the deep cervical fascia enveloping the vertebrae and the deep cervical muscles of the neck.

Principal lymph node of the tongue. A large lymph node of the deep cervical chain, responsible for draining the tip of the tongue and the region of the lingual frenulum.

Protrusion. A motion that juts away from its normal resting place, such as the motion possible with the mandible.

Proximal. Closer to the origin.

Pterygopalatine fossa. Small, pyramidal space enclosed by the maxilla, sphenoid, and palatine bones.

Pupil. Circular orifice in the middle of the iris through which light enters the eye.

Rathke pouch. A diverticulum of oral ectoderm in the roof of the developing oral cavity, destined to give rise to a portion of the pituitary gland.

Reflex arc. The simplest form of functional neurologic pathway, bypassing many connecting neurons.

Regional anatomy. Study approach in which individual anatomic regions of the body are considered as units.

Reichert cartilage. A cartilage developed in the second pharyngeal arch that later becomes obscured.

Retraction. A motion that causes a structure to be drawn back, such as the motion possible with the mandible.

Right lymphatic duct. Major vessel of the lymphatic system delivering lymph to the right subclavian vein.

Rods. Light-sensitive cells of the retina concerned with vision in dim light.

Rostral. Cephalad. Toward the cephalic (head) end of the organism.

Rotation. To move about an axis.

Rotatory motion. One of the motions possible at the temporomandibular joint, involving the mandibular condyle and articular disc.

Sacral outflow. Parasympathetic outflow to the viscera of the pelvic region from the sacral spinal cord.

Sagittal suture. A suture of the skull, located in the midline, that separates the parietal bones.

Sclera. White of the eye.

Sesamoid bones. Bones developed in tendons, providing extra leverage or reducing friction at the joint.

Sialography. Radiologic examination of salivary glands and their ducts subsequent to introduction of a radio-opaque dye.

Sinusitis. Inflammation of the mucosa of the paranasal sinuses.

Special somatic afferent. Sensation traveling to the brain from the special senses of vision and hearing.

Special visceral afferent. Sensation traveling to the brain via cranial nerves from the special visceral senses of taste and smell.

Special visceral efferent. Motor innervation from the brain via cranial nerves to the muscles of branchiomeric origin.

Sphenomandibularis muscle. A newly discovered muscle of the deep face, originally believed to be a portion of the deep temporalis muscle. Recent careful dissections have demonstrated it to be a separate entity with its own vascular and nerve supply. It is believed to assist in mastication.

Stellate ganglion. Fused inferior cervical and first thoracic sympathetic ganglia.

Stenson duct. Parotid duct.

Striated muscle. Skeletal muscle. Voluntary muscle.

Subarachnoid space. Space between the arachnoid and pia mater, containing the cerebrospinal fluid.

Subclavian triangle. One of the subdivisions of the posterior triangle, bounded by the inferior belly of the omohyoid muscle, the sternocleidomastoid muscle, and the middle one third of the clavicle.

Subcutaneous connective tissue. Hypodermis. Loose, connective tissue deep to the dermis. Superficial fascia.

Subdural space. Potential space between the dura mater and the arachnoid layers of the meninges.

Sublingual caruncula. Opening of the submandibular duct at the base of the lingual frenulum.

Submandibular triangle. One of the subdivisions of the anterior triangle of the neck, bounded by both bellies of the digastric muscle and the inferior border of the mandible.

Submental triangle. The only unpaired subdivision of the neck. It is bounded by the anterior bellies of the digastric muscles and the hyoid bone.

Suboccipital triangle. A triangular area in the back of the neck, circumscribed by three muscles: rectus capitis posterior major, obliquus capitis superior, and inferior.

Sulcus. 1. A depression on the bone housing a structure. 2. A depression or groove located between gyri on the surface of the cerebral hemispheres.

Sulcus terminalis. A posteriorly directed, V-shaped groove separating the anterior two thirds and posterior one third of the tongue.

Superficial. Relative position near the surface of the body from any respect.

Superficial cervical lymph nodes. Chain of lymph nodes aligned along the external jugular vein.

Superficial fascia. Subcutaneous connective tissue deep to the dermis.

Superior. Toward the head, or cranial.

Superior cervical ganglion. The superior-most ganglion of the cervical sympathetic trunk, located at the level of the second and third cervical vertebrae.

Superior laryngeal aperture. The superior inlet of the larynx.

Suture. A type of fibrous joint found in bones of the skull.

Sympathetic nervous system. Division of the autonomic nervous system originating in the thoracic and first few lumbar spinal cord segments. The system prepares for "fight or flight."

Sympathetic trunk. The sympathetic chain ganglia and their connections.

Symphysis. A cartilaginous bony joint between two continuous bones.

Synapse. A place where a neuron cell communicates with another cell.

Synchondrosis. A temporary cartilaginous joint that will be ossified later.

Syndesmosis. Bony joint with fibrous connective tissue union permitting little movement.

Synovial fluid. Fluid produced within the synovial sheath to bathe the muscle tendon joint and bursa, thus reducing friction.

Synovial joint. A bony joint surrounded by synovial cavities.

Synovial sheath. A saclike covering over a muscle tendon or joint, producing synovial fluid to bathe the tendon and joint, thus reducing friction.

Systemic anatomy. Study approach in which each system of the body is considered separately.

Temporal fossa. A depression on the lateral aspect of the skull, containing the temporalis muscle and its fascia, vessels, and nerves.

Tentorium cerebelli. Meningeal reflection of the dura mater, intervening between the cerebellum and the occipital lobe of the cerebrum.

Terminal ganglia. Parasympathetic ganglia usually located very near the viscera or glands to be innervated.

Thalamus. Largest portion of the diencephalon. Functions to relay sensory impulses to the cerebral cortex.

Thoracic duct. Major vessel of the lymphatic system delivering lymph to the left subclavian vein.

Thoracolumbar outflow. Region of spinal cord from which sympathetic system originates.

Thyroglossal duct. Remnants of the embryologic origins and migratory path of the tissue destined to be the thyroid.

Tracheotomy. A surgical procedure whereby an incision is made in the anterior aspect of the trachea to provide an airway passage to relieve dyspnea.

Translatory motion. One of the motions possible at the temporomandibular joint, involving the temporal bone and the articular disc (a sliding motion).

Transverse plane. Horizontal plane at right angles to sagittal and frontal planes.

Trigeminal nerve. Fifth cranial nerve.

Trochlear nerve. Fourth cranial nerve.

Turbinate bones. Conchae. Three mucosa-covered, scroll-like bones on the lateral nasal wall jutting into the nasal fossa.

Tympanic plexus. Plexus of nerves derived from cranial nerve IX and the sympathetic plexus. It serves the mucous membranes of the middle ear.

Tympanum. Middle ear cavity; also eardrum.

Vagus nerve. Tenth cranial nerve.

Vallate papillae. Circumvallate papillae. A row of large, mushroom-shaped papillae anterior to the sulcus terminalis on the tongue.

Venous pterygoid plexus. A venous plexus receiving tributaries from many areas of the head. It is located between the temporalis and the pterygoid muscles.

Venous sinus. Large, venous channel not possessing the normal histologic complement of veins.

Ventral. Equal to anterior but usually reserved for quadrupeds.

Ventral horn. Gray matter of the spinal cord, containing motor neurons.

Ventral root. Motor axons exiting the ventral root of the spinal cord.

Vermilion zone. Red area of the lips.

Vestibule. Cleft or space between lips and cheeks and the teeth and gingiva.

Vestibulocochlear nerve. Eighth cranial nerve.

Vidian nerve. Nerve of the pterygoid (vidian) canal. It is composed of the greater petrosal nerve (of cranial nerve VII) accompanied by the deep petrosal nerve (of the carotid plexus) as they pass through the pterygoid canal.

Vocal cord. A fold of mucous membrane on the lateral wall of the larynx, responsible for the formation of sound.

Voluntary muscle. Striated or skeletal muscle. Contraction occurs by conscious control.

Wharton duct. Duct of the submandibular gland.

White matter. Region of the central nervous system consisting mainly of fiber tracts.

White rami communicantes. Myelinated fibers (preganglionic) connecting spinal nerves with a sympathetic ganglion.

Wormian bones. Additional bones that may be found in suture lines of the skull.

Zygomatic arch. Malar arch. The arch formed by the temporal process of the zygoma and the zygomatic process of the temporal bone.

Figure Credits

Chapter 2

2-1   Cohen BJ. *Memmler's The Human Body in Health and Disease.* 10th ed. Baltimore: Lippincott Williams & Wilkins, 2005:9, Fig. 1.8.

Chapter 3

3-1   Gartner LP, Hiatt JL. *Color Atlas of Histology.* 4th ed. Philadelphia: Lippincott Williams & Wilkins, 2006:224, Graphic 11.1.

3-3   Moore KL, Dalley AF. *Clinically Oriented Anatomy.* 5th ed. Baltimore: Lippincott Williams & Wilkins, 2006:27, Fig. I.16.

3-4   Moore KL, Dalley AF. *Clinically Orientated Anatomy.* 5th ed. Baltimore: Lippincott Williams & Wilkins, 2006:985, Fig. 7-43E.

3-6   McConnell TH. *The Nature of Disease.* Baltimore: Lippincott Williams & Wilkins, 2007:272, Fig.12-1.

3-7   Cohen BJ. *Memmler's The Human Body in Health and Disease.* 10th ed. Baltimore: Lippincott Williams & Wilkins, 2005:318, Fig. 15.11.

3-8   Agur AMR, Dalley AF. *Grant's Atlas of Anatomy.* 11th ed. Baltimore: Lippincott Williams & Wilkins, 2005:736, Fig. 8.6A.

3-9   Moore KL, Dalley AF. *Clinically Oriented Anatomy.* 5th ed. Baltimore: Lippincott Williams & Wilkins, 2006:522, Fig. 4-23.

3-10   Gartner LP, Hiatt JL. *Color Atlas of Histology.* 4th ed. Baltimore: Lippincott Williams & Wilkins, 2006:133, Graphic 7.2.

3-12   Gartner LP, Hiatt JL. *Color Textbook of Histology.* 3rd ed. Philadelphia: WB Saunders, 2007:207, Fig. 9-23.

3-13   Moore KL, Dalley AF. *Clinically Oriented Anatomy.* 5th ed. Baltimore: Lippincott Williams & Wilkins, 2006:63,65, Figs. 1.41A and 1.43B.

Chapter 4

4-15   Courtesy of Dr. R. Jaynes, Ohio State University, College of Dentistry, Department of Radiology.

4-16   Redrawn and colorized with permission from the American Dental Association.

4-17   Courtesy of Dr. Jon Park, DDS, Department of Oral Diagnosis, Dental School, University of Maryland, Baltimore.

4-19   Adapted and colorized from Hollinshead WH. *Textbook of Anatomy.* 3rd ed. Hagerstown, MD: Harper & Row, 1974:930–931.

4-20   Moore KL, Dalley AF. *Clinically Oriented Anatomy.* 5th ed. Baltimore: Lippincott Williams & Wilkins, 2006:997, Fig. 7.49.

Chapter 5

5-1   Redrawn and colorized after Sadler, TW. *Langman's Medical Embryology.* 10th ed. Baltimore: Lippincott Williams & Wilkins, 2006:272, Fig. 16.21B.

5-2, A–D Redrawn and colorized after Langman, J. *Medical Embryology.* 3rd ed. Baltimore: Williams & Wilkins, 1975.

5-3, A–C Reprinted with permission from Hinrichsen K. The early development of morphology: Patterns of the face in the human embryo. *Adv Anat Embryol* 1987;98:1.

5-10, A–F Sadler TW. *Langman's Medical Embryology.* 10th ed. Baltimore: Lippincott Williams & Wilkins, 2006:276, Fig. 16.28A–F.

5-11   Courtesy Dr. SD Josell, Department of Orthodontics, Dental School, University of Maryland.

5-12   Courtesy Dr. SD Josell, Department of Orthodontics, Dental School, University of Maryland.

Chapter 6

6-11   Wicke L. *Atlas of Radiographic Anatomy.* 4th ed. Munich: Urban & Schwarzenberg, 1978.

6-12   Wicke L. *Atlas of Radiographic Anatomy.* 4th ed. Munich: Urban & Schwarzenberg, 1978.

6-13   Courtesy of Dr. C. Ferrel, Department of Orthodontics, Dental School, University of Maryland.

6-14   Grossman, CB. *Magnetic Resonance Imaging and Computed Tomography of the Head and Spine.* 2nd ed. Baltimore: Lippincott Williams & Wilkins, 1996, Fig. 6-28.

Chapter 7

7-2   Agur AMR, Dalley AF. *Grant's Atlas of Anatomy.* 11th ed. Baltimore: Lippincott Williams & Wilkins, 2005:731, Fig. 8.3II.

7-3   Moore KL, Agur AMR. *Essential Clinical Anatomy.* 3rd ed. Philadelphia: Lippincott Williams & Wilkins, 2007:585, Fig. 8.2C.

7-4   Moore KL, Agur AMR. *Essential Clinical Anatomy.* 3rd ed. Philadelphia: Lippincott Williams & Wilkins, 2007:585, Fig. 8.2A.

7-5   Agur AMR, Dalley AF. *Grant's Atlas of Anatomy.* 11th ed. Baltimore: Lippincott Williams & Wilkins, 2005:316, Fig. 4.35.

7-7   Moore KL, Agur AMR. *Essential Clinical Anatomy.* 3rd ed. Philadelphia: Lippincott Williams & Wilkins, 2007:585, Fig. 8.2A,B.

7-8   Agur AMR, Dalley AF. *Grant's Atlas of Anatomy.* 11th ed. Baltimore: Lippincott Williams & Wilkins, 2005:732, Fig. 8.3III.

7-10   Redrawn and colorized after Agur AMR, Dalley AF. *Grant's Atlas of Anatomy.* 11th ed. Baltimore: Lippincott Williams & Wilkins, 2005:756, Fig. 8.20.

7-12   Redrawn and colorized after Netter FH. *Atlas of Human Anatomy.* 4th ed. Philadelphia: WB Saunders, 2006, Plate 69.

7-13   Redrawn and colorized after Netter FH. *Atlas of Human Anatomy.* 4th ed. Philadelphia: WB Saunders, 2006, Plate 71.

Chapter 8

8-4   Agur AMR, Dalley AF. *Grant's Atlas of Anatomy.* 11th ed. Baltimore: Lippincott Williams & Wilkins, 2005:652, Fig. 7-43B.

8-5   *Stedman's Medical Dictionary.* 27th ed. Arteries of the Head and Neck. Baltimore: Lippincott, Williams & Wilkins, 2002.

8-6   *Stedman's Medical Dictionary.* 27th ed. Veins of the Head and Neck. Baltimore: Lippincott, Williams & Wilkins, 2002.

Chapter 9

9-1   Agur AMR, Dalley AF. *Grant's Atlas of Anatomy.* 11th ed. Baltimore: Lippincott Williams & Wilkins, 2005:612, Fig. 7.15A.

9-2   Moore KL, Dalley AF. *Clinically Oriented Anatomy.* 5th ed. Baltimore: Lippincott Williams & Wilkins, 2006:1131, Fig. 9.1.

Chapter 10

10-4   McConnell TH. *The Nature of Disease.* Baltimore: Lippincott Williams & Wilkins, 2007:680, Fig. 25.2.

10-5   McConnell TH. *The Nature of Disease.* Baltimore: Lippincott Williams & Wilkins, 2007:681, Fig. 25.3.

Chapter 11

11-2   Agur AMR, Dalley AF. *Grant's Atlas of Anatomy.* 11th ed. Baltimore: Lippincott Williams & Wilkins, 2005:652, Fig. 7-43B.

Chapter 12

12-6   Redrawn and colorized from Agur AMR, Dalley AF. *Grant's Atlas of Anatomy.* 11th ed. Baltimore: Lippincott Williams & Wilkins, 2005:659, Fig. 7.47.

12-7   Redrawn and colorized from Agur AMR, Dalley AF. *Grant's Atlas of Anatomy.* 11th ed. Baltimore: Lippincott Williams & Wilkins, 2005:658, Fig. 7.47.

12-9   Agur AMR, Dalley AF. *Grant's Atlas of Anatomy.* 11th ed. Baltimore: Lippincott Williams & Wilkins, 2005:660, Fig. 7.48.

12-10   Moore KL, Dalley AF. *Clinically Oriented Anatomy.* 5th ed. Baltimore: Lippincott Williams & Wilkins, 2006:911, Fig. 7.10B.

Chapter 13

13-1,   Redrawn and colorized from Agur AMR, Dalley
B and C   AF. *Grant's Atlas of Anatomy.* 11th ed. Baltimore: Lippincott Williams & Wilkins, 2005:665, Figs. 7.51B and C, respectively.

13-4   CT and MRI scans from Langland OE, Langlais RP, Preece JW. *Principles of Dental Imaging.* 2nd ed. Baltimore: Lippincott Williams & Wilkins 2002:278, Figs. 1132A, B and 1133A, B.

Chapter 14

14-1   Agur AMR, Dalley AF. *Grant's Atlas of Anatomy.* 11th ed. Baltimore: Lippincott Williams & Wilkins, 2005:660, Fig. 7.48.

14-2   Agur AMR, Dalley AF. *Grant's Atlas of Anatomy.* 11th ed. Baltimore: Lippincott Williams & Wilkins, 2005:688, Fig. 7.70A.

14-5   Asset provided by Anatomical Chart Company. Baltimore: Lippincott Williams & Wilkins.

14-7   Agur AMR, Dalley AF. *Grant's Atlas of Anatomy.* 11th ed. Baltimore: Lippincott Williams & Wilkins, 2005:687, Fig. 7.69A.

Chapter 15

15-1   Redrawn and colorized after Netter FH. *Atlas of Human Anatomy.* 4th ed. Philadelphia: WB Saunders, 2006, Plate 59.

15-2   Redrawn and colorized after Putz R, Pabst R. Translated by Taylor AN. *Sobotta Atlas of Human Anatomy*. Vol. 1. Baltimore: Williams & Wilkins, 1997:112, Fig. 203.

15-4   Moore KL, Dalley AF. *Clinically Oriented Anatomy*. 5th ed. Baltimore: Lippincott Williams & Wilkins, 2006:1004, Table 7-16 A,B.

15-5   Redrawn and colorized after Agur AMR, Dalley AF. *Grant's Atlas of Anatomy*. 11th ed. Baltimore: Lippincott Williams & Wilkins, 2005:670, Fig. 7.55A.

15-6   Redrawn and colorized after Agur AMR, Dalley AF. *Grant's Atlas of Anatomy*. 11th ed. Baltimore: Lippincott Williams & Wilkins, 2005:821, Table 9-14, lateral view.

15-7   Moore KL, Dalley AF. *Clinically Oriented Anatomy*. 5th ed. Baltimore: Lippincott Williams & Wilkins, 2006:1005, Fig. 7.56.

15-8   Redrawn, modified, and colorized after Netter FH. *Atlas of Human Anatomy*. 4th ed. Philadelphia: WB Saunders, 2006, Plate 59.

Chapter 16

16-1   Redrawn and colorized after Putz R, Pabst R. Translated by Taylor AN. *Sobotta Atlas of Human Anatomy*. Vol. 1. Baltimore: Williams & Wilkins, 1997, Plate 103, Fig. 185.

16-2   Redrawn and colorized after Netter FH. *Atlas of Human Anatomy*. 4th ed. Philadelphia: WB Saunders, 2006, Plate 65.

16-3   Adapted and colorized from Hollinshead WH. *Textbook of Anatomy*. 3rd ed. Hagerstown, MD: Harper & Row, 1974:930–931.

16-5   Agur AMR, Dalley AF. *Grant's Atlas of Anatomy*. 11th ed. Baltimore: Lippincott Williams & Wilkins, 2005:775, Fig. 8.32C.

16-6   Redrawn and colorized after Putz R, Pabst R. Translated by Taylor AN. *Sobotta Atlas of Human Anatomy*. Vol. 1. Baltimore: Williams & Wilkins, 1997:123, Fig. 228.

16-8   Asset provided by Anatomical Chart Company. Baltimore: Lippincott Williams & Wilkins.

16-9   Modified and colorized after Moore KL, Dalley AF. *Clinically Oriented Anatomy*. 5th ed. Baltimore: Lippincott Williams & Wilkins, 2006:1097, Fig. 8.33.

Chapter 17

17-6   Agur AMR, Dalley AF. *Grant's Atlas of Anatomy*. 11th ed. Baltimore: Lippincott Williams & Wilkins, 2005:612, Fig. 7.15A.

17-7   Moore KL, Dalley AF. *Clinically Oriented Anatomy*. 5th ed. Baltimore: Lippincott Williams & Wilkins, 2006:929, Table 7.3C.

17-8   Agur AMR, Dalley AF. *Grant's Atlas of Anatomy*. 11th ed. Baltimore: Lippincott Williams & Wilkins, 2005:322, Fig. 4.40.

17-10   Gartner LP, Hiatt JL. *Color Textbook of Histology*. 3rd ed. Philadelphia: WB Saunders, 2007:207, Fig. 9-23.

Chapter 18

18-13   Redrawn, modified, and colorized after Netter FH. *Atlas of Human Anatomy*. 4th ed. Philadelphia: WB Saunders, 2006, Plate 59.

Chapter 21

21-2   Redrawn and colorized after Netter FH. *Atlas of Human Anatomy*. 4th ed. Philadelphia: WB Saunders, 2006, Plate 69.

21-3   Moore KL, Dalley AF. *Clinically Oriented Anatomy*. 5th ed. Baltimore: Lippincott Williams & Wilkins, 2006:1005, Fig. 7.56.

21-6   Redrawn and colorized from Agur AMR, Dalley AF. *Grant's Atlas of Anatomy*. 11th ed. Baltimore: Lippincott Williams & Wilkins, 2005:659, Fig. 7.47.

21-7   Redrawn and colorized from Agur AMR, Dalley AF. *Grant's Atlas of Anatomy*. 11th ed. Baltimore: Lippincott Williams & Wilkins, 2005:658, Fig. 7.47.

21-8   Redrawn and colorized after Putz R., Pabst R. Translated by Taylor AN. *Sobotta Atlas of Human Anatomy*. Vol. 1. Baltimore: Williams & Wilkins, 1997, Plate 103, Fig. 185.

21-9   Redrawn and colorized after Agur AMR, Dalley AF. *Grant's Atlas of Anatomy*. 11th ed. Baltimore: Lippincott Williams & Wilkins, 2005:756, Fig. 8.20.

21-10   Agur AMR, Dalley AF. *Grant's Atlas of Anatomy*. 11th ed. Baltimore: Lippincott Williams & Wilkins, 2005:613, Fig. 7.16.

21-11   Moore KL, Dalley AF. *Clinically Oriented Anatomy*. 5th ed. Baltimore: Lippincott Williams & Wilkins, 2006:911, Fig. 7.10B.

Chapter 22

22-1   Moore KL, Agur AMR. *Essential Clinical Anatomy*. 3rd ed. Baltimore: Lippincott Williams & Wilkins, 2007:585, Fig. 8.2C.

22-2   Moore KL, Agur AMR. *Essential Clinical Anatomy*. 3rd ed. Baltimore: Lippincott Williams & Wilkins, 2007:585, Fig. 8.2A.

22-3   Agur AMR, Dalley AF. *Grant's Atlas of Anatomy*. 11th ed. Baltimore: Lippincott Williams & Wilkins, 2005:731, Fig. 8.3II.

Suggested Readings

Gross Anatomy Textbooks

Hall-Craggs ECB. *Anatomy as a Basis for Clinical Medicine.* 3rd ed. Baltimore: Lippincott Williams & Wilkins, 1995.

Moore KL, Agur AMR. *Essential Clinical Anatomy.* 3rd ed. Baltimore: Lippincott Williams & Wilkins, 2007.

Moore KL, Dalley AF. *Clinically Oriented Anatomy.* 5th ed. Baltimore: Lippincott Williams & Wilkins, 2006.

Rosse C, Gaddum-Rosse P, Hollinshead WH. *Hollinshead's Textbook of Anatomy.* 5th ed. Baltimore: Lippincott Williams & Wilkins, 1997.

Slaby, FJ, McCune, SK, Summers RW. *Gross Anatomy in the Practice of Medicine.* Philadelphia: Lea & Febiger, 1994.

Snell, RS. *Clinical Anatomy.* 7th ed. Baltimore: Lippincott Williams & Wilkins, 2004.

Standring, S. *Gray's Anatomy: The Anatomical Basis of Clinical Practice.* 39th ed. New York, Churchhill Livingstone, 2004.

Standring, S, ed. *Gray's Anatomy,* 39th British ed. Philadelphia: Elsevier, 2008

Developmental Anatomy Textbooks

Sadler TW. *Langman's Medical Embryology.* 10th ed. Baltimore: Lippincott Williams & Wilkins, 2006.

Bath-Balogh M, Fehrenbach MJ. *Illustrated Dental Embryology, Histology, and Anatomy.* 2nd ed. Philadelphia, W.B. Saunders Company, 2006.

Moore KL, Persaud TVN. *Before We are Born: Essentials of Embryology and Birth Defects.* 7th ed. Philadelphia: W.B. Saunders Company, 2007.

Moore KL, Persaud TVN. *The Developing Human: Clinically Oriented Embryology.* 8th ed. Philadelphia. W.B. Saunders Company. 2007.

Neuroanatomy Textbooks

Bergman RA, Afifi A. *Functional Neuroanatomy.* 2nd ed. St. Louis: McGraw-Hill Medical, 2005.

Kiernan JA. *Barr's The Human Nervous System.* 8th ed. Baltimore: Lippincott Williams &Wilkins, 2005.

Gartner LP, Patesta MA. *Essentials of Neuroanatomy*: Baltimore: Jen House Publishing Company, 2003.

Haines DE. *Fundamental Neuroscience for Basic and Clinical Applications.* 3rd ed. New York: Churchill Livingstone, 2005.

Kandel ER, Schwartz JH, Jessell TM. *Principles of Neural Science.* 4th ed. St. Louis: McGraw-Hill, 2000.

Martin JH. *Neuroanatomy: Text and Atlas.* 3rd ed. St. Louis: McGraw-Hill Medical, 2003.

Patestas MA, Gartner LP. *A Textbook of Neuroanatomy.* Wiley-Blackwell, 2006.

Snell RS. *Clinical Neuroanatomy for Medical Students.* 6th ed. Baltimore: Lippincott Williams & Wilkins, 2005.

Young PA, Young PH, Tolbert DI. *Basic Clinical Neuroscience.* 2nd ed. Baltimore: Lippincott Williams & Wilkins, 2007.

Wilson-Pauwels LW, Akesson EJ, Stewart PA, Spacey SD. *Cranial Nerves in Health and Disease.* 2nd ed. Toronto: BC Decker, Inc., 2002.

Head and Neck Anatomy Textbooks

Brand RW, Iselhard DE. *Anatomy of Orofacial Structures.* 7th ed. St. Louis: C.V. Mosby Co., 2003.

Febrenbach MJ, Herring SW. *Illustrated Anatomy of the Head and Neck.* 3rd ed. Philadelphia: W.B. Saunders Company, 2007.

Norton NS. *Netter's Head and Neck Anatomy for Dentistry.* Philadelphia: W.B. Saunders Company, 2006.

Atlases

Abrahams PH, Marks SC, Hutchings RT. *McMinn's Color Atlas of Human Anatomy.* 5th ed. Philadelphia: C.V. Mosby Co., 2002.

Agur AMR, Dalley AF. *Grant's Atlas of Anatomy.* 11th ed. Baltimore: Lippincott Williams & Wilkins, 2005.

Clemente CD. *Anatomy A Regional Atlas of the Human Body.* 5th ed. Baltimore: Lippincott Williams & Wilkins, 2006.

Netter FH. *Atlas of Human Anatomy.* 4th ed. Philadelphia: W.B. Saunders Company, 2006.

Olson TR, Pawlina W. *A.D.A.M. Student Atlas of Anatomy.* 2nd ed. Cambridge University Press, 2008.

Rohen JW, Yokochi C, Lutjen-Drecoll E. *Color Atlas of Anatomy.* 5th ed. Baltimore: Lippincott Williams & Wilkins, 2002.

Taylor AN. *Sabotta Atlas of Human Anatomy, vol, I,* 12th English ed. *Head, Neck, Upper Limbs.* Baltimore: Williams & Wilkins, 1997.

Index

Page numbers in *italics* denote figures; those followed by a "*t*" denote tables.